Henke's Med-Math

Dosage Calculation, Preparation and Administration

FIFTH EDITION

Henke's Med-Math

Dosage Calculation, Preparation and Administration

Susan Buchholz, RN, MSN
Associate Professor
Georgia Perimeter College
Lawrenceville, Georgia

Sister Grace Henke, SC, RN, MSN, EdD
Ethics Associate
Department of Ethics
Saint Vincent Catholic Medical Centers of New York
New York, New York

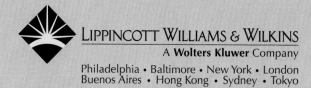

LIPPINCOTT WILLIAMS & WILKINS
A **Wolters Kluwer** Company

Philadelphia • Baltimore • New York • London
Buenos Aires • Hong Kong • Sydney • Tokyo

Acquisitions Editor: Margaret Zuccarini
Managing Editor: Helen Kogut
Senior Project Editor: Tom Gibbons
Senior Production Manager: Helen Ewan
Managing Editor / Production: Erika Kors
Creative Director: Doug Smock
Manufacturing Manager: Karin Duffield
Indexer: Victoria Boyle
Compositor: Circle Graphics
Printer: R. R. Donnelley-Willard

ISBN: 0-7817-6264-2

Fifth Edition

LWW.com

Reviewers

Anita Au
Sessional Instructor for the Undergraduate and the
    After-Degree Programs
University of Alberta
Edmonton, Alberta
Canada

Beryl K. Broughton, MSN, CRNP, CS, FNP, C.
Level 100 Chairperson, Nursing Faculty
Frankford Hospital School of Nursing
Philadelphia, Pennsylvania

Gina S. Brown, PhD, RN
Chair and Professor
Columbia Union College
Takoma Park, Maryland

Frances H. Davis
Assistant Professor
Ohio University—Zanesville
Zanesville, Ohio

Charlene Gagliardi, RN, BSN, MSN
Instructor—Faculty, BSN Programs—
    Accelerated and Traditional
Mount Saint Mary's College
Los Angeles, California

Mary Goolik, MS, RN
Instructor—Associate and Baccalaureate Degree
Indiana University School of Nursing
Bloomington, Indiana

Karen Hoffman, RN, BS, MS
Assistant Professor
Indiana Wesleyan University
Marion, Indiana

Gail C. Kost, RN, MSN
Clinical Lecturer
Indiana University
Indianapolis, Indiana

Adrianne D. Linton, PhD, RN
Associate Professor
University of Texas Health Science Center at
    San Antonio School of Nursing
San Antonio, Texas

Susan Stoner, RN, MSN
Assistant Professor
Ohio University—Zanesville
Zanesville, Ohio

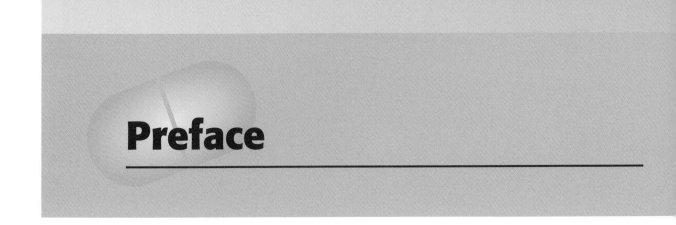

Preface

A humorous look at dosage calculations:

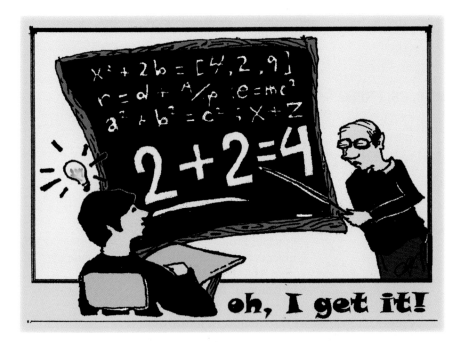

oh, I get it!

It's true that in arithmetic, mathematics, geometry, calculus and most importantly dosage calculations, the more you practice and solve problems, the more it starts to make sense!

This book is to help you "get it" and understand dosage calculations.

Text Organization

Henke's Med-Math: Dosage Calculation, Preparation and Administration, Fifth Edition, has been designed to meet the needs of students in every type of nursing program. This text has also been widely used by other health care professionals who administer drugs and is recommended to practicing nurses in need of review or nurses who wish to return to practice. Students in introductory courses should complete the chapters in order. Practicing nurses may wish to do the proficiency tests at the end of each dosage chapter to target areas of weakness for content review.

The first five chapters of this workbook lay the foundation for further study.

Chapter 1 concentrates on the arithmetic needed to calculate doses.

Chapter 2 identifies abbreviations used in prescriptions and explains how to interpret them.

Chapter 3 clarifies information printed on drug labels and types of drug packaging.

Chapter 4 explains dosage measurement systems and teaches students how to convert among systems when the physician or health care provider order differs from the available stock medication.

Chapter 5 defines the forms in which drugs are manufactured and the equipment used in administration.

Chapters 6 to 10 concentrate on calculating doses through the application of simple rules for

- oral solid and liquid problems
- injections from liquids and powders
- intravenous medications and pediatric doses

Chapter 11 explains the dimensional analysis method of drug calculation.

Chapters 12 and 13 present information and techniques for safe administration, including universal precautions, pregnancy categories, and legal and ethical considerations. Also included is information on how to administer drugs orally, parenterally, and topically.

Numerous examples, self-tests, and proficiency tests enable students to achieve mastery of the material.

Key Features of the Text

- Dosage problems simulate actual clinical experience
- Simple to complex organization of the text
- Easy-to-learn formulas and a step-by-step approach in solving problems
- Self-tests and proficiency tests offer varied opportunities to translate text into clinical application
- "Learning Aid" feature provides key strategies to promote understanding
- Rule and Example style of presentation highlights important rules of thumb, followed by their application to clarify student learning
- In-chapter self-tests with answers at the end of each chapter
- Proficiency tests in every chapter provide ready-made material for student assignments. These tests are perforated and three-hole punched for easy removal
- Easy-to-locate answer key for proficiency tests in Appendix A
- Calculations for meters squared and milliunits, body surface nomogram, and patient controlled analgesia (PCA) are included
- Glossary with definitions and common abbreviations
- Enclosed CD-ROM contains math problems for students to practice calculations
- Intravenous calculations in two chapters provide content on basic, advanced, and special types of intravenous administration
- Principles of Drug Administration chapter

New to This Edition

- Current drug labels for the most common and most relevant drugs
- Approved JCAHO (Joint Commission on Accreditation of Healthcare Organizations) abbreviations
- Colorful labels and tables

- Shows three methods of calculation (formula, ratio, proportion)
- New chapter on Dimensional Analysis Method
- Four methods of calculation are shown with proficiency tests (formula, ratio, proportion, and dimensional analysis)
- Handy quick-reference plastic card with common conversions and formulas
- Critical thinking questions, using clinical situations/case studies with "What If" questions

Aids for Students and Faculty

- **Free CD-ROM**
  includes over 15 minutes of video clips on safe medication administration, a dosage calculation tool, and access to free additional dosage calculation quizzes.
- **Connection web site**
  Go online! Visit the Lippincott Connection web site (http://connection.lww.com/) for more content and learning resources.
- **Instructor's Resource CD-ROM**
  includes a fully updated Instructor's Manual and Testbank, and is available for teachers to help you optimize your teaching of dosage calculations and medication administration.

Clinical Accuracy

The right dose is one of the five rights in medication administration. The more you work with the medication dosages and the formulas, the more you become an expert at dosage calculations. This is the goal of the book.

Susan Buchholz, RN, MSN

Acknowledgments

I dedicate this edition to my parents, Herman and Helen Buchholz, who taught me to set goals and complete them.

It takes a village to write a book. I want to thank the following members of that village:

Margaret Zuccarini, Senior Acquisitions Editor, Lippincott Williams & Wilkins

Sister Grace Henke, the original author

Tom Gibbons, Senior Production Editor, Lippincott Williams & Wilkins

Helen Kogut, Senior Managing Editor, Lippincott Williams & Wilkins

Joe Morita, Managing Editor, Lippincott Williams & Wilkins

Pharmaceutical companies that provided the labels for this text

Colleagues and nursing students (past and present) at Georgia Perimeter College, Atlanta, Georgia

Oakhurst Baptist Church, my faith community in Decatur, Georgia

Laura Lacey Bordeaux, photographer

Mia Merlin, illustrator

Emily Harrison, artist

Ken Moss, photographer and educational technologist

Laura Wallace, contributing author, Chapters 12 and 13

DeKalb Medical Center, supplier of drug packaging

Donna Woolf, pharmacist, supplier of drug labels

Shirley Tyldesley, proofreader

Mary, Andrew and Chelsea, my greatest blessings

Contents

CHAPTER 13
Administration Procedures   354

Arithmetic Needed for Dosage

When a medication order differs from the fixed amount at which a drug is supplied, the dose needed must be calculated. Calculation requires knowledge of the systems of dosage measurements (see Chapter 4) and the ability to solve arithmetic. This chapter covers those common arithmetic functions needed for the safe administration of drugs.

Beginning students invariably express anxiety that they will miscalculate a dose and cause harm. Although *everyone* is capable of error, no one has to cause one. The surest way to prevent a mistake is to exercise care in performing basic arithmetic operations.

Do not skip this chapter!

Students who believe their skills are satisfactory should complete the self-tests and the proficiency exam. Answers to all problems are located at the end of the chapter.

Students with math anxiety and those with deficiencies in performing arithmetic should work through this chapter page by page. Examples and learning aids demonstrate how calculations are performed; self-tests provide practice and drill. The proficiency exam should be taken after mastering the content.

Why perform arithmetic operations when calculators are readily available? Solving the arithmetic forces one to think logically about the amount ordered and to evaluate the answer in relation to the dose. Mentally solving dose problems increases speed and efficiency in preparing medications. One must also know what numbers and functions to enter when using a calculator. There may be occasions when a problem that requires a calculator arises in the clinical area; however, all arithmetic problems in this chapter can be completed without a calculator.

▷ Multiplying Whole Numbers

The multiplication table (Fig. 1-1) is provided for review. Study the table for the numbers 1 through 12. You should achieve 100% accuracy without referring to the table.

Example Multiply 8 by 7 (8×7).

1. Find row number 8.

2. Find column number 7.

3. Read across row 8 until you intersect column number 7. The answer is 56.

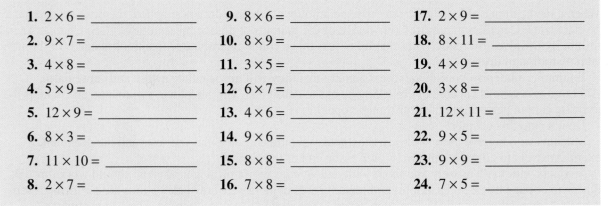

	1	2	3	4	5	6	⑦	8	9	10	11	12
	2	4	6	8	10	12	14	16	18	20	22	24
	3	6	9	12	15	18	21	24	27	30	33	36
	4	8	12	16	20	24	28	32	36	40	44	48
	5	10	15	20	25	30	35	40	45	50	55	60
	6	12	18	24	30	36	42	48	54	60	66	72
	7	14	21	28	35	42	49	56	63	70	77	84
→	⑧	16	24	32	40	48	㊹	64	72	80	88	96
	9	18	27	36	45	54	63	72	81	90	99	108
	10	20	30	40	50	60	70	80	90	100	110	120
	11	22	33	44	55	66	77	88	99	110	121	132
	12	24	36	48	60	72	84	96	108	120	132	144

FIGURE 1-1

The multiplication table. The numbers going down the left side (from 1 to 12) are the row numbers. The numbers going across the top (from 1 to 12) are the column numbers. To multiply any two numbers from 1 to 12, find the column for one number, find the row for the other number, and read across the row until you intersect the column.

SELF-TEST 1   Multiplication

After studying the multiplication table, write the answers to these problems. Answers are given at the end of the chapter; if you do not achieve 100%, you need more study time.

1. $2 \times 6 =$ _____
2. $9 \times 7 =$ _____
3. $4 \times 8 =$ _____
4. $5 \times 9 =$ _____
5. $12 \times 9 =$ _____
6. $8 \times 3 =$ _____
7. $11 \times 10 =$ _____
8. $2 \times 7 =$ _____

9. $8 \times 6 =$ _____
10. $8 \times 9 =$ _____
11. $3 \times 5 =$ _____
12. $6 \times 7 =$ _____
13. $4 \times 6 =$ _____
14. $9 \times 6 =$ _____
15. $8 \times 8 =$ _____
16. $7 \times 8 =$ _____

17. $2 \times 9 =$ _____
18. $8 \times 11 =$ _____
19. $4 \times 9 =$ _____
20. $3 \times 8 =$ _____
21. $12 \times 11 =$ _____
22. $9 \times 5 =$ _____
23. $9 \times 9 =$ _____
24. $7 \times 5 =$ _____

▶ Dividing Whole Numbers

The multiplication table is also helpful when dividing large numbers by smaller ones. Study the table for the division of numbers 2 through 12 (Fig. 1-2). Again, you should be able to achieve 100% accuracy without referring to the table; if not, study it again.

Example

Divide 108 by 12 ($108 \div 12$).

1. Find 12 (the smaller number) in the left row.
2. Read across that row until you find 108 (the larger number).
3. The number at the top of that column is the answer: 9.

Remember, because $9 \times 12 = 108$, then $108 \div 12 = 9$ (see Fig. 1-2).

1	2	3	4	5	6	7	8	⑨	10	11	12
2	4	6	8	10	12	14	16	18	20	22	24
3	6	9	12	15	18	21	24	27	30	33	36
4	8	12	16	20	24	28	32	36	40	44	48
5	10	15	20	25	30	35	40	45	50	55	60
6	12	18	24	30	36	42	48	54	60	66	72
7	14	21	28	35	42	49	56	63	70	77	84
8	16	24	32	40	48	56	64	72	80	88	96
9	18	27	36	45	54	63	72	81	90	99	108
10	20	30	40	50	60	70	80	90	100	110	120
11	22	33	44	55	66	77	88	99	110	121	132
⑫	24	36	48	60	72	84	96	(108)	120	132	144

FIGURE 1-2
Division table. The numbers going down the left side (from 1 to 12) are the row numbers. The numbers going across the top (from 1 to 12) are the column numbers. To divide, find the divisor (the number performing the division) in the row. Read across the row to the dividend (the number to be divided). The number at the top of that column is the answer.

SELF-TEST 2 Division

After studying the division of larger numbers by smaller numbers, write the answers to the following problems. Answers are given at the end of the chapter.

1. $63 \div 7 =$ _____
2. $24 \div 6 =$ _____
3. $36 \div 12 =$ _____
4. $42 \div 6 =$ _____
5. $35 \div 5 =$ _____
6. $96 \div 12 =$ _____
7. $12 \div 3 =$ _____
8. $27 \div 9 =$ _____
9. $49 \div 7 =$ _____
10. $18 \div 3 =$ _____
11. $72 \div 8 =$ _____
12. $48 \div 8 =$ _____
13. $28 \div 7 =$ _____
14. $21 \div 7 =$ _____
15. $24 \div 8 =$ _____
16. $84 \div 12 =$ _____
17. $81 \div 9 =$ _____
18. $32 \div 8 =$ _____
19. $36 \div 6 =$ _____
20. $18 \div 9 =$ _____
21. $21 \div 3 =$ _____
22. $48 \div 4 =$ _____
23. $144 \div 12 =$ _____
24. $56 \div 8 =$ _____

Fractions

A *fraction* is a portion of a whole number. The top number is called the *numerator*. The bottom number is called the *denominator*.

Example

$\dfrac{1}{4}$ → numerator → denominator

Learning Aid

The line between the numerator and the denominator is a division sign. Therefore, the fraction can be read as one divided by four.

Types of Fractions

In a *proper* fraction, the numerator is smaller than the denominator.

Example $\frac{2}{5}$ (Read as two fifths.)

In an *improper* fraction, the numerator is larger than the denominator.

Example $\frac{5}{2}$ (Read as five halves.)

A *mixed number* has a whole number plus a fraction.

Example $1\frac{2}{3}$ (Read as one and two thirds.)

In a *complex* fraction, both the numerator and the denominator are already fractions.

Example $\frac{\frac{1}{2}}{\frac{1}{4}}$ (Read as one half divided by one fourth.)

RULE   **REDUCING FRACTIONS**

Find the largest number that can be divided evenly into the numerator *and* the denominator.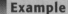

Example   *EXAMPLE 1*

Reduce $\frac{4}{12}$

$$\frac{\overset{1}{\cancel{4}}}{\underset{3}{\cancel{12}}} = \frac{1}{3}$$

EXAMPLE 2

Reduce $\frac{7}{49}$

$$\frac{\overset{1}{\cancel{7}}}{\underset{7}{\cancel{49}}} = \frac{1}{7}$$

Learning Aid

Check to see if the denominator is evenly divisible by the numerator. The number 7 can be evenly divided into 49.

Sometimes fractions are more difficult to reduce because the answer is not obvious.

Example   *EXAMPLE 1*

Reduce $\frac{56}{96}$

$$\frac{56}{96} = \frac{\overset{1}{\cancel{8}} \times 7}{\underset{1}{\cancel{8}} \times 12} = \frac{7}{12}$$

Learning Aid

Your knowledge of the multiplication table can help you. Change the numbers to their multiples.

EXAMPLE 2

Reduce $\frac{54}{99}$

$$\frac{54}{99} = \frac{\overset{1}{\cancel{9}} \times 6}{\underset{1}{\cancel{9}} \times 11} = \frac{6}{11}$$

Patience is required to reduce a very large fraction. It may be difficult to find the largest number that will divide evenly into the numerator and the denominator, and you may have to reduce several times.

Example

EXAMPLE 1

Reduce $\frac{189}{216}$

Try to divide both by 3 $\dfrac{\overset{63}{\cancel{189}}}{\underset{72}{\cancel{216}}} = \frac{63}{72}$

Then use multiples $\frac{63}{72} = \dfrac{\overset{1}{\cancel{9}} \times 7}{\underset{1}{\cancel{9}} \times 12} = \frac{7}{8}$

EXAMPLE 2

Reduce $\frac{27}{135}$

Try to divide both by 3 $\dfrac{\overset{\overset{1}{\cancel{9}}}{\cancel{27}}}{\underset{\underset{5}{\cancel{45}}}{\cancel{135}}} = \frac{\cancel{9}}{\cancel{45}} = \frac{1}{5}$

Learning Aid

Certain numbers are called prime numbers because they cannot be reduced further. Examples are 2, 3, 5, 7, and 11.

When reducing, if the last number is even or a zero; try 2.

If the last number is a zero, or 5, try 5.

If the last number is odd, try 3, 7, or 11.

SELF-TEST 3 Reducing Fractions

Reduce these fractions to their lowest terms. Answers are given at the end of the chapter. Be patient!

1. $\frac{16}{24}$

2. $\frac{36}{216}$

3. $\frac{18}{96}$

4. $\frac{70}{490}$

5. $\frac{18}{81}$

6. $\frac{8}{48}$

7. $\frac{12}{30}$

8. $\frac{68}{136}$

9. $\frac{55}{121}$

10. $\frac{15}{60}$

Multiplying Fractions

There are two ways to multiply fractions.

First Way

Multiply the numerators across. Multiply denominators across. Reduce the answer to its lowest terms.

Example

$\frac{2}{7} \times \frac{3}{4} = \frac{2 \times 3}{7 \times 4} = \frac{6}{28}$

$\frac{6}{28} = \dfrac{3 \times \overset{1}{\cancel{2}}}{14 \times \underset{1}{\cancel{2}}} = \frac{3}{14}$

Learning Aid

When multiplying fractions, sometimes one way will be easier. Use whichever method is more comfortable for you.

Second Way (When There Are Several Fractions)

Reduce by dividing numerators into denominators evenly. Multiply the remaining numerators across. Multiply the remaining denominators across. Check to see if further reductions can be made.

| **Example** | *EXAMPLE 1* |

$$\frac{3}{14} \times \frac{7}{10} \times \frac{5}{12} = \frac{\overset{1}{\cancel{3}}}{\underset{2}{\cancel{14}}} \times \frac{\overset{1}{\cancel{7}}}{\underset{2}{\cancel{10}}} \times \frac{\overset{1}{\cancel{5}}}{\underset{4}{\cancel{12}}} = \frac{1}{16}$$

Learning Aid

$12 \div 3 = 4$

$14 \div 7 = 2$

$10 \div 5 = 2$

EXAMPLE 2

$$1\frac{1}{2} \times \frac{4}{6} = \frac{\overset{1}{\cancel{3}}}{\underset{1}{\cancel{2}}} \times \frac{\overset{2}{\cancel{4}}}{\underset{2}{\cancel{6}}} = \frac{2}{2} = 1$$

Learning Aid

Mixed numbers must be changed to improper fractions. Multiply the whole number by the denominator and add the numerator.

$$1\frac{1}{2} = 1 \times 2 + 1 = \frac{3}{2}$$

EXAMPLE 3

$$\frac{4}{5} \times 6\frac{2}{3} = \frac{4}{\underset{1}{\cancel{5}}} \times \frac{\overset{4}{\cancel{20}}}{3} = \frac{16}{3}$$

Learning Aid

Change the mixed number to an improper fraction.

$$6 \times 3 = 18 + 2 = \frac{20}{3}$$

SELF-TEST 4   **Multiplying Fractions**

Multiply these fractions. Answers are given at the end of the chapter.

1. $\frac{1}{6} \times \frac{4}{5} \times \frac{5}{2} =$

2. $\frac{4}{15} \times \frac{3}{2} =$

3. $1\frac{1}{2} \times 4\frac{2}{3} =$

4. $\frac{1}{5} \times \frac{15}{45} =$

5. $3\frac{3}{4} \times 10\frac{2}{3} =$

6. $\frac{7}{20} \times \frac{2}{14} =$

7. $\frac{9}{2} \times \frac{3}{2} =$

8. $6\frac{1}{4} \times 7\frac{1}{9} \times \frac{9}{5} =$

Dividing Fractions

Fractions can be divided by inverting the number after the division sign then changing the division sign to a multiplication sign.

| **Example** | *EXAMPLE 1* |

$$\frac{1}{75} \div \frac{1}{150} = \frac{1}{\underset{1}{\cancel{75}}} \times \frac{\overset{2}{\cancel{150}}}{1} = 2$$

EXAMPLE 2

$$\frac{\frac{1}{4}}{\frac{3}{8}} = \frac{1}{4} \div \frac{3}{8} = \frac{1}{\underset{1}{4}} \times \frac{\overset{2}{8}}{3} = \frac{2}{3}$$

EXAMPLE 3

$$\frac{1\frac{1}{5}}{\frac{2}{3}} = \frac{6}{5} \div \frac{2}{3} = \frac{\overset{3}{6}}{5} \times \frac{3}{\underset{1}{2}} = \frac{9}{5}$$

Learning Aid

Complex fractions such as

$$\frac{\frac{1}{4}}{\frac{3}{8}} \text{ may be read as } \frac{1}{4} \div \frac{3}{8}$$

Remember, the long line represents a division sign.

SELF-TEST 5 **Dividing Fractions**

Divide these fractions. This operation is important in calculating doses correctly. Answers are given at the end of the chapter.

1. $\frac{1}{75} \div \frac{1}{150} =$

2. $\frac{1}{8} \div \frac{1}{4} =$

3. $2\frac{2}{3} \div \frac{1}{2} =$

4. $75 \div 12\frac{1}{2} =$

5. $\frac{7}{25} \div \frac{7}{75} =$

6. $\frac{1}{2} \div \frac{1}{4} =$

7. $\frac{3}{4} \div \frac{8}{3} =$

8. $\frac{1}{60} \div \frac{7}{10} =$

Changing Fractions to Decimals

This can be accomplished by dividing the numerator by the denominator. Remember that the line between the numerator and the denominator is a division sign; hence, $\frac{1}{4}$ can be read as $1 \div 4$.

In division, the number being divided is called the *dividend;* the number that does the dividing is called the *divisor;* the answer is called the *quotient.*

$$\text{divisor} \rightarrow 16\overline{)640.} \quad \begin{array}{l} \leftarrow \text{quotient} \\ \leftarrow \text{dividend} \end{array}$$
$$\underline{64}$$
$$0$$

1. Look at the fraction $\frac{1}{4}$

   $\frac{1}{4} \quad \begin{array}{l} \leftarrow \text{numerator} = \text{dividend} \\ \leftarrow \text{denominator} = \text{divisor} \end{array}$

2. Write

   $4\overline{)1}$

3. If you have difficulty setting this up, you can continue the line for the fraction and place the number above the line into the box.

   $$\frac{1}{4} = \frac{1}{4\overline{)1}}$$

4. Once the division problem is set up, place a decimal point immediately after the dividend and also bring the decimal point up to the quotient.

$$\frac{\cancel{1}}{4} \overline{)1.} \quad \begin{array}{l} \cdot \leftarrow \text{quotient} \\ \leftarrow \text{dividend} \end{array}$$

Important! Failure to place decimal points carefully can lead to serious dose errors.

5. Carry out the division.

$$\frac{\cancel{1}}{4} \overline{\smash{\big)}\begin{array}{l} .25 \\ 1.00 \\ \underline{8} \\ 20 \\ \underline{20} \\ 0 \end{array}} = 0.25$$

> **Learning Aid**
>
> If the answer does not have a whole number; place a zero before the decimal. This prevents misreading the answer; .25 is incorrect; 0.25 is correct.
>   The number of places to report your answer will vary depending on the way the stock drug comes and the equipment you use. For these exercises, carry answers to three decimal places.

Example   *EXAMPLE 1*

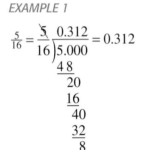

$$\frac{5}{16} = \frac{\cancel{5}}{16} \overline{\smash{\big)}\begin{array}{l} 0.312 \\ 5.000 \\ \underline{4\,8} \\ 20 \\ \underline{16} \\ 40 \\ \underline{32} \\ 8 \end{array}} = 0.312$$

EXAMPLE 2

$$\frac{640}{8} = \frac{\cancel{640}}{8} \overline{\smash{\big)}\begin{array}{l} 80. \\ 640. \end{array}} = 80$$

> **Learning Aid**
>
> Note that there is a space between the 8 and the decimal point in the answer. When this occurs, place a zero in the space to complete the answer.

EXAMPLE 3

$$\frac{1}{75} = \frac{\cancel{1}}{75} \overline{\smash{\big)}\begin{array}{l} 0.013 \\ 1.000 \\ \underline{75} \\ 250 \\ \underline{225} \\ 25 \end{array}} = 0.013$$

SELF-TEST 6   **Converting Fractions to Decimals**

Divide these fractions to produce decimals. Answers are given at the end of the chapter. Carry decimal places to three if necessary.

1. $\frac{1}{6}$

2. $\frac{6}{8}$

3. $\frac{4}{5}$

4. $\frac{9}{40}$

5. $\frac{1}{8}$

6. $\frac{1}{7}$

Decimals

Most medication orders are written in the metric system, which uses decimals.

Reading Decimals

Count the number of places after the decimal point. As you read the decimal, you also create a fraction.

0.1 is read as one tenth $\left(\frac{1}{10}\right)$.

0.01 is read as one hundredth $\left(\frac{1}{100}\right)$.

0.001 is read as one thousandth $\left(\frac{1}{1000}\right)$.

Learning Aid

The first number after the decimal point is the tenth place.
The second number after the decimal point is the 100th place.
The third number after the decimal point is the 1000th place.

Example

$0.56 =$ fifty-six hundredths $\left(\frac{56}{100}\right)$

$0.2 =$ two tenths $\left(\frac{2}{10}\right)$

$0.194 =$ one hundred ninety-four thousandths $\left(\frac{194}{1000}\right)$

$0.31 =$ thirty-one hundredths $\left(\frac{31}{100}\right)$

$1.6 =$ one and six tenths $\left(1\frac{6}{10}\right)$

$17.354 =$ seventeen and three hundred fifty-four thousandths $\left(17\frac{354}{1000}\right)$.

Learning Aid

When reading decimals, read the number first, then count off the decimal places.
Whole numbers preceding decimals are read in the usual way.

SELF-TEST 7 Reading Decimals

Write these decimals in longhand and as fractions. Answers are given at the end of the chapter.

1. 0.25 _____

2. 0.004 _____

3. 1.7 _____

4. 0.5 _____

5. 0.334 _____

6. 136.75 _____

7. 0.1 _____

8. 0.150 _____

Dividing Decimals

Again, in division the number that is being divided is called the *dividend;* the number that does the dividing is called the *divisor;* and the answer is called the *quotient.*

$$\text{divisor} \rightarrow 16\overline{)5.000} \rightarrow \text{dividend}$$
$$\qquad\qquad 0.312 \rightarrow \text{quotient}$$

Note that a decimal point is placed immediately after the dividend is written and is moved up to the quotient as well.

Example

$$\frac{13}{16}\,16\overline{)13.}$$

Division is then completed.

Example

$$16\overline{)13.000}\quad\frac{0.812}{}$$
$$\underline{12\ 8}$$
$$20$$
$$\underline{16}$$
$$40$$
$$\underline{32}$$
$$8$$

Clearing the Divisor of Decimal Points

Before dividing one decimal by another, clear the divisor of decimal points. To do this, move the decimal point to the far right. Move the decimal point in the dividend *the same number of places* and bring the decimal point up to the quotient in the same place.

Example

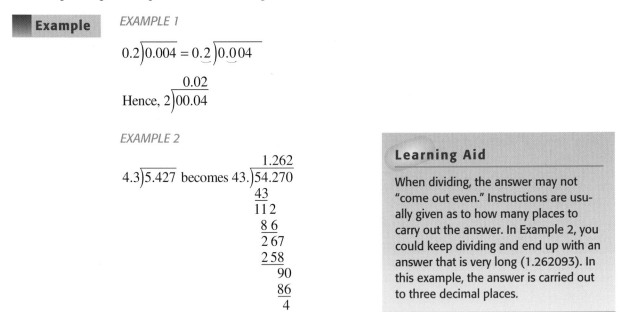

EXAMPLE 1

$$0.2\overline{)0.004}=0.2\overline{)0.004}$$

Hence, $2\overline{)00.04}\quad\frac{0.02}{}$

EXAMPLE 2

$$4.3\overline{)5.427}\text{ becomes }43.\overline{)54.270}\quad\frac{1.262}{}$$
$$\underline{43}$$
$$11\ 2$$
$$\underline{8\ 6}$$
$$2\ 67$$
$$\underline{2\ 58}$$
$$90$$
$$\underline{86}$$
$$4$$

Learning Aid

When dividing, the answer may not "come out even." Instructions are usually given as to how many places to carry out the answer. In Example 2, you could keep dividing and end up with an answer that is very long (1.262093). In this example, the answer is carried out to three decimal places.

SELF-TEST 8 | **Division of Decimals**

Do these problems in division of decimals. The answers are given at the end of this chapter. If necessary, carry the answer to three places.

1. $24\overline{)0.0048}$

2. $0.004\overline{)0.1}$

3. $0.02\overline{)0.2}$

4. $7.8\overline{)140}$

5. $6\overline{)140}$

6. $0.025\overline{)10}$

Rounding Off Decimals

How do you determine the number of places to carry out division? The answer depends on the way the drug is dispensed and the equipment needed to administer the drug. Some tablets can be broken into halves or fourths. Some liquids are prepared in units of measurement in tenths, hundredths, or thousandths. Some syringes are marked to the nearest tenth, hundredth, or thousandth place. Intravenous rates are usually rounded to the nearest whole number. As you become familiar with dosage, you will learn how far to round off answers. First, let us review the general rule for rounding off decimals.

RULE **ROUNDING OFF DECIMALS**

When the number to be dropped is 5 or more, drop the number and add 1 to the previous number. When the last number is 4 or less, drop the number.

Example
0.864 becomes 0.86

1.55 becomes 1.6

0.33 becomes 0.3

4.562 becomes 4.56

2.38 becomes 2.4

Suppose you want answers to the nearest tenth. Look at the number in the hundredth place and follow the rules for rounding off.

Example
0.12 becomes 0.1

0.667 becomes 0.7

1.46 becomes 1.5

Suppose you want answers to the nearest hundredth. Look at the number in the thousandth place and follow the rules for rounding off.

Example
0.664 becomes 0.66

0.148 becomes 0.15

2.375 becomes 2.38

Suppose you want answers to the nearest thousandth. Look at the number in the ten-thousandth place and follow the rules for rounding off.

Example
1.3758 becomes 1.376

0.0024 becomes 0.002

4.5555 becomes 4.556

SELF-TEST 9 | Rounding Decimals

Round off these decimals as indicated. Answers are given at the end of the chapter.

Nearest Tenth

1. 0.25 = _____
2. 1.84 = _____
3. 3.27 = _____
4. 0.05 = _____
5. 0.63 = _____

Nearest Hundredth

6. 1.268 = _____
7. 0.750 = _____
8. 0.677 = _____
9. 4.539 = _____
10. 1.222 = _____

Nearest Thousandth

11. 1.3254 = _____
12. 0.0025 = _____
13. 0.4520 = _____
14. 0.7259 = _____
15. 0.3482 = _____

Comparing the Value of Decimals

Understanding which decimal is larger or smaller is often a help in solving dosage problems. For example, will I need more than one tablet or less than one tablet?

RULE **DETERMINING THE VALUE OF DECIMALS**

The decimal with the higher number in the tenth place has the greater value. ■

Example Compare 0.25 with 0.5.

It is clear that 0.5 is greater because the number 5 is higher than the number 2.

SELF-TEST 10 | Value of Decimals

In each pair, underline the decimal with the greater value. Answers are given at the end of the chapter.

1. 0.125 and 0.25
2. 0.04 and 0.1
3. 0.5 and 0.125

4. 0.1 and 0.2
5. 0.825 and 0.44
6. 0.9 and 0.5

7. 0.25 and 0.4
8. 0.7 and 0.350

Percent

Percent means parts per hundred. Percent is a fraction, with the number becoming the numerator and 100 becoming the denominator. Whole numbers, fractions, and decimals may be written as percents. Percents may be changed to decimals or to fractions.

Example Whole number: 4% (four percent)

Decimal: 0.2% (two-tenths percent)

Fraction: $\frac{1}{4}$% (one-fourth percent)

Percents That Are Whole Numbers

> **Example**

EXAMPLE 1

Change to a fraction.

$$4\% = \frac{4}{100} = \frac{1}{25}$$

EXAMPLE 2

Change to a decimal.

$$4\% = \frac{4}{100} \quad \frac{.04}{100\overline{)4.00}} = 0.04$$

> **Learning Aid**
>
> Note that 4% means four parts per 100. The one hundredth place has two decimal points. A quick rule to change a percent to a decimal is to move the decimal point two places to the left.
>
> 4% = 0.04
>
> 25% = 0.25

Percents That Are Decimals

These may be changed in three ways:

1. By using the quick rule (see Learning Aid)

   $$0.2\% = 00.2 = 0.002$$

> **Learning Aid**
>
> Quick rule: To remove a percent sign, move the decimal point two places to the left.

2. By keeping the decimal (see Learning Aid)

   $$0.2\% = \frac{0.2}{100} \quad \frac{0.002}{100\overline{)0.200}} = 0.002$$

> **Learning Aid**
>
> Method 2: Place the number over 100.

3. By changing to a complex fraction

   $$0.2\% = \frac{\frac{2}{10}}{100} =$$

   $$\frac{2}{10} \div \frac{100}{1} =$$

   $$\frac{2}{10} \times \frac{1}{100} = \frac{2}{1000}$$

   $$\frac{\frac{1}{2}}{\frac{1000}{500}} = \frac{1}{500}$$

> **Learning Aid**
>
> Remember that the number after a division sign is inverted. The sign is changed to a multiplication sign.
> Every whole number is understood to have a denominator of 1.
>
> $$\frac{2}{10} \div 100 = \frac{2}{10} \times \frac{1}{100}$$

Percents That Are Fractions

> **Example**

EXAMPLE 1

$$\frac{1}{4}\% = \frac{\frac{1}{4}}{100} = \frac{1}{4} \div \frac{100}{1} = \frac{1}{4} \times \frac{1}{100} = \frac{1}{400}$$

EXAMPLE 2

$$\tfrac{1}{2}\% = \frac{\tfrac{1}{2}}{100} = \tfrac{1}{2} \div \tfrac{100}{1} = \tfrac{1}{2} \times \tfrac{1}{100} = \tfrac{1}{200}$$

ALTERNATIVE WAY. Because $\tfrac{1}{2} = 0.5$, $\tfrac{1}{2}\%$ could also be written as 0.5%. By using the quick rule of moving the decimal point two places to the left to clear a percent, you have $00.5\% = 0.005$. Note that 0.005 is $\tfrac{5}{1000} = \tfrac{1}{200}$. You could also write $\tfrac{0.5}{100}$.

SELF-TEST 11   Conversion of Percents

*Change these percents to both a **fraction** and a **decimal**. Answers are given at the end of the chapter.*

1. 10% _____ _____

2. 0.9% _____ _____

3. $\tfrac{1}{5}\%$ _____ _____

4. 0.01% _____ _____

5. 2/3% _____ _____

6. 0.45% _____ _____

7. 20% _____ _____

8. 0.4% _____ _____

9. $\tfrac{1}{10}\%$ _____ _____

10. 2 1/2% _____ _____

11. 33% _____ _____

12. 50% _____ _____

► Ratio and Proportion

A ratio indicates the relationship between two numbers. Ratios can be written as a fraction $\left(\tfrac{1}{10}\right)$ or as two numbers separated by a colon (1:10). (Read as *one is to ten.*)

Proportion indicates a relationship between two ratios. Proportions can be written as fractions or as two ratios separated by a double colon.

Example $\tfrac{2}{8} = \tfrac{10}{40}$ (Read as *two is to eight as ten is to forty.*)

5:30 :: 6:36 (Read as *five is to thirty as six is to thirty-six.*)

Proportions written with colons can be written as fractions; therefore 5:30 :: 6:36 becomes

$$\tfrac{5}{30} = \tfrac{6}{36}$$

Solving Proportion with an Unknown

When one of the numbers in a proportion is unknown, the letter x is substituted. There are three steps in determining the value of x in a proportion.

Step 1.   Cross-multiply.

Step 2.   Clear x.

Step 3.   Reduce.

Let's see how this is done.

Proportions Expressed as Decimals

Suppose you had to solve this proportion:

$\frac{1}{0.125} = \frac{x}{0.25}$

Step 1. Cross-multiply the numerators and denominators.

$0.125x = 0.25$

> **Learning Aid**
>
> How to cross-multiply
>
> $\frac{1}{0.125} \times \frac{x}{0.25}$

Step 2. Clear x by dividing both sides of the equation with the number preceding x.

$x = \frac{0.25}{0.125}$

> **Learning Aid**
>
> $\frac{0.125x}{0.125} = \frac{0.25}{0.125}$

Step 3. Reduce the number.

$0.125 \overline{)0.250.}$ with $2.$ above

$x = 2$

> **Learning Aid**
>
> Remember, the line between the two numbers in a fraction is a division sign.
>
> $\frac{0.25}{0.125}$
>
> This can be read as 0.25 divided by 0.125.

Proportions Expressed as Two Ratios Separated by Colons

Suppose you had this proportion:

$4 : 3.2 :: 7 : x$

Step 1. Cross-multiply the two outside numbers (called *extremes*) and the two inside numbers (called *means*).

$4 : 3.2 :: 7 : x$

$4x = 22.4$

Step 2. Clear x by dividing both sides of the equation with the number preceding x.

$x = \frac{22.4}{4}$

> **Learning Aid**
>
> $\frac{4x}{4} = \frac{22.4}{4}$
>
> Remember that the line between two numbers in a fraction is a division sign. This can be read as 22.4 divided by 4.

Step 3.   Reduce the number.

$x = 5.6$

Learning Aid

$$4\overline{)22.4}$$
$$5.6$$

Example $\dfrac{45}{180} \bowtie \dfrac{3}{x}$

$45x = 540$

$x = 12$

Learning Aid

$$45\overline{)540.}$$
$$12.$$
$$45$$
$$\overline{90}$$
$$90$$

Example $11x = 363$

$x = 33$

$11 : 121 :: 3 : x$

Learning Aid

$$11\overline{)363.}$$
$$33.$$
$$33$$
$$\overline{33}$$
$$33$$

SELF-TEST 12   Solving Proportions

Solve these proportions. Answers are given at the end of the chapter.

1. $\dfrac{120}{4.2} = \dfrac{16}{x}$

2. $750 : 250 :: x : 5$

3. $\dfrac{14}{140} = \dfrac{22}{x}$

4. $2 : 5 :: x : 10$

5. $\dfrac{81}{3} = \dfrac{x}{15}$

6. $0.125 : 0.5 :: x : 10$

Ratio and Proportion in Dosage

When the amount of drug ordered by a physician differs from the supply, ratio and proportion are used to solve the problem.

Example   Order: 0.5 mg of a drug

Supply: A liquid labeled 0.125 mg per 4 mL

We know the liquid comes as 0.125 mg in 4 mL. We want 0.5 mg. We don't know what amount of liquid will contain 0.5 mg. We have three pieces of information. We need the fourth, which is *X*.

This arithmetic operation can be set up and solved as a fraction–ratio or as two ratios separated by colons.

Fraction–Ratio

$$\frac{0.5}{0.125} \diagdown \frac{X}{4}$$

$$0.125X = 2$$

$$\downarrow$$

$$\frac{0.125X}{0.125} = \frac{2}{0.125}$$

$$\downarrow$$

$$X = \frac{2}{0.125}$$

$$\downarrow$$

$$X = \frac{2}{0.125} \quad 0.125\overline{)2.000.}^{16.}$$
$$\underline{1\ 25}$$
$$750$$
$$\underline{750}$$

$$X = 16$$

Two Ratios Using Colons

$$0.5 : 0.125 :: X : 4$$

$$0.125X = 2$$

$$\downarrow$$

$$\frac{0.125X}{0.125} = \frac{2.0}{0.125}$$

$$\downarrow$$

$$X = \frac{2}{0.125}$$

$$\downarrow$$

$$X = \frac{2}{0.125} \quad 0.125\overline{)2.000.}^{16.}$$
$$\underline{1\ 25}$$
$$750$$
$$\underline{750}$$

Learning Aid

Clear *X* by dividing both sides of the equation with the number preceding *X*.

Learning Aid

Notice both methods eventually become the same calculation.

Learning Aid

Remember, the line between the two numbers in a fraction is a division sign. This is read as 2.0 divided by 0.125.

In the previous examples, several steps are needed to solve ratio and proportion. This procedure can be simplified.

In Chapter 6 we will learn the formula method, which is derived from ratio and proportion. In Chapter 11, the dimensional analysis method is explained and proficiency test problems are solved that show all four methods of calculations.

Name: _____

These arithmetic operations are needed to calculate doses. Answers are on page 391. If you have diffi-culty in any area, study the related materials again. Your instructor can provide other practice tests if necessary from the Instructors' Manual.

A. Multiply

   a) $\begin{array}{r} 647 \\ \times\,38 \\ \hline \end{array}$ **b)** $\frac{8}{9} \times \frac{12}{32}$ **c)** $\begin{array}{r} 0.56 \\ \times\,0.17 \\ \hline \end{array}$

B. Divide. If necessary, report to two decimal places.

   a) $82\overline{)793}$ **b)** $5\frac{1}{4} \div \frac{7}{4}$ **c)** $0.015\overline{)0.3}$

C. Change to a decimal. If necessary, report to two decimal places.

   a) $\frac{1}{18}$ **b)** $\frac{3}{8}$

D. Change to a fraction and reduce to lowest terms.

   a) 0.35   **b)** 0.08

E. In each set, which number has the greater value?

   a) _____ 0.4 and 0.162

   b) _____ 0.76 and 0.8

   c) _____ 0.5 and 0.83

   d) _____ 0.3 and 0.25

F. Reduce these fractions to their lowest terms as decimals. Report to two decimal places.

   a) $\frac{20}{12}$ **b)** $\frac{7}{84}$ **c)** $\frac{6}{13}$

G. Round off these decimals as indicated.

   a) nearest tenth   5.349 _____

   b) nearest hundredth   0.6284 _____

   c) nearest thousandth   0.9244 _____

H. Change these percents to a fraction.

   a) $\frac{1}{3}\%$ **b)** 0.8%

I. Solve these ratios.

   a) $\frac{32}{128} = \frac{4}{X}$

   b) $8 : 72 :: 5 : X$

   c) $\frac{0.4}{0.12} = \frac{X}{8}$ (nearest whole number)

Answers

Self-Test 1 Multiplication

1. 12	**5.** 108	**9.** 48	**13.** 24	**17.** 18	**21.** 132
2. 63	**6.** 24	**10.** 72	**14.** 54	**18.** 88	**22.** 45
3. 32	**7.** 110	**11.** 15	**15.** 64	**19.** 36	**23.** 81
4. 45	**8.** 14	**12.** 42	**16.** 56	**20.** 24	**24.** 35

Self-Test 2 Division

1. 9	**5.** 7	**9.** 7	**13.** 4	**17.** 9	**21.** 7
2. 4	**6.** 8	**10.** 6	**14.** 3	**18.** 4	**22.** 12
3. 3	**7.** 4	**11.** 9	**15.** 3	**19.** 6	**23.** 12
4. 7	**8.** 3	**12.** 6	**16.** 7	**20.** 2	**24.** 7

Self-Test 3 Reducing Fractions

1. $\frac{16}{24} = \frac{4}{6} = \frac{2}{3}$ (Divide by 4, then 2.)

Alternatively: $\frac{16}{24} = \frac{2}{3}$ (Divide by 8.)

2. $\frac{36}{216} = \frac{6}{36} = \frac{1}{6}$ (Divide by 6, then 6.)

3. $\frac{18}{96} = \frac{9}{48} = \frac{3}{16}$ (Divide by 2, then 3.)

4. $\frac{70}{490} = \frac{7}{49} = \frac{1}{7}$ (Divide by 10, then 7.)

5. $\frac{18}{81} = \frac{2}{9}$ (Divide by 9.)

6. $\frac{8}{48} = \frac{1}{6}$ (Divide by 8.)

7. $\frac{12}{30} = \frac{6}{15} = \frac{2}{5}$ (Divide by 2, then 3.)

Alternatively: $\frac{12}{30} = \frac{2}{5}$ (Divide by 6.)

8. $\frac{68}{136} = \frac{34}{68} = \frac{1}{2}$ (Divide by 2, then 34.)

9. $\frac{55}{121} = \frac{5}{11}$ (Divide by 11.)

10. $\frac{15}{60} = \frac{1}{4}$ (Divide by 15.)

Alternatively: $\frac{15}{60} = \frac{3}{12} = \frac{1}{4}$ (Divide by 5, then 3.)

Self-Test 4 Multiplying Fractions (Two Ways to Solve)

First Way

1. $\frac{1}{6} \times \frac{4}{5} \times \frac{5}{2} = \frac{20}{60} = \frac{1}{3}$

2. $\frac{4}{15} \times \frac{3}{2} = \frac{\overset{2}{12}}{\underset{5}{30}} = \frac{2}{5}$

(Divide by 6)

3. $1\frac{1}{2} \times 4\frac{2}{3} = \frac{3}{2} \times \frac{14}{3} = \frac{\overset{7}{42}}{\underset{1}{6}} = 7$

4. $\frac{1}{5} \times \frac{15}{45} = \frac{\overset{3}{15}}{\underset{45}{225}} = \frac{3}{45} = \frac{1}{15}$

(Divide by 5.)

Second Way

1. $\frac{1}{\underset{3}{6}} \times \frac{\overset{1}{4}}{\underset{1}{5}} \times \frac{\overset{1}{5}}{\underset{1}{2}} = \frac{\overset{1}{2}}{\underset{3}{6}} = \frac{1}{3}$

2. $\frac{\overset{2}{4}}{\underset{5}{15}} \times \frac{\overset{1}{3}}{\underset{1}{2}} = \frac{2}{5}$

3. $1\frac{1}{2} \times 4\frac{2}{3} = \frac{\overset{1}{3}}{\underset{1}{2}} \times \frac{\overset{7}{14}}{\underset{1}{3}} = 7$

4. $\frac{1}{5} \times \frac{\overset{1}{15}}{\underset{3}{45}} = \frac{1}{15}$

5. $3\frac{3}{4} \times 10\frac{2}{3} = \frac{15}{4} \times \frac{32}{3}$

(Too confusing! Use the second way.)

6. $\frac{7}{20} \times \frac{2}{14}$

(Too difficult. Use the second way.)

7. $\frac{9}{2} \times \frac{3}{2} = \frac{27}{4}$

(Cannot reduce.)

8. $6\frac{1}{4} \times 7\frac{1}{9} \times \frac{9}{5} = \frac{25}{4} \times \frac{64}{9} \times \frac{9}{5}$

(Too difficult. Use the second way.)

5. $\dfrac{\overset{5}{\cancel{15}}}{\underset{1}{\cancel{4}}} \times \dfrac{\overset{8}{\cancel{32}}}{\underset{1}{\cancel{3}}} = 40$

6. $\dfrac{\overset{1}{\cancel{7}}}{\underset{10}{\cancel{20}}} \times \dfrac{\overset{1}{\cancel{2}}}{\underset{2}{\cancel{14}}} = \dfrac{1}{20}$

8. $\dfrac{\overset{5}{\cancel{25}}}{\underset{1}{\cancel{4}}} \times \dfrac{\overset{16}{\cancel{64}}}{\underset{1}{\cancel{9}}} \times \dfrac{\overset{1}{\cancel{9}}}{\underset{1}{\cancel{5}}} = 80$

Self-Test 5 Dividing Fractions

1. $\frac{1}{75} \div \frac{1}{150} = \frac{1}{\cancel{75}} \times \frac{\overset{2}{\cancel{150}}}{1} = 2$

2. $\frac{1}{8} \div \frac{1}{4} = \frac{1}{\cancel{8}} \times \frac{\overset{1}{\cancel{4}}}{1} = \frac{1}{2}$

3. $2\frac{2}{3} \div \frac{1}{2} = \frac{8}{3} \times \frac{2}{1} = \frac{16}{3}$

4. $75 \div 12\frac{1}{2} = 75 \div \frac{25}{2} = \frac{\overset{3}{\cancel{75}}}{} \times \frac{2}{\underset{1}{\cancel{25}}} = 6$

5. $\frac{7}{25} \div \frac{7}{75} = \frac{\overset{1}{\cancel{7}}}{\underset{1}{\cancel{25}}} \times \frac{\overset{3}{\cancel{75}}}{\underset{1}{\cancel{7}}} = 3$

6. $\frac{1}{2} \div \frac{1}{4} = \frac{1}{\cancel{2}} \times \frac{\overset{2}{\cancel{4}}}{1} = 2$

7. $\frac{3}{4} \div \frac{8}{3} = \frac{3}{4} \times \frac{3}{8} = \frac{9}{32}$

8. $\frac{1}{60} \div \frac{7}{10} = \frac{1}{\underset{6}{\cancel{60}}} \times \frac{\overset{1}{\cancel{10}}}{7} = \frac{1}{42}$

Self-Test 6 Converting Fractions to Decimals

1. $\dfrac{1}{6} \quad 6\overline{)1.000}^{\,.166} = 0.166$

$\dfrac{6}{40}$

$\dfrac{36}{40}$

$\dfrac{36}{4}$

2. $\dfrac{\overset{3}{\cancel{6}}}{\underset{4}{\cancel{8}}} = \dfrac{3}{4} \quad 4\overline{)3.00}^{\,.75} = 0.75$

$\dfrac{2\,8}{20}$

$\dfrac{20}{0}$

3. $\dfrac{4}{5} \quad 5\overline{)4.0}^{\,.8} = 0.8$

$\dfrac{4\,0}{0}$

4. $\dfrac{9}{40} \quad 40\overline{)9.000}^{\,.225} = 0.225$

$\dfrac{8\,0}{1\,00}$

$\dfrac{80}{200}$

$\dfrac{200}{0}$

5. $\dfrac{1}{8} \quad 8\overline{)1.000}^{\,.125} = 0.125$

$\dfrac{8}{20}$

$\dfrac{16}{40}$

$\dfrac{40}{0}$

6. $\dfrac{1}{7} \quad 7\overline{)1.000}^{\,.145} = 0.142$

$\dfrac{7}{30}$

$\dfrac{28}{20}$

$\dfrac{14}{6}$

Self-Test 7 Reading Decimals

1. Twenty-five hundredths $\left(\frac{25}{100}\right)$

2. Four thousandths $\left(\frac{4}{1000}\right)$

3. One and seven tenths $\left(1\frac{7}{10}\right)$

4. Five tenths $\left(\frac{5}{10}\right)$

5. Three hundred thirty-four thousandths $\left(\frac{334}{1000}\right)$

6. One hundred thirty-six and seventy-five hundredths $\left(136\frac{75}{100}\right)$

7. One tenth $\left(\frac{1}{10}\right)$

8. One hundred fifty thousandths $\left(\frac{150}{1000}\right)$. The zero at the end of 0.150 is not necessary. The number could be read as fifteen hundredths $\left(\frac{15}{100}\right)$.

Self-Test 8 Division of Decimals

1. $24\overline{)0.0048}$ $\;\;0.0002$ No decimals in the divisor, so no need to move the decimal in the dividend.

2. $0.004\overline{)0.100}$ Now it is $4\overline{)100.}$ $25.$

3. $0.02\overline{)0.20}$ Now it is $2\overline{)20.}$ $10.$

4. $7.8\overline{)140.0}$ Now it is $78\overline{)1400.000}$ 17.948

$$
\begin{array}{r}
17.948 \\
78\overline{)1400.000} \\
\underline{78} \\
620 \\
\underline{546} \\
74\,0 \\
\underline{70\,2} \\
3\,80 \\
\underline{3\,12} \\
680 \\
\underline{624} \\
56
\end{array}
$$

5. $6\overline{)140.000}$

$$
\begin{array}{r}
23.333 \\
6\overline{)140.000} \\
\underline{12} \\
20 \\
\underline{18} \\
20 \\
\underline{18} \\
20 \\
\underline{18} \\
20 \\
\underline{18} \\
2
\end{array}
$$

6. $0.025\overline{)10.000}$ Now it is $25\overline{)10000.}$ $400.$

Note that because there are two places between the 4 and the decimal, you had to add two zeros.

Self-Test 9 Rounding Decimals

Nearest Tenth	*Nearest Hundredth*	*Nearest Thousandth*
1. 0.3	6. 1.27	11. 1.325
2. 1.8	7. 0.75	12. 0.003
3. 3.3	8. 0.68	13. 0.452
4. 0.1	9. 4.54	14. 0.726
5. 0.6	10. 1.22	15. 0.348

Self-Test 10 Value of Decimals

1. 0.25	4. 0.2	7. 0.4
2. 0.1	5. 0.825	8. 0.7
3. 0.5	6. 0.9	

Self-Test 11 Conversion of Percents

1. Fraction $10\% = \dfrac{\frac{1}{10}}{\frac{100}{10}} = \frac{1}{10}$

   Decimal $10\% = \dfrac{10}{100}\ \overset{.1}{100)\overline{10.0}} = 0.1$

   Quick-rule decimal $\underset{\smile}{10.}\% = 0.1$

2. Fraction $0.9\% = \dfrac{\frac{9}{10}}{100} = \frac{9}{10} \div 100 = \frac{9}{10} \times \frac{1}{100} = \frac{9}{1000}$

   Decimal $0.9\% = \dfrac{0.9}{100}\ \overset{.009}{100)\overline{0.900}} = 0.009$

   Quick-rule decimal $\underset{\smile}{00.9}\% = 0.009$

3. Fraction $\frac{1}{5}\% = \dfrac{\frac{1}{5}}{100} = \frac{1}{5} \div 100 = \frac{1}{5} \times \frac{1}{100} = \frac{1}{500}$

   Decimal $\dfrac{1}{5}\% = \dfrac{1}{5} \div 100 = \dfrac{1}{500}\ \overset{.002}{500)\overline{1.000}} = 0.002$

   Quick-rule decimal $\dfrac{1}{5}\% = \dfrac{1}{5}\ \overset{.2}{5)\overline{1.0}} = 0.2\%$

   $\underset{\smile}{00.2} = 0.002$

4. Fraction $0.01\% = \dfrac{\frac{1}{100}}{100} = \frac{1}{100} \div \frac{100}{1} = \frac{1}{100} \times \frac{1}{100} = \frac{1}{10000}$

   Decimal $0.1\% = \dfrac{0.01}{100}\ \overset{0.0001}{100)\overline{.0100}} = 0.0001$

   Quick-rule decimal $\underset{\smile}{00.01} = 0.0001$

5. Fraction $\frac{2}{3}\% = \dfrac{\frac{2}{3}}{100} = \frac{2}{3} \div \frac{100}{1} = \frac{2}{3} \times \frac{1}{100} = \frac{2}{300} = \frac{1}{150}$

   Decimal $\dfrac{2}{3}\% = \dfrac{2}{3} \div \dfrac{100}{1} = \dfrac{2}{3} \times \dfrac{1}{100} = \dfrac{2}{300}\ \overset{.0066}{300)\overline{2.000}} = 0.0066$

   Quick-rule decimal $\dfrac{2}{3}\% = \dfrac{2}{3}\ \overset{.66}{3)\overline{2.00}} = 0.66\% = \underset{\smile}{00.66} = 0.0066$

6. Fraction $0.45\% = \dfrac{\frac{45}{100}}{100} = \frac{45}{100} \div \frac{100}{1} = \frac{45}{100} \times \frac{1}{100} = \frac{45}{10000} = \frac{9}{2000}$

   Decimal $0.45\% = \dfrac{.45}{100}\ \overset{.0045}{100)\overline{0.4500}} = 0.0045$

   Quick-rule decimal $\underset{\smile}{00.45}\% = 0.0045$

7. Fraction $\dfrac{\overset{1}{\cancel{20}}}{\underset{5}{\cancel{100}}} = \dfrac{1}{5}$

Decimal $20\% = \dfrac{20}{100}\ \overset{0.2}{\overline{)20.0}}$

Quick-rule decimal $\underset{\smile}{20}.\% = 0.2$

8. Fraction $0.4\% = \dfrac{\frac{4}{10}}{100} = \dfrac{4}{10} \div \dfrac{100}{1} = \dfrac{\overset{1}{\cancel{4}}}{10} \times \dfrac{1}{\underset{25}{\cancel{100}}} = \dfrac{1}{250}$

Decimal $0.4\% = \dfrac{0.4}{100}\ \overset{0.004}{\overline{)0.400}} = 0.004$

Quick-rule decimal $\underset{\smile}{00}.4\% = 0.004$

9. Fraction $\dfrac{1}{10}\% = \dfrac{\frac{1}{10}}{100} = \dfrac{1}{10} \div \dfrac{100}{1} = \dfrac{1}{10} \times \dfrac{1}{100} = \dfrac{1}{1000}$

Decimal $\dfrac{1}{10}\% = \dfrac{1}{10} \div \dfrac{100}{1} = \dfrac{1}{10} \times \dfrac{1}{100} = \dfrac{1}{1000}\ \overset{0.001}{\overline{)1.000}} = 0.001$

Quick-rule decimal $\dfrac{1}{10}\% = \dfrac{1}{10}\ \overset{0.1}{\overline{)1.0}} = 0.1\% = \underset{\smile}{00}.1 = 0.001$

10. Fraction $2\tfrac{1}{2}\% = 2.5\% = \dfrac{\frac{25}{10}}{100} = \dfrac{25}{10} \div \dfrac{100}{1} = \dfrac{25}{10} \times \dfrac{1}{100} = \dfrac{25}{1000} = \dfrac{1}{40}$

Decimal $2.5\% = \dfrac{2.5}{100}\ \overset{0.025}{\overline{)2.50}} = 0.025$

Quick-rule decimal $\underset{\smile}{000}.2.5\% = 0.025$

11. Fraction $33\% = \dfrac{33}{100}$

Decimal $33\% = \dfrac{33}{100}\ \overset{.33}{\overline{)33.00}} = 0.33$

Quick-rule decimal $\underset{\smile}{33}.\% = 0.33$

12. Fraction $50\% = \dfrac{50}{100} = \dfrac{1}{2}$

Decimal $50\% = \dfrac{50}{100}\ \overset{.5}{\overline{)50.0}} = 0.5$

Quick-rule decimal $\underset{\smile}{50}.\% = 0.5$

Self-Test 12 Solving Proportions

1. $\frac{120}{4.2} = \frac{16}{x}$

$120x = 67.2$

$x = 0.56$

$$\begin{array}{r} 0.56 \\ 120\overline{\smash{)}67.20} \\ \underline{60\ 0} \\ 7\ 20 \\ \underline{7\ 20} \end{array}$$

4. $2:5::x:10$

$5x = 20$

$x = 4$

2. $750:250::x:5$

$250x = 750 \times 5$

$x = 15$

$\dfrac{\overset{3}{\cancel{750}} \times 5}{\underset{1}{\cancel{250}}} = 15$

5. $\frac{81}{3} = \frac{x}{15}$

$3x = 81 \times 15$

$x = 405$

$\dfrac{81 \times \overset{5}{\cancel{15}}}{\underset{1}{\cancel{3}}} = 405$

3. $\frac{14}{140} = \frac{22}{x}$

$14x = 22 \times 140$

$x = 220$

$\dfrac{22 \times \overset{10}{\cancel{140}}}{\underset{1}{\cancel{14}}} = 220$

6. $0.125:0.5::x:10$

$0.5x = 0.125 \times 10 = \dfrac{\overset{1}{\cancel{0.125}}}{\underset{4}{\cancel{0.500}}} \times 10 = \dfrac{10}{4}\,\overline{\smash{)}10.0}^{\,2.5}$

$x = 2.5$

Interpreting the Language of Prescriptions

Misreading abbreviations leads to medication errors. When you are unsure of the abbreviation or the handwriting, or have a question regarding a medication order, do not attempt to prepare the dose. *Clarify the order with the person who wrote the order.*

Here are three medication orders that will make sense to you after studying material in this chapter:

Morphine sulfate 15 mg sub Q stat and 10 mg q4h prn

Chloromycetin 0.01% Ophth Oint OS bid

Ampicillin 1 g IVPB q6h

In 2004, the Joint Commission on Accreditation of Healthcare Organizations issued a list of "do not use" abbreviations. These abbreviations were often misread and led to medication errors. In this text, these abbreviations will be mentioned and noted as "Do Not Use." A complete list of the "do not use" abbreviations may be accessed on the JCAHO Web site (www.jcaho.org) and by doing a search on "prohibited abbreviations."

Time of Administration of Drugs

The abbreviations for times of drug administration are based on Latin words. They are included in the following table for your information, but it is not necessary for you to study or learn the Latin words. Learn the abbreviations, their meanings, and the sample times that indicate how the abbreviations are interpreted.

Time Abbreviation	Meaning	Learning Aid
ac	Before meals	Latin, *ante cibum* **Sample Time** 7:30 AM, 11:30 AM, 4:30 PM
pc	After meals	Latin, *post cibum* **Sample Time** 10 AM, 2 PM, 6 PM

(continued)

(Continued)

Time Abbreviation	Meaning	Learning Aid		Do Not Use
daily	Every day, daily	Latin, *quaque die*		q.d.
		Sample Time	10 AM	qd
bid	Twice a day	Latin, *bis in die*		
		Sample Time	10 AM, 6 PM	
tid	Three times a day	Latin, *ter in die*		
		Sample Time	10 AM, 2 PM, 6 PM	
qid	Four times a day	Latin, *quater in die*		
		Sample Time	10 AM, 2 PM, 6 PM, 10 PM	
qh	Every hour	Latin, *quaque hora* Because the drug is given every hour, it will be given 24 times in one day.		
at bedtime	At bedtime, hour of sleep	Latin, *hora somni*.		hs
		Sample Time	10 PM	h.s.
qn	Every night	Latin, *quaque nocte*		
		Sample Time	10 PM	
stat	Immediately	Latin, *statim*		
		Sample Time	Now!	

The time abbreviations in the following table are based on a 24-hour day. To determine the number of times a medication is given in a day, divide 24 by the number given in the abbreviation.

Time Abbreviation	Meaning	Learning Aid	
q2h or q2°	Every 2 hours	The drug will be given 12 times in a 24-hour period (24 ÷ 2).	
		Sample Times	even hours at 2 AM, 4 AM, 6 AM, 8 AM, 10 AM, 12 noon, 2 PM, 4 PM, 6 PM, 8 PM, 10 PM, 12 midnight
q4h or q4°	Every 4 hours	The drug will be given six times in a 24-hour period (24 ÷ 4)	
		Sample Times	2 AM, 6 AM, 10 AM, 2 PM, 6 PM, 10 PM
q6h or q6°	Every 6 hours	The drug will be given four times in a 24-hour period (24 ÷ 6)	
		Sample Times	6 AM, 12 noon, 6 PM, 12 midnight
q8h or q8°	Every 8 hours	The drug will be given three times in a 24-hour period (24 ÷ 8)	
		Sample Times	6 AM, 2 PM, 10 PM
q12h or q12°	Every 12 hours	The drug will be given twice in a 24-hour period (24 ÷ 12)	
		Sample Times	6 AM, 6 PM

There are four additional time abbreviations that require explanation. They are as follows:

Time Abbreviation	Meaning	Learning Aid	Do Not Use
every other day	Every other day	Latin, *quaque otra die* This abbreviation is interpreted by the days of the **month:** the nurse writes on the medication record: qod odd days of the month **Sample Time** — 10 AM on the first, third, fifth day, and so on The nurse might write: qod even days of the month **Sample Time** — 10 AM on the second, fourth, sixth day, and so on	qod q.o.d.
pm	As needed	Latin, *pro re nata* **This abbreviation is usually combined with a time abbreviation.** **Example** — q4h prn (every 4 hours as needed) This permits the nurse to assess the patient and make a nursing judgment about whether to administer the medication. **Sample** — acetaminophen 650 mg po q4h prn (650 milligrams acetaminophen by mouth, every 4 hours as needed for pain) The nurse assesses the patient for pain every 4 hours. If the patient has pain, the nurse may administer the drug. This abbreviation has three administration implications: 1. The nurse **must wait** 4 hours before giving the next dose. 2. Once 4 hours have elapsed, the dose may be given any time thereafter. 3. Sample times are not given because the nurse does not know when the patient will need the drug.	
3 times weekly	Three times per week	Latin, *ter in vicis* Time relates to days of the **week.** **Sample Time** — 10 AM on Monday, Wednesday, Friday Do not confuse with tid (three times per **day**).	tiw t.i.w.
biw	Twice per week	Latin, *bis in vicis* Time relates to days of the **week.** **Sample Time** — 10 AM on Monday, Thursday Do not confuse with bid (twice per **day**).	

SELF-TEST 1 Abbreviations

After studying the abbreviations for times of administration, give the meaning of the following terms. Include sample times. Indicate if the abbreviation is not to be used, and the words to substitute for it. Answers are given at the end of the chapter.

1. tid_____
2. qn_____
3. pc_____
4. qod_____
5. bid_____
6. hs_____
7. stat_____
8. qid_____

9. q4h_____
10. ac_____
11. qd_____
12. q8h_____
13. qh_____
14. prn_____
15. q4h prn_____

Military Time: The 24-Hour Clock

Confusion about times of administration can arise by misinterpreting handwriting as AM or PM. To prevent error, many institutions have converted from the traditional 12-hour clock to a 24-hour clock, referred to as *military time.*

The 24-hour clock begins at midnight as 0000. The hours from 1 AM to 12 noon are the same as traditional time; colons and the terms AM and PM are omitted. For example:

Traditional	*Military*
12 midnight	0000
1 AM	0100
5 AM	0500
7:30 AM	0730
11:45 AM	1145
12:00 noon	1200

The hours from 1 PM continue numerically; 1 PM becomes 1300. For example:

Traditional	*Military*
1 PM	1300
2:30 PM	1430
5 PM	1700
7:15 PM	1915
10:45 PM	2245
11:59 PM	2359

Learning Aid

To change traditional time to military time from 1 PM on, add 12.

SELF-TEST 2 | **Military Time**

A. *Change these traditional times to military time. Answers are given at the end of the chapter.*

1. 2 PM _____   **5.** 1:30 AM _____

2. 9 AM _____   **6.** 9:15 PM _____

3. 4 PM _____   **7.** 4:50 AM _____

4. 12 noon _____   **8.** 6:20 PM _____

B. *Change these military times to traditional times. Answers are given at the end of the chapter.*

1. 0130 _____   **5.** 1910 _____

2. 1745 _____   **6.** 0600 _____

3. 1100 _____   **7.** 0050 _____

4. 2015 _____   **8.** 1000 _____

> **Learning Aid**
>
> To change military time to traditional
> time from 1300 on, subtract 12.

▶ Routes of Administration

Some of the following abbreviations are based on Latin words, whereas others are not. Again, the Latin words are included for your information, but it is not necessary to study them. Alternative abbreviations are given in parentheses.

Route Abbreviation	Meaning	Learning Aid	Do Not Use
Write out	Right ear	Latin, *aures dextra*	AD
Write out	Left ear	Latin, *aures laeva*	AL
Write out	Each ear	Latin, *aures utrae*	AU
HHN	Hand-held nebulizer	Medication is placed in a device that produces a fine spray for inhalation.	
IM	Intramuscularly	The injection is given at a 90° angle into a muscle.	
IV	Intravenously	The injection is given into a vein.	
IVP	Intravenous push	Medication is injected directly in a vein.	
IVPB	Intravenous piggyback	Medication prepared in a small volume of fluid is attached to an IV (which is already infusing fluid into a patient's vein) at specified times.	
MDI	Metered-dose inhaler	An aerosol device delivers medication by inhalation.	
NEB	Nebulizer	Medication is placed in a device that produces a fine spray for inhalations.	
NGT (ng)	Nasogastric tube	Medication is placed in the stomach through a tube in the nose.	
OD*	In the right eye	Latin, *oculus dextra*	
OS*	In the left eye	Latin, *oculus sinister*	
OU*	In both eyes	Latin, *oculi utrique*	
po (PO)	By mouth	Latin, *per os*	
pr (PR)	In the rectum	Latin, *per rectum*	
Sub-Q or Sub Q	Subcutaneously	The injection is usually given at a 45° angle into subcutaneous tissue.	sc sq s.c. s.q.
SL	Sublingual, under the tongue	Latin, *sub lingua*	
S & S	Swish and swallow	By using tongue and cheek muscles, the patient coats his/her mouth with a liquid medication.	

*Although not included on the "Do Not Use" list, it is considered safer to write out "right eye," "left eye," and "both eyes."

1 mL   **Carpuject®**
                                  with Luer Lock

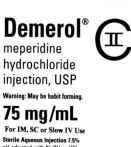

Demerol®
meperidine
hydrochloride
injection, USP

Warning: May be habit forming.

75 mg/mL

For IM, SC or Slow IV Use

Sterile Aqueous Injection 7.5%
pH adjusted with NaOH or HCl.
For usual dosage and route of administration, see
package insert.
Store at room temperature up to 25°C (77°F).
Caution: Federal (USA) law prohibits dispensing
without prescription.
Demerol® is a registered trademark of Sanofi
Pharmaceuticals, Inc.

©Abbott 1997   08-8409-2/R1-11/97   Printed in USA
Abbott Laboratories, North Chicago, IL 60064, USA

FIGURE 2-1

Label states the routes of administration. Meperidine HCL may be administered intramuscularly (IM), subcutaneously, or slowly intravenous (IV). (Courtesy of Abbott Laboratories)

SELF-TEST 3   **Abbreviations (Routes)**

After studying the abbreviations for routes of administration, give the meaning of the following terms. Indicate if the abbreviation is not to be used and the words to substitute for it. Answers are given at the end of the chapter.

1. SL_____   6. OD _____   11. S&S _____

2. OU _____   7. IVPB _____   12. SC_____

3. NGT_____   8. OS _____   13. AU _____

4. IV _____   9. IM_____   14. AL _____

5. po _____   10. pr _____

▶ Metric and SI Abbreviations

Metric abbreviations in dosage relate to a drug's weight or volume and are the most common measures in dosage. The International System of Units (Système International d'Unités; SI) was adapted from the metric system in 1960. Most developed countries except the United States have adopted SI nomenclature to provide a standard language of measurement.

Differences between metric and SI systems do not occur in dosage. The meaning and abbreviations for weight and volume are the same. Weight measures are based on the gram; volume measures are based on the liter.

Study the meaning of the abbreviations listed in the following table. Under Learning Aid, one equivalent is given for each abbreviation to help you understand what kinds of quantities are involved. It is not yet necessary to study the equivalents (equivalents are discussed in Chapter 4). The preferred abbreviation is listed first; variations are given in parentheses.

Metric Abbreviation	Meaning	Learning Aid	Do Not Use
cc	Cubic centimeter	This is a measure of volume usually reserved for measuring gases. However, you may still find it used as a liquid measure. (One cubic centimeter is approximately equal to 16 drops from a medicine dropper.)	Substitute mL.
g (gm, Gm)	Gram	This is a solid measure of weight. (One gram is approximately equal to the weight of two paper clips.)	
kg (Kg)	Kilogram	This is a weight measure. (One kilogram equals 2.2 pounds.)	
L	Liter	This is a liquid measure. (One liter is a little more than a quart.)	
mcg	Microgram	This is a measure of weight. (One thousand micrograms make up 1 milligram: 1000 mcg = 1 mg.)	μg
mEq	Milliequivalent	No equivalent necessary. Drugs are prepared and ordered in this weight measure.	
mg	Milligram	This is a measure of weight. (One thousand milligrams make up 1 gram: 1000 mg = 1 g.)	
mL (ml)	Milliliter	This is a liquid measure. The terms *cubic centimeter* (cc) and *milliliter* (mL) are interchangeable in dosage (1 cc = 1 mL).	
unit	Unit	This is a measure of biologic activity. Nurses do not calculate this measure. ■ **Example** penicillin potassium 300,000 units *Important:* It is considered safer to write the word *unit* rather than use the abbreviation, because the *U* could be read as a zero and a medication error might result.	U

SELF-TEST 4   Abbreviations (Metric)

After studying metric abbreviations, write the meaning of the following terms. Indicate if the abbreviation is not to be used and the words to substitute for it. Answers are given at the end of the chapter.

1. 0.3 g_____
2. 150 mcg_____
3. 80 U_____
4. 0.5 mL_____
5. 1.7 cc_____

6. 0.25 mg_____
7. 14 kg_____
8. 20 mEq_____
9. 1.5 L_____
10. 50 μg_____

▶ Apothecary Abbreviations

Apothecary measures were common in the United States as far back as colonial times. Today apothecary measures are discouraged for several reasons: equivalency with the metric system is not exact, the system requires Roman numbers and fractions, and apothecary symbols can be misinterpreted. These apothecary terms are in minimal use:

Minim   Abbreviated m, it is about the size of one drop. The term is found on some syringes. In Figure 2-2, note two sets of marks. The upper lines indicate doses to 3 cubic centimeters. The lower lines indicate minims. On this syringe, 1 cubic centimeter = 16 minims. Substitute "mL" for "cc," although many syringes are marked "cc."

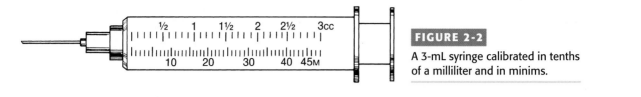

FIGURE 2-2

A 3-mL syringe calibrated in tenths of a milliliter and in minims.

Dram	Abbreviated dr, it is a liquid measure slightly less than a household teaspoon. 1 dr = 4 mL. In Figure 2-3, note that the medication cup has measures in metric, household, and apothecary systems. If the answer to a dosage calculation was 12 mL, one could pour 3 drams.
Grain	Abbreviated gr, it derives from the Latin word *granum*. This solid measure was based on the weight of a grain of wheat in medieval times. There is no commonly accepted equivalent to the grain in the metric system. Generally, 60 mg equals 1 gr, except with acetaminophen (Tylenol) and aspirin: 65 mg = 1 gr. See Figure 2-4. In written prescriptions, the metric gram (g; gm; Gm) can be confused with the apothecary grain (gr).
Drop	Abbreviated gtt, it derives the Latin word *guttae*. This liquid measure was based on a drop of water; 1 gtt = 1 m. The term *gtt* is used in ordering eye medications. For example, Timoptic 0.25% Ophth Sol 1 gtt ou bid.
i	Means one in Roman numerals, which are represented by using letters of the alphabet. Roman numbers never have more than three of the same digit in a row. For example, ii = 2, iii = 3, V = 5, and X = 10.

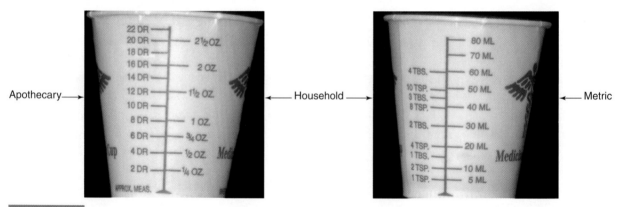

FIGURE 2-3

A medicine cup with metric, household, and apothecary equivalents. Two sides of the cup are shown. (© 2004 Lacey-Bordeaux Photography.)

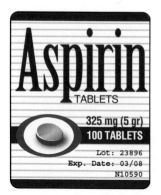

FIGURE 2-4

Aspirin tablet labeled in both metric and apothecary measures with additional type.

| SELF-TEST 5 | Abbreviations (Apothecary) |

After studying apothecary abbreviations still used in prescriptions, write the meaning of the following terms. Answers are given at the end of the chapter.

1. m x _____   **6.** gr i _____

2. ii dr _____   **7.** 2 gtt _____

3. 5 gr _____   **8.** 10 gr _____

4. gtt iii _____   **9.** m v _____

5. dr i _____

Household Abbreviations

Physicians may use these common household measures to order drugs, especially if the drug is to be administered at home. Metric equivalents are included in the Learning Aid column for your information.

Household Abbreviation	Meaning	Learning Aid
pt	Pint	One pint is approximately equal to 500 milliliters (1 pt ≅ 500 mL). One quart is approximately equal to 1 liter, which is equal to 1000 milliliters (1 qt ≅ 1 L = 1000 mL).
qt	Quart	One half of a quart is approximately equal to 1 pint ($\frac{1}{2}$ qt ≅ 1 pt = 500 mL).
tbsp	Tablespoon	One tablespoon equals 15 milliliters (1 tbsp = 15 mL).
tsp	Teaspoon	One teaspoon equals 5 milliliters (1 tsp = 5 mL).
oz	Ounce	One ounce equals 30 milliliters (1 oz = 30 mL).

Example   6 tsp = 1 oz = 30 mL
3 tsp = $\frac{1}{2}$ oz = 15 mL
2 tbsp = 1 oz = 30 mL = 6 tsp (see Fig. 2-3)

| SELF-TEST 6 | Abbreviations (Household) |

After studying household measures, write the meaning of the following terms. Answers are given at the end of the chapter.

1. 3 tsp _____   **3.** $\frac{1}{2}$ qt _____   **5.** 1 pt _____

2. 1 oz _____   **4.** 1 tsp _____   **6.** 2 tbsp _____

Terms and Abbreviations for Drug Preparations

The following abbreviations and terms are used to describe selected drug preparations.

Term Abbreviation	Meaning	Learning Aid
cap, caps	Capsule	Medication is encased in a gelatin shell.
CR LA SA SR DS	Controlled release Long acting Sustained action Slow release Double strength	These abbreviations indicate that the drug has been prepared in a form that allows extended action. Therefore, the drug is given less frequently.
EC	Enteric coated	The tablet is coated with a substance that will not dissolve in the acid secretions of the stomach; instead, it dissolves in the more alkaline secretions of the intestines.
el, elix	Elixir	A drug is dissolved in a hydroalcoholic sweetened base.
sol	Solution	The drug is contained in a clear liquid preparation.
sp	Spirit	This is an alcoholic solution of a volatile substance (eg, spirit of ammonia).
sup, supp	Suppository	This is a solid, cylindrically shaped drug that can be inserted into a body opening (eg, the rectum or vagina).
susp	Suspension	Small particles of drug are dispersed in a liquid base and must be shaken before being poured; gels and magmas are also suspensions.
syr	Syrup	A sugar is dissolved in a liquid medication and flavored to disguise the taste.
tab, tabs	Tablet	Medication is compressed or molded into a solid form; additional ingredients are used to shape and color the tablet.
tr, tinct.	Tincture	This is a liquid alcoholic or hydroalcoholic solution of a drug.
ung, oint.	Ointment	This is a semisolid drug preparation that is applied to the skin (for external use only).
KVO	Keep vein open	**Example order** 1000 mL dextrose 5% in water IV KVO. The nurse is to continue infusing this fluid.
TKO	To keep open	
Discontinue	Discontinue	**Example order** Discontinue ampicillin (do not use D/C)
NKA	No known allergies	This is an important assessment that is noted on the medication record of a patient.
NKDA	No known drug allergies	This is an important assessment that is noted on the medication record of a patient.

SELF-TEST 7   Abbreviations (Drug Preparations)

After studying the abbreviations for drug preparations, write out the meaning of the following terms. Answers are given at the end of the chapter.

1. elix
2. DS
3. NKA
4. caps
5. susp

6. tab
7. SR
8. LA
9. supp
10. tr

You should now be able to interpret the orders that were presented at the beginning of this chapter.

Original: Morphine sulfate 15 mg Sub Q stat and 10 mg q4h prn

Interpretation: Morphine sulfate 15 mg subcutaneously immediately and 10 mg every 4 hours as needed.

Original: Chloromycetin 0.01% Opth Oint OS bid

Interpretation: Chloromycetin 0.01% ophthalmic ointment left eye twice a day.

Original: Ampicillin 1 g IVPB q6h

Interpretation: Ampicillin 1 gram intravenous piggyback every 6 hours.

PROFICIENCY TEST 1 Abbreviations

Name: _____

Aim for 90% or better on this test. There are 50 items and each is worth 2 points. If you have any difficulty, study the content again. Indicate if the abbreviation is not to be used and the words to substitute for it. Answers are given on page 393.

1. bid _____
2. hs _____
3. prn _____
4. OU _____
5. po _____
6. pr _____
7. SL_____
8. S&S _____
9. tiw _____
10. mL _____
11. q4h _____
12. cc _____
13. SC_____
14. AU _____
15. g _____
16. PC_____
17. qd _____

18. stat _____
19. q12h_____
20. tid_____
21. OS _____
22. kg _____
23. qn _____
24. qh _____
25. OD _____
26. mEq _____
27. AC _____
28. qid _____
29. mg _____
30. IM_____
31. qod _____
32. biw _____
33. NGT_____
34. q8h _____

35. L_____
36. mcg_____
37. q6h _____
38. µg _____
39. U_____
40. tsp_____
41. AD _____
42. gr _____
43. IV _____
44. susp _____
45. tbsp_____
46. IVPB _____
47. m _____
48. Gm _____
49. q2h _____
50. q3h _____

Name: _____

Now that you have studied the language of prescriptions, you are ready to interpret medication orders. Write the following orders in longhand. Give sample times. Answers are given on page 393.

1. Nembutal 100 mg at bedtime prn po _____

2. Propranolol hydrochloride 40 mg po bid _____

   _____

3. Ampicillin 1 g IVPB q6h _____

   _____

4. Demerol 50 mg IM q4h prn for pain _____

   _____

5. Tylenol 325 mg tabs ii po stat _____

   _____

6. Pilocarpine gtt ii OU q3h _____

   _____

7. Scopolamine 0.8 mg subcutaneously stat _____

   _____

8. Digoxin el 0.25 mg po qd _____

   _____

9. Kaochlor 30 mEq po bid _____

   _____

10. Liquaemin sodium 6000 units subcutaneously q4h _____

    _____

11. Tobramycin 70 mg IM q8h _____

    _____

12. Prednisone 10 mg po every other day _____

    _____

13. Milk of magnesia 1 tbsp po at bedtime qn _____

    _____

14. Septra DS tab i every day po _____

    _____

15. Morphine sulfate 15 mg subcutaneously stat and 10 mg q4h prn _____

    _____

Name: _____

These are actual prescriptions written by physicians. Interpret each in longhand. Remember that if an order is not clear, you must check with the person who wrote the order. Note any "do not use" abbreviation. Answers are given on page 394.

1. Colace 100 mg po TID	1.
2. Ativan 1mg IVP x 1 now	2.
3. 10 meq KCl in 100cc NS over 1h X1	3.
4. Tylenol #3 II tabs po q4° prn pain	4.
5. Heparin 25,000 IU in 250ª D5W @ 500 u/hr.	5.
6. Ticlid 250mg I PO BID.	6.
7. lopресsor 25 mg po BID.	7.
8. Benadryl 25 mg po qhs	8.

Answers

Self-Test 1 Abbreviations

1. Three times a day (**sample times:** 10 AM, 2 PM, 6 PM)

2. Every night (**sample time:** 10 PM)

3. After meals (**sample times:** 10 AM, 2 PM, 6 PM)

4. Every other day (**sample times:** odd days of month at 10 AM). Do not use "qod" (write out "every other day").

5. Twice a day (**sample times:** 10 AM, 6 PM)

6. Do not use hs. Use "at bedtime." (**sample time:** 10 PM)

7. Immediately (**sample time:** whatever the time is now)

8. Four times a day (**sample times:** 10 AM, 2 PM, 6 PM, 10 PM)

9. Every 4 hours (**sample times:** 2 AM, 6 AM, 10 AM, 2 PM, 6 PM, 10 PM)

10. Before meals (**sample times:** 7:30 AM, 11:30 AM, 4:30 PM)

11. Do not use qd; use "every day." (**sample time:** 10 AM)

12. Every 8 hours (**sample times:** 6 AM, 2 PM, 10 PM)

13. Every hour

14. Whenever necessary (**sample times:** No time routine can be written.)

15. Every 4 hours as needed (**sample times:** No time routine is written because we do not know when the drug will be needed.)

Self-Test 2 Military Time

A.
1. 1400
2. 0900
3. 1600
4. 1200
5. 0130
6. 2115
7. 0450
8. 1820

B.
1. 1:30 AM
2. 5:45 PM
3. 11 AM
4. 8:15 PM
5. 7:10 PM
6. 6 AM
7. 12:50 AM
8. 10 AM

Self-Test 3 Abbreviations (Routes)

1. Sublingual; under the tongue
2. Both eyes
3. Nasogastric tube
4. Intravenously
5. By mouth
6. Right eye
7. Intravenous piggyback
8. Left eye
9. Intramuscularly
10. Rectally
11. Swish and swallow
12. Do not use SC; use "subcutaneously."
13. Do not use au; use "both ears."
14. Do not use al; use "left ear."

Self-Test 4 Abbreviations (Metric)

1. Three tenths of a gram
2. One hundred fifty micrograms
3. Eighty units. Do not use U; use "unit."
4. Five tenths of a milliliter
5. One and seven tenths of a milliliter. Do not use cc; use "milliliter."
6. Twenty-five hundredths of a milligram
7. Fourteen kilograms
8. Twenty milliequivalents
9. One and five tenths of a liter
10. Fifty micrograms. Do not use μg; use "microgram."

Self-Test 5 Abbreviations (Apothecary)

1. 10 minims
2. 2 drams
3. 5 grains
4. 3 drops
5. 1 dram
6. 1 grain
7. 2 drops
8. 10 grains
9. 5 minims

Self-Test 6 Abbreviations (Household)

1. Three teaspoons
2. One ounce
3. One-half quart
4. One teaspoon
5. One pint
6. Two tablespoons

Self-Test 7 Abbreviations (Drug Preparations)

1. Elixir
2. Double strength
3. No known allergies
4. Capsules
5. Suspension
6. Tablet
7. Slow release
8. Long acting
9. Suppository
10. Tincture

Drug Labels and Packaging

▶ Drug Labels

An understanding of drug labels and the ways in which drugs are packaged provides a background for dosage and administration. This information can be self-taught and does not require class time.

Labels that contain specific facts are found on drugs to be administered in the form in which they are packaged. This form may be solid or liquid. Occasionally some information such as route of administration, usual dose, and storage may not be on the label because the container is too small. When further information is needed, a professional reference should be consulted. Figure 3-1 shows a sample drug label.

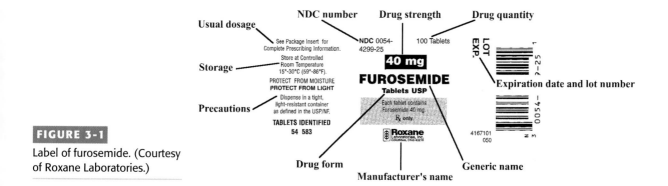

FIGURE 3-1

Label of furosemide. (Courtesy of Roxane Laboratories.)

NDC NUMBER. The National Drug Code (NDC) is a number used by the pharmacist to identify the drug and the method of packaging. The NDC in Figure 3-1 is 0054-4299-25. The letters NSN (not shown) mean national supply number, a code for ordering the drug.

TOTAL AMOUNT OF DRUG IN THE CONTAINER. This information is found at the top of the label to the left or the right, or at the bottom. Figure 3-1 indicates 100 tablets.

TRADE NAME. The term *trade name,* which is also referred to as *brand name* or *proprietary name,* may be identified by the symbol ® that follows the name. Several companies may manufacture the same drug using different trade names. Trade names may be capitalized on the labels or they may have an initial capital only. *They are always written with the first letter capitalized.* In Figure 3-1, Lasix® is the trade or brand name. It is not on this label.

GENERIC NAME. The generic name is the official accepted name of a drug, as listed in the United States Pharmacopeia (USP). A drug may have several trade names but only one official generic name. The generic name is not capitalized. The generic name given in Figure 3-1 is furosemide.

STRENGTH OF THE DRUG. Solid drugs are given in metric weights; liquids are stated as a solution of drug in solvent. In Figure 3-1, the strength is 40 mg.

FORM OF THE DRUG. The label specifies the type of preparation in the container. Figure 3-1 indicates the drug is dispensed in tablets.

USUAL DOSAGE. This states how much drug is given at a single time or during a 24-hour period and identifies who should receive the drug. Figure 3-1 label states: See Package Insert for Prescribing Information.

ROUTE OF ADMINISTRATION. The label specifies how the drug is to be given: orally, parenterally (an injection of some type), or topically (applied to skin or mucous membranes). *When the label does not specify the route, the drug is in an oral form.* In Figure 3-1, the route is oral.

STORAGE. This information describes the conditions necessary to protect the drug from losing its potency (effectiveness). Some drugs come in a dry form and must be dissolved—that is, reconstituted. The drug may be stored one way when dry and another way after reconstitution. Figure 3-1 states to store the drug at controlled room temperature of 15 to 30°C (59–86°F).

PRECAUTIONS. These are specific instructions related to safety, effectiveness, and/or administration that must be noted and followed. In Figure 3-1: Federal law prohibits dispensing without prescription. Protect from moisture. Protect from light. Dispense in a tight, light-resistant container.

MANUFACTURER'S NAME. Any questions about the drug should be directed to this company. In Figure 3-1, the company is Roxane Laboratories, Inc.

EXPIRATION DATE. The drug cannot be used after the last day of the month indicated (not shown in Fig. 3-1).

LOT NUMBER. This number indicates the batch of drug from which this stock came (not shown in Fig. 3-1).

ADDITIVES. The manufacturer may have used substances to bind the drug, to aid in dissolving the drug, to produce a specific pH, and so on. This information may be found on the label or in the literature accompanying the drug (not shown in Fig. 3-1).

- Some drugs are dispensed in a dry (powder) form and must be reconstituted (dissolved).
- The drug label or drug insert provides specific directions about dissolving the powder.
- The amount and type of liquid to be used to dissolve the drug and the resulting solution are stated by the manufacturer.

Example   Amoxicillin (Polymox) comes in powder form. Prepare suspension at time of dispensing. Add 88 mL water to the bottle. For ease in preparation, add the water in two portions. Shake well after each addition. This provides 150 mL suspension. Dosage is 125 mg amoxicillin per 5 mL solution.

SELF-TEST 1   Drug Labels

Read the label in Figure 3-2 and give the information requested. Answers are given at the end of the chapter.

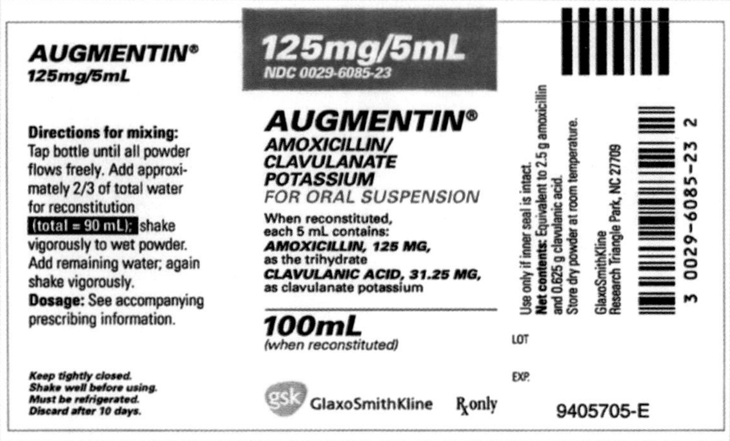

FIGURE 3-2

Label of Augmentin for oral suspension. (Reproduced with permission of Glaxo-SmithKline.)

1. NDC number _____

2. Total amount of drug in the container _____

3. Trade name _____

4. Generic name _____

5. Strength of the drug _____

6. Form of the drug _____

7. Usual dosage _____

8. Route of administration _____

9. Storage _____

   _____

10. Directions for preparation _____

    _____

11. Precautions _____

    _____

12. Manufacturer _____

13. Expiration date _____

Drug Labels (Continued)

Read the label in Figure 3-3 and answer the following questions. Answers are given at the end of the chapter.

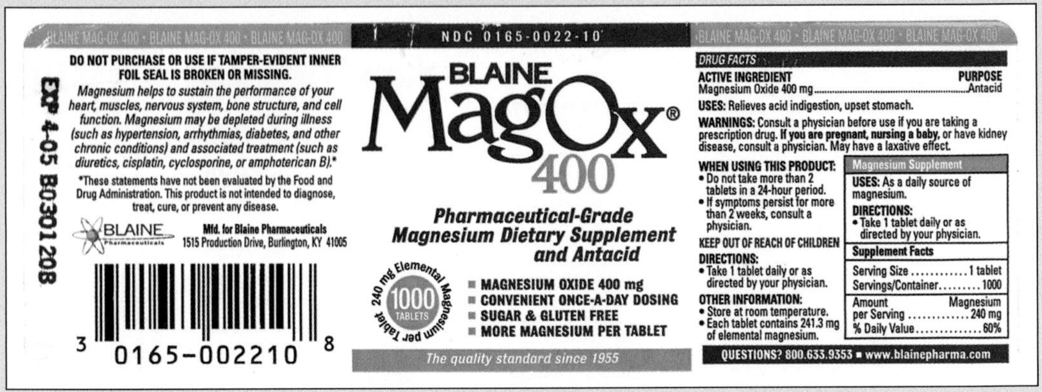

FIGURE 3-3

Label of MagOx 400. (Courtesy of Blaine Pharmaceuticals.)

14. What is the trade name? _____

15. What is the generic name? _____

16. By what route(s) may this drug be given?_____

17. In what form is the drug dispensed? _____

18. What is the strength of the drug? _____

19. What is the total amount of drug in the container? _____

20. What is the usual adult dose? _____
_____

21. List seven cautions identified on the label regarding this drug. _____
_____
_____
_____
_____

When a medication container holds a single drug, the written prescription indicates the dose in milligrams or grams, and calculation may be necessary.

Example

a. Tylenol 0.6 g po q 4 h prn for temperature ↑ 101°
Label: Tylenol 325 mg tablets

b. Prednisone 20 mg po bid
Label: Prednisone 10 mg tablets

c. Digoxin 0.5 mg po daily
Label: Digoxin 0.25 mg

d. Cefozil 0.5 g po q 8°
Label: 125 mg/5 mL

Some medication labels indicate more than one drug in the dose form. These combination drugs are ordered by the number of tablets to give or the amount of liquid to pour.

Example a. Order: Tylenol #3 tabs ii po q 4 h prn for pain

Label: acetaminophen 300 mg/codeine 30 mg tablet

b. Order: Robitussin DM 1 tsp po qid

Label: guaifenesin 100 mg/dextromethorphan 10 mg per 5 mL

c. Order: Talwin Compound 1 tab po q 6 h

Label: aspirin 325 mg/pentazocine 12.5 mg

d. Order: Phenergan VC Syrup 2 tsp po q 6 h while awake

Label: phenylephrine 5 mg/promethazine 6.25 mg per 5 mL

Drug Packaging

In the future, innovative delivery systems will revolutionize the ways in which drugs are administered. In this chapter, however, we focus on the common types of containers that nurses handle as they prepare medications.

There are two types of packaging: *unit dose* and *multidose*. Each type may contain a solid or liquid form of the drug for oral, parenteral, or topical use. Most institutions use a combination of unit dose and multidose.

Unit-Dose Packaging

In an institutional setting, each dose is individually wrapped and labeled, and a 24-hour supply is prepared by the pharmacy and dispensed. A major value of unit-dose packaging is that two professionals check the drug and the dose—the pharmacist and the nurse—thereby decreasing the possibility of error.

It should be stressed that unit-dose packaging does not relieve responsibility to *check the label three times* and to calculate the amount of drug needed. Unit-dose drugs come in different strengths, and there is always a chance of error when trade names are ordered instead of generic names. A dose may consist of one unit packet, two or more unit packets, or a fraction of one packet.

Example A nurse has a unit-dose 100-mg tablet. If an order calls for 50 mg, only half the tablet would be administered.

A nurse may have an order for 75 mg. Unit packets contain 25-mg tablets. The nurse would administer three tablets.

FOR THE ORAL ROUTE. For oral administration, unit-dose packaging may consist of

1. Plastic bubble, foil, or paper wrappers containing tablets or capsules (Fig. 3-4A)

2. Plastic or glass containers that hold a single dose of a liquid or powder. The powder is reconstituted to a liquid form by following the directions given on the label (Fig. 3-4B).

3. A sealed medication cup containing one dose of a liquid. The nurse removes the cover and the dose is ready to administer (Fig. 3-4C).

FOR THE PARENTERAL ROUTE. These drugs are given by injection. The route must be specified in the order (eg, IM, Sub-Q, IVPB). Drugs in such containers are sterile, and sterile technique is used for their preparation and administration. The drugs may come in a solid or liquid form.

1. An *ampule* (ampoule) is a glass container that holds a single sterile dose of drug (Fig. 3-5). The container has a narrow neck that must be broken to reach the drug. A sterile syringe is used to withdraw the medication. The drug in the ampule may come as a liquid, a powder, or a crystal. Directions must

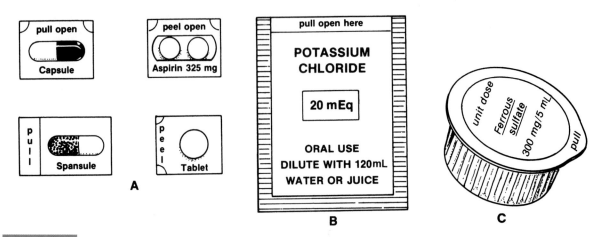

FIGURE 3-4

(**A**) Unit-dose tablets and capsules in foil wrappers. (**B**) Unit-dose powder in a sealed packet; it is placed in a container and diluted before giving. (**C**) Sealed cup containing one dose of a liquid medication ready to administer.

be followed to reconstitute the solid forms. Once the glass is broken, any portion of the drug not used must be discarded, because the drug cannot be kept sterile.

2. A *vial* is a glass or plastic container with a sealed rubber top (Fig. 3-5). Medication in the container can be kept sterile. The container may have a sterile liquid or a sterile powder that must be reconstituted with a sterile diluent and syringe. *Single-dose vials* do not contain a preservative or a bacteriostatic agent. Therefore, any medication remaining after the dose is prepared should be discarded.

3. Flexible *plastic bags* or *glass vials* may hold sterile medication for intravenous use (Fig. 3-6). The fluid is administered with the use of IV tubing that is connected to a needle or catheter placed in the patient's blood vessel.

4. *Prefilled syringes* contain sterile liquid medication that is ready to administer without further preparation. This type of unit-dose packaging is expensive but life-saving in an emergency when speed is essential.

5. *Prefilled cartridges* are actually small vials with a needle attached that fit into a metal or plastic holder and eject one unit dose of a sterile drug in liquid form (Fig. 3-7).

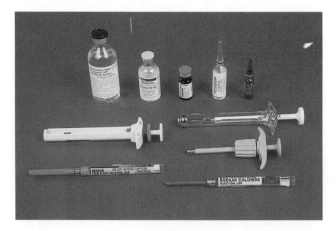

FIGURE 3-5

Parenteral route: (*top row*) vials and ampules; (*middle-bottom row*) prefilled cartridges and holders.

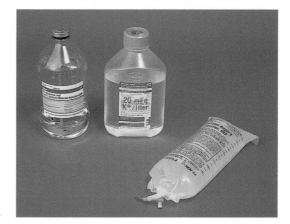

FIGURE 3-6

Plastic or glass containers hold medication for IV use.

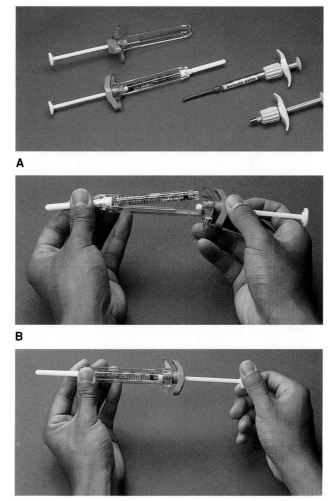

FIGURE 3-7

(**A**) Prefilled cartridges. (**B**) Inserting cartridge into injector device. (**C**) Cartridge is screwed into device, ready to administer drug.

FOR TOPICAL ADMINISTRATION. Drugs are applied to the skin or mucous membranes to achieve a local effect. They may be absorbed into the circulation, thereby achieving a systemic effect.

1. *Transdermal patches* or *pads* are adhesive bandages placed on the skin (Fig. 3-8). They hold a drug form that is slowly absorbed into the circulation over a period ranging from hours to several days.

2. *Lozenges and pastilles* are disklike solids that are slowly dissolved in the mouth (eg, cough drops). Some drugs are prepared in a gum and are released by chewing (eg, nicotine).

3. *Suppositories* in foil or plastic wrappers are molded forms that can be inserted into the rectum or vagina (Fig. 3-9). They hold medication in a substance, such as cocoa butter, that melts at body temperature and releases the drug. Suppositories may be used for unconscious patients or those unable to swallow.

4. *Plastic, disposable, squeezable containers* hold prepared solutions for the vagina (douches) or enema solutions that are administered rectally (Fig. 3-10). The containers for enemas have a lubricated nozzle for ease in insertion. As the container is squeezed, the solution is forced out.

Multidose Packaging

In the institutional setting, each unit may receive large stock containers of medications from which doses are poured. This type of packaging reduces the pharmacy's workload but requires more time to prepare and increases the possibility of error.

FOR THE ORAL ROUTE. Stock bottles contain a liquid or a solid form such as tablets, capsules, or powders. When powders are reconstituted, the date and time of preparation must be written on the label, and storage directions and expiration must be carefully noted. Powders, once dissolved, begin losing potency. Large stock bottles hold medication that is dispensed over a period of days (Fig. 3-11A).

FOR THE PARENTERAL ROUTE. Large-volume vials contain a sterile liquid or powder to be reconstituted using sterile technique. The date and time of preparation must be written on the label, and the expiration and storage noted (Fig. 3-11B).

FOR TOPICAL ADMINISTRATION. Care must be exercised to avoid contaminating these containers because they will be used over an extended period. Whenever possible, label the container with the patient's name and reserve its use for that one patient. The following types of containers may be used:

1. *Metal or plastic tubes* that contain ointments or creams to be applied to the skin or mucous membranes are squeezed to release the medication (Fig. 3-12A).

2. To avoid contamination, medication is removed from *jars for creams, ointments, and pastes* by using a sterile tongue blade or sterile glove.

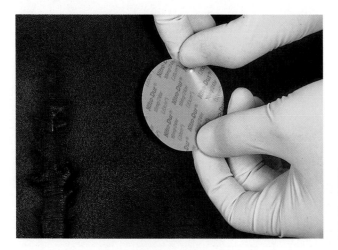

FIGURE 3-8

Transdermal patches or pads are placed on the skin. Drugs prepared in this manner include estrogen, fentanyl, testosterone, and nitroglycerin.

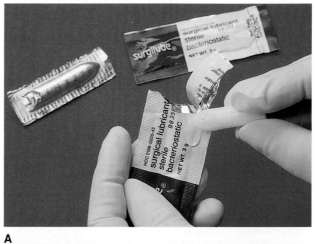

A

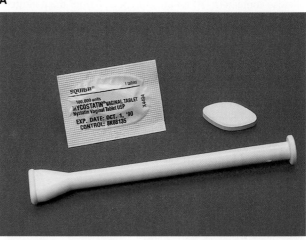

B

FIGURE 3-9

(**A**) Rectal suppository. (**B**) Vaginal suppository and applicator.

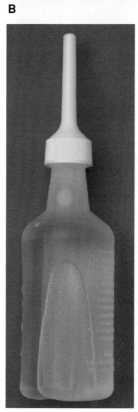

A

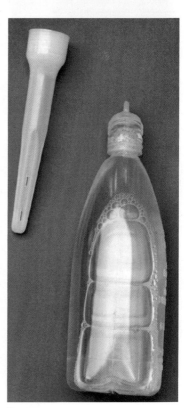

B

FIGURE 3-10

Unit-dose containers for rectal enema (**A**) and vaginal irrigation (**B**). (© 2004 Lacey-Bordeaux Photography.)

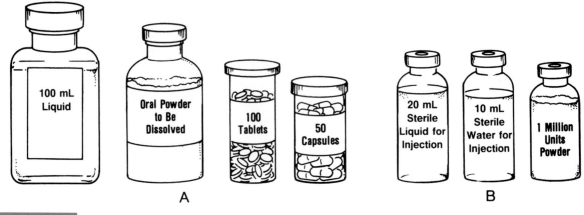

FIGURE 3-11

Multidose containers: (**A**) for the oral route; (**B**) for the parenteral route.

3. To prevent cross-contamination, *dropper bottles* for eye, ear, or nose medications should be labeled with the patient's name. The nurse must be careful to avoid touching mucous membranes with the dropper, because contamination of the dropper could result in the growth of pathogens. There are two kinds of droppers: monodrop containers that are squeezed to release the medication and those in which the dropper can be removed from the bottle. Separate, packaged droppers are available to administer medications. These are sometimes calibrated (that is, marked in milliliters; Fig. 3-12B, C).

Eye medications are labeled "ophthalmic" or "for the eye." Ear drugs are labeled "otic" or "auric" or "for the ear." Drugs for nasal administration are labeled "nose drops." Routes must never be interchanged.

4. *Lozenges and pastilles* may be packaged in multidose as well as unit-dose containers.

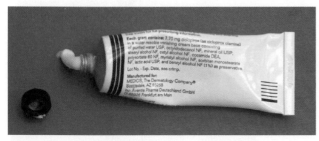

A

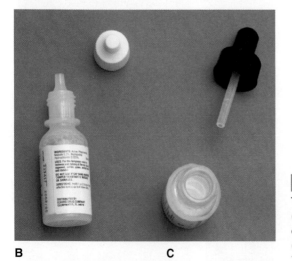

B   C

FIGURE 3-12

Topical multidose containers. (**A**) Tubes for creams or ointments. (**B**) Monodrop containers—the dropper is attached. (**C**) Removable dropper is sometimes calibrated for liquid measures. (© 2004 Lacey-Bordeaux Photography.)

5. *Metered-dose inhalers* (MDIs; Fig. 3-13) are aerosol devices that consist of two parts: a canister under pressure and a mouthpiece. The canister contains multiple drug doses in a liquid form or as a microfine powder or crystal. The mouthpiece fits on the canister. Finger pressure on the mouthpiece opens a valve on the canister that discharges one dose. The physician's order will state the number of inhalations or "puffs" to be taken. Medications for inhalation also may be packaged as liquids in vials or bottles or as capsules containing powder to be used with a hand-held nebulizer (HHN) or with an intermittent positive-pressure breathing apparatus (IPPB).

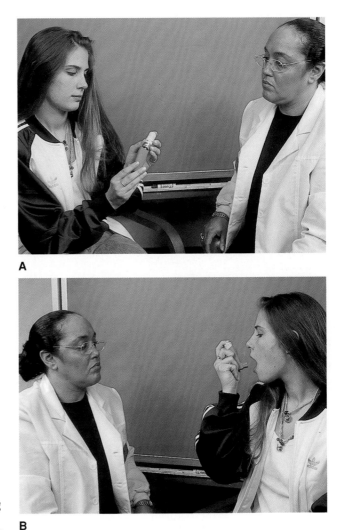

A

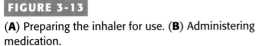

FIGURE 3-13

(**A**) Preparing the inhaler for use. (**B**) Administering medication.

B

SELF-TEST 2   **Drug Packaging**

Match Column A with the letters in Column B to identify the meaning of terms used in drug packaging.
Answers are given at the end of the chapter.

Column A

1. _____ Unit dose
2. _____ Ampule
3. _____ Parenteral
4. _____ Prefilled cartridge
5. _____ Reconstitution
6. _____ Topical
7. _____ Transdermal patch
8. _____ Vial
9. _____ Lozenge
10. _____ Cocoa butter

Column B

a. Dissolving a powder into solution

b. Glass container with a sealed rubber top

c. Route of administration to skin or mucous membranes

d. Individually wrapped and labeled drugs

e. Disklike solid that dissolves in the mouth

f. Suppository ingredient that melts at body temperature

g. General term for an injection route

h. Adhesive bandage applied to the skin that gradually releases a drug

i. Small vial, with a needle attached, that fits into a syringe holder

j. Glass container that must be broken to obtain the drug

Complete these statements related to drug packaging. Answers are given at the end of the chapter.

11. Date and time of reconstitution must be written _____

_____

_____

12. The best way to avoid cross-contamination of a multidose tube of ointment is to _____

_____

13. To remove medication from a jar of paste, the nurse should use _____

_____

14. Dropper bottles for eye medications will be labeled _____

_____

15. Doses of medication that require use of a metered-dose inhaler are ordered in _____

_____

16. Medications for the ear will be labeled _____

_____

17. The term *multidose* refers to _____

_____

(continued)

SELF-TEST 2   **Drug Packaging (Continued)**

18. The type of drug packaging that decreases the possibility of error is termed _____

_____

19. Drugs administered topically for a local effect may be absorbed and produce another effect
that is called _____

_____

_____

20. The word *lozenge* describes _____

_____

_____

Labels and Packaging

Name: _____

Complete these questions. Answers are given on page 394.

1. Explain the difference between each of these pairs.

   a. 1. Unit dose _____

       2. Multidose _____

   b. 1. Ampule _____

       2. Vial _____

   c. 1. Topical _____

       2. Parenteral _____

   d. 1. Trade name _____

       2. Generic name _____

   e. 1. Prefilled _____

       2. Reconstituted _____

2. Choose the correct answer.

   _____ **a.** A major advantage of the unit-dose system of drug administration is that

       1. The drug supply is always available

       2. No error is possible

       3. Drugs are less expensive than stock bottles

       4. The pharmacist provides a second professional check

   _____ **b.** A major disadvantage of ampules over vials is that ampules

       1. Are only glass

       2. When opened cannot be kept sterile

       3. Contain only liquids

       4. Cannot be used for injections

   _____ **c.** Which information is not found on the label for a drug to be given IVPB?

       1. Expiration date

       2. Indications (uses)

       3. Generic name

       4. Average dose

   _____ **d.** An order reads Valium 5 mg po now. A nurse correctly chooses diazepam. What name does diazepam represent?

       1. Generic

       2. Chemical

       3. Trade

       4. Proprietary

   _____ **e.** Which drug form is safest to administer to an unconscious patient?

       1. Suppository

       2. Syrup

       3. Capsule

       4. Aerosol

(continued)

5. In the equivalent 1 g = 1000 mg, the gram is the larger measure. It takes 1000 mg to make 1 g.

Example

EXAMPLE 1

Order: 0.25 g

Supply: 125 mg

You want to convert grams to milligrams.

0.25 g > _250_ mg

The arrow is telling you to move the decimal point three places to the right.

0.250 = 250

Hence, 0.25 g = 250 mg

EXAMPLE 2

Order: 1.5 g   1500

Supply: 500 mg

You want to convert grams to milligrams.

1.5 g > _____ mg

1.500 = 1500

Hence, 1.5 g = 1500 mg

SELF-TEST 1   Grams to Milligrams

Try these conversions from grams to milligrams. Answers are given at the end of the chapter.

1. 0.3 g = _____ mg
2. 0.001 g = _____ mg
3. 0.02 g = _____ mg
4. 1.2 g = _____ mg
5. 5 g = _____ mg
6. 0.4 g = _____ mg

7. 0.08 g = _____ mg
8. 0.275 g = _____ mg
9. 0.04 g = _____ mg
10. 0.325 g = _____ mg
11. 2 g = _____ mg
12. 0.0004 g = _____ mg

RULE   **CHANGING MILLIGRAMS TO GRAMS**

To divide by 1000, move the decimal point three places to the left. ■

Example

EXAMPLE 1

100 mg = _0.1_ g

100. = 0.1

100 mg = 0.1 g

EXAMPLE 2

8 mg = <u>0.008</u> g

$\underset{\frown}{008.} = 0.008$

8 mg = 0.008 g

Milligrams to Grams Quick Rule: The arrow method also works to convert milligrams to grams. Remember the steps:

1. Write the order first.
2. Write the equivalent measure needed.
3. Use an arrow to show which way the decimal point should move.
4. The open part of the arrow always faces the *larger* measure.
5. In the equivalent 1 g = 1000 mg, the gram is the larger measure.

Example

EXAMPLE 1

Order: 15 mg

Supply: 0.03 g

You want to convert milligrams to grams.

15 mg < g

The arrow tells you to move the decimal point three places to the left.

$\underset{\frown}{015.} = 0.015$

15 mg = 0.015 g

EXAMPLE 2

Order: 500 mg

Supply: 1 g

You want to convert mg to g.

500 mg = _____ g

500 mg < g

The arrow tells you to move the decimal point three places to the left.

$\underset{\frown}{500.} = 0.5$

500 mg = 0.5 g

SELF-TEST 2   Milligrams to Grams

Try these conversions from milligrams to grams. Answers are given at the end of the chapter.

1. 4 mg = _____ g
2. 120 mg = _____ g
3. 40 mg = _____ g
4. 75 mg = _____ g
5. 250 mg = _____ g
6. 1 mg = _____ g
7. 50 mg = _____ g
8. 600 mg = _____ g
9. 5 mg = _____ g
10. 360 mg = _____ g
11. 10 mg = _____ g
12. 0.1 mg = _____ g

Answers

Self-Test 1 Grams to Milligrams

1. 300	**4.** 1200	**7.** 80	**10.** 325
2. 1	**5.** 5000	**8.** 275	**11.** 2000
3. 20	**6.** 400	**9.** 40	**12.** 0.4

Self-Test 2 Milligrams to Grams

1. 0.004	**4.** 0.075	**7.** 0.05	**10.** 0.36
2. 0.12	**5.** 0.25	**8.** 0.6	**11.** 0.01
3. 0.04	**6.** 0.001	**9.** 0.005	**12.** 0.0001

Self-Test 3 Milligrams to Micrograms

1. 300	**4.** 80	**7.** 5000	**10.** 10000
2. 1	**5.** 1200	**8.** 700	**11.** 900
3. 20	**6.** 400	**9.** 40	**12.** 10

Self-Test 4 Micrograms to Milligrams

1. 0.8	**4.** 0.025	**7.** 0.05	**10.** 0.075
2. 0.004	**5.** 0.001	**8.** 0.75	**11.** 0.0001
3. 0.014	**6.** 0.2	**9.** 0.325	**12.** 0.15

Self-Test 5 Mixed Conversions

1. 0.0003	**4.** 100	**7.** 14	**9.** 200
2. 30	**5.** 0.1	**8.** 0.2	**10.** 650
3. 0.015	**6.** 0.05		

Self-Test 6 Common Equivalents

1. 1	**5.** 0.2	**9.** 0.015	**12.** 400
2. 0.6	**6.** 0.1	**10.** 0.01	**13.** 300
3. 0.5	**7.** 0.06	**11.** 600	**14.** 250
4. 0.3	**8.** 0.03		

Self-Test 7 Review of Grams to Milligrams

1. Multiply grams by 1000, move decimal point three places to the right, or use an arrow with the open part toward gram to show movement of decimal point three places.

2. 1000

3. 10

4. 200

5. 120

6. 1000

7. 600

8. 500

9. 300

10. 200

11. 100

12. 60

13. 30

14. 15

15. 10

Self-Test 8 Converting Grains to mg

1. 100 mg
2. 300 mg
3. 0.4 mg
4. 900 or 1000 mg
5. 240 mg
6. 15 mg
7. 650 mg
8. 325 mg
9. gr 45 or gr 50
10. gr 5
11. gr ¼
12. gr $\frac{1}{120}$
13. gr 135
14. gr 10
15. gr 5

Self-Test 9 Liquid Equivalents

1. 30
2. 15
3. 15
4. 60
5. 16
6. 1
7. 5
8. 2
9. 2.5
10. 1000
11. 1
12. 45
13. 45
14. 1
15. 1
16. 2
17. 1
18. 500
19. 1000
20. 1
21. 1
22. 1
23. 1
24. 1
25. 1
26. 1
27. 1000
28. 15
29. 1
30. 2.2

Drug Preparations and Equipment to Measure Doses

Drugs are manufactured in different forms for oral, parenteral, and topical administration. This chapter focuses on the more common drug preparations used in the clinical area and on the equipment that nurses use to prepare accurate doses.

▶ Drug Preparations

Oral Route

Oral drug forms are generally the easiest for the patient to take and the most convenient for the nurse to administer.

Tablets are powdered drugs that are compressed or molded into solid shapes. Tablets may contain ingredients that bind the powder or aid in its gastrointestinal absorption (Fig. 5-1A). Plain tablets for oral administration may be crushed if a patient has difficulty swallowing. There are several types of pill or tablet crushers available:

Scored tablets have a line down the center so that the tablet can be broken into halves. Unscored tablets should not be broken because there is no certainty that the drug is evenly distributed (Fig. 5-1A). When in doubt, check with the pharmacist.

Coated tablets or film-coated tablets are smooth and easy to swallow because of their coating. If necessary, some tablets may be crushed.

Enteric-coated tablets dissolve in the more alkaline secretions of the intestine rather than in the highly acidic stomach juices. The enteric coating protects the drug from being inactivated in the stomach and reduces the chance that the drug will irritate the gastric mucosa. Enteric-coated tablets should *not* be crushed (Fig. 5-1B).

Prolonged-release or *extended-release tablets* (also abbreviated XL, extended length; CD, controlled dose; SR, sustained release) disintegrate more slowly and have a longer duration of action. The use of these preparations decreases the number of doses needed to only one or two tablets each day. Prolonged-release tablets should not be crushed.

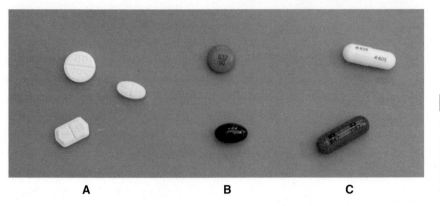

FIGURE 5-1
(**A**) Tablets that may be crushed or broken on the scored line. (**B**) Tablets that may not be crushed. (**C**) Capsules. (© 2004 Lacey-Bordeaux Photography.)

Sublingual tablets dissolve quickly under the tongue. Medication is absorbed through the capillaries and reaches the circulation without passing through the gastrointestinal tract.

Coded tablets have a number or letter, or both, that make them easily identifiable (Fig. 5-1).

Capsules are gelatin containers that hold a drug in solid or liquid form. Nurses should avoid opening capsules; the drug is encased in the capsule for a reason—possibly because contact with gastric juices will decrease drug potency or because the drug could irritate the stomach lining. Occasionally, however, if a patient has difficulty swallowing, the nurse may open a capsule and combine the contents with a semi-solid such as applesauce or custard. Before doing this, always check with the pharmacist to find out if the drug is available as a liquid or if there is an alternative (Fig. 5-1C). Some capsules are enteric-coated. Others (called *spansule, timespan, time release,* or *sustained release*) contain particles of the drug that are coated to dissolve at different times. These capsules are long acting and should not be opened.

Syrups are solutions of sugar in water that disguise the medication's unpleasant taste. Because they contain sugar, syrups may be contraindicated in patients with diabetes mellitus.

Elixirs are clear hydroalcoholic liquids that are sweetened. Elixirs may be contraindicated in patients with a history of alcoholism.

Fluidextracts and *tinctures* are alcoholic, liquid concentrations of a drug. They are potent and, consequently, are ordered in small amounts. Tinctures are ordered in drops. The average dose of a fluid-extract is 2 tsp or less. Fluidextracts are the most concentrated of all liquids.

Solutions are clear liquids that contain a drug dissolved in water.

Suspensions are solid particles of a drug dispersed in a liquid. The particles settle to the bottom of the container upon standing and must be resuspended to obtain an accurate dose; therefore, oral preparations must be shaken before being poured.

Magmas contain large bulky particles—for example, milk of magnesia.

Gels have small particles—for example, magnesium hydroxide gel.

Emulsions are creamy, white suspensions of fats or oils in an agent that reduces surface tension and makes the oil easier to swallow—for example, emulsified castor oil.

Powders are dry, finely ground drugs that are reconstituted according to directions. Oral antibiotics are frequently supplied as powders. In liquid form these preparations become oral suspensions. Powders must be dissolved according to the manufacturer. When the nurse reconstitutes a powder, four facts should be written on the label: the date, the time, the nurse's initials, and the solution made.

Parenteral Route

The drug forms for parenteral administration include solutions, suspensions, and powders (as defined previously). The term *parenteral* does not indicate a specific route; it is a general term that means *by injection.* Four common parenteral routes are IM, Sub Q, IV, and IVPB. Drug forms for parenteral use are sterile, and aseptic technique is used to prepare and administer them.

Topical Route

Commonly ordered preparations include aerosol powders or liquids, creams, ointments, pastes, suppositories, and transdermal medications. The health provider's orders will indicate application to the skin, eye, ear, nose, vagina, or rectum.

Aerosol powders and liquids are combined with a propellant and are used for sprays on the skin or in nebulizers and inhalers to reach the mucous membranes of the lower respiratory tract.

Powders may be applied to the skin in dry form.

Creams are semisolid drug preparations applied externally to the skin or mucous membranes. Vaginal creams require a special applicator for insertion.

Ointments are semisolid preparations in a petroleum or lanolin base for topical use. Ointments used for the eye must be labeled "ophthalmic."

Pastes are thick ointments used to protect the skin. They absorb secretions and soften the skin.

Suppositories contain medication molded with a firm base, such as cocoa butter, that melts at body temperature. Suppositories are shaped for insertion into the rectum, vagina, and, less commonly, the urethra.

Transdermal medications are drug molecules contained in a unique polymer patch that is applied to the skin as one would an ordinary plastic bandage. The medication is easy to apply and is effective for hours or days at a time as it is slowly released and absorbed through the skin.

SELF TEST 1 | Terms

Match Column A with the letters in Column B to identify the meaning of the terms used for drug preparations. Answers are given at the end of the chapter.

Column A
1. _____ Scored tablet
2. _____ Enteric coated
3. _____ Spansule
4. _____ Sublingual tablet
5. _____ Capsule
6. _____ Syrup
7. _____ Elixir
8. _____ Fluidextract
9. _____ Tincture
10. _____ Magma
11. _____ Gel
12. _____ Topical
13. _____ Suppository

Column B
a. Coated drug particles dissolve at different times
b. The most concentrated of all liquids
c. Hydroalcoholic liquid ordered in drops
d. Large particles suspended in a liquid
e. A solid that can be broken in half
f. Route applied to skin or mucous membrane
g. Small particles suspended in a liquid
h. Medication that dissolves under the tongue
i. Gelatin containers for a solid or liquid drug
j. Molded solid inserted into the rectum
k. Drug dissolves in the more alkaline secretions of the intestine
l. Sweetened hydroalcoholic liquid
m. Solution of sugar in water to improve the taste of a drug

Equipment to Measure Doses

Nurses do not use a scale to weigh oral solid doses such as the gram and the grain. Solids for oral administration come in tablets and capsules. The nurse calculates the number to give and pours the amount needed into a small container or cup that is discarded once the medication has been given.

Liquids may be prepared as unit doses ready to administer or may be found in stock bottles, which require calculation and measurement. Liquids must be measured accurately. Two practices will aid in achieving this goal:

1. *Pour liquids to a line.* Never estimate a dose between two lines.

2. *Pour liquids at eye level* (Fig. 5-2). The surface of a liquid has a natural curve called the *meniscus*. At eye level, the center of the curve should be on the measurement line. The fluid at the sides of the container will appear to be above the line (Fig. 5-3).

The pieces of equipment used most often by nurses to measure liquids are the medicine cup and syringes.

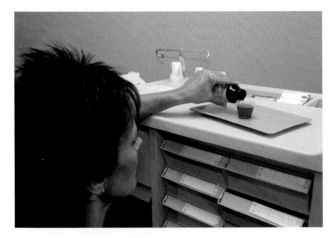

FIGURE 5-2

Liquids are poured at eye level. (Used with permission from Evans-Smith, P. [2005] *Taylor's clinical nursing skills.* Philadelphia: Lippincott, Williams & Wilkins, p. 117.)

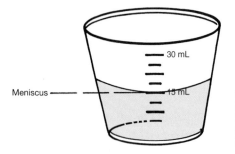

FIGURE 5-3

When viewing the liquid from eye level, the meniscus (lower curve of the fluid) should be on the line.

Medicine Cup

The medicine cup is a plastic or paper disposable container that has equivalent measures for metric doses in milliliters, for apothecary doses in drams, and for household doses in tablespoons and teaspoons (Fig. 5-4).
   The following exercise will help you apply your knowledge of liquid equivalents.

SELF TEST 2 | **Medicine Cup Measurements**

Look at the medicine cup in Figure 5-4. Two sides are shown. Fill in answers related to this measuring device. Check your answers at the end of the chapter.

1. Find 30 mL. What other measures are equivalent to this?

   _____   _____   _____   _____

2. Find 5 mL. Is a dram equal to 5 mL? _____

3. If an order reads dram ii, what line would you use to pour the dose? _____

4. Find 15 mL. What other equivalents equal this?

   _____   _____   _____

5. Consider the following answers to oral liquid dosage problems. What measurement line would you use?

   a. 10 mL   Pour _____

   b. 4 tsp   Pour _____

   c. ½ oz   Pour _____

6. Suppose an answer to an oral liquid problem is 2 mL. Could you pour this dose into a medicine cup?

   Explain what you would do. _____

   _____

   _____

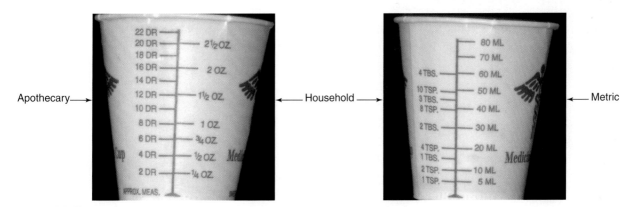

FIGURE 5-4

A medicine cup for measurement of apothecary, household, or metric dose units.
(© 2004 Lacey-Bordeaux Photography.)

Syringes

There are several types of syringes used by nurses to prepare routine parenteral doses. Each is different from the other. Understanding these differences will help you to prepare doses (Fig. 5-5).

The 3-mL syringe, 1-mL syringe, and insulin 100-unit and insulin 50-unit syringes are presented.

SYRINGE. The syringe shown in Figure 5-6 is routinely used for injections. (Note: cc is used on this syringe. Remember—cc = mL.) It has a 22-gauge needle, 1½ inches long. The term *gauge* indicates the diameter (width) of the needle.

Note the following on the 3-mL syringe:

- The markings on one side are in mL to the nearest tenth. Each line indicates 0.1 mL.

- The markings on the opposite side are in minims. Each line indicates 1 minim. Note: Some syringes no longer show minims.

- When preparing a dose, hold the syringe with the needle up, and draw down the medication into the barrel. Suppose a dose were calculated to be 1.1 mL or 18 minims. Look at Figure 5-6 and count the lines to reach the dose.

SELF TEST 3	3-mL Syringe Amounts

Use an arrow to indicate these amounts on the 3-mL syringe in Figure 5-6. Check your answers at the end of this chapter.

0.3 mL

25 m

1.2 mL

½ mL

2.7 mL

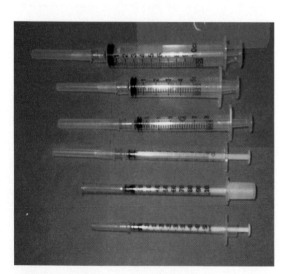

(*Top to bottom*) 10-mL syringe, 5-mL syringe, 3-mL syringe, 1-mL syringe (often called a *tuberculin syringe*), insulin 100-unit syringe, and insulin 50-unit syringe.

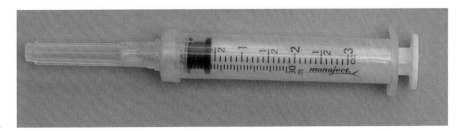

FIGURE 5-6

A 3-mL syringe with metric and apothecary measures. (© 2004 Lacey-Bordeaux Photography.)

The 3-mL syringe has markings for 0.7 mL and 0.8 mL. What would you do if a dosage answer were 0.75 mL? Nurses do not approximate doses between lines. There are two ways to handle this problem:

1. Round off 0.75 mL to the nearest tenth. The answer would be 0.8 mL, which can be drawn up to a line. (Rounding off numbers was discussed in Chapter 1 and is discussed again in this chapter.)

2. Use a different syringe with markings to the nearest hundredth. There is a precision syringe that has markings to the nearest hundredth.

PRECISION SYRINGE. The 1-mL precision syringe with a 25-gauge, ⅝-inch needle is the most accurate of the syringes nurses use. It is sometimes called a *tuberculin syringe.* This syringe is marked in hundredths of a milliliter and in half minims (Fig. 5-7).

Note the following on the 1-mL precision syringe:

- The markings on one side are in minims. There is a short line between each half minim and a long line for a whole minim.

- The markings on the other side are in milliliters. There are nine lines before 0.10. Each line is 0.01 mL.

- To prepare an injection, hold the syringe with the needle up then draw down the medication into the barrel. Suppose a dose was calculated to be 0.25 mL. Look at Figure 5-7 and count the lines to reach the dose.

SELF TEST 4 1-mL Syringe Amounts

Use arrows to mark the following doses on the 1-mL precision syringe in Figure 5-7. Check your answers at the end of this chapter.

0.3 mL

0.45 mL

0.61 mL

0.95 mL

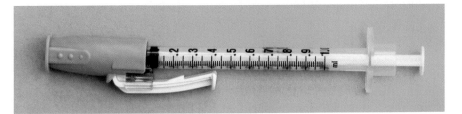

FIGURE 5-7

A 1-mL precision syringe with metric and apothecary measures. (© 2004 Lacey-Bordeaux Photography.)

Rounding Off Numbers in Liquid Dosage Answers

For solving liquid injection problems, answers are in milliliters or minims. The answer may not be an even number and the nurse must decide the degree of accuracy to be obtained. *The degree of accuracy depends on the syringe chosen to give the dose.*

RULE	ROUNDING OFF NUMBERS

1. When the last number is 5 or more, add 1 to the previous number.
2. When the number is 4 or less, drop the number. ■

Example

0.864 becomes 0.86	4.562 becomes 4.56
1.55 becomes 1.6	2.38 becomes 2.4
0.33 becomes 0.3	0.25 becomes 0.3

With the *3-mL syringe,* carry out decimals two places and round off to the *nearest tenth for milliliters.* Carry out answers in *minims* to the nearest tenth and *round off to the nearest whole number.*

With the *1-mL precision syringe,* carry out decimals three places and round off to the *nearest 100th* for milliliters. Carry out answers in *minims* to the nearest 100th and *round off to the nearest tenth.*

SELF TEST 5   3-mL Syringe—Rounding Answers

The following are possible answers to dosage problems that require use of a 3-mL syringe. Put a check (✓) next to the answer if it is acceptable. If it is not acceptable, change the answer to a correct form. Check your answers at the end of this chapter.

a. 0.1 mL _____   e. 0.2 mL _____   i. 0.4 mL _____

b. 1½ mL _____   f. 8½ minims _____   j. 0.65 mL _____

c. 0.83 mL _____   g. 1.7 mL _____   k. 3 minims _____

d. 0.98 minims _____   h. ½ mL _____   l. 5.5 minims _____

SELF TEST 6   1-mL Syringe—Rounding Answers

The following are possible answers to dosage problems that require the use of a 1-mL precision syringe. Put a check (✓) next to the answer if it is acceptable. If not acceptable, change the answer to a correct form. Check your answers at the end of this chapter.

a. 0.65 mL _____   d. 12.8 m _____   g. 0.758 mL _____

b. 12.5 minims _____   e. 0.346 mL _____   h. 5 minims _____

c. 0.04 mL _____   f. 0.290 mL _____

INSULIN SYRINGE. The 1-mL insulin syringe (for unit 100 insulin) is marked in units rather than in milliliters or minims. It is used to prepare only unit 100 insulins. The physician orders the type of insulin, the strength of insulin, and the number of units (Fig. 5-8).

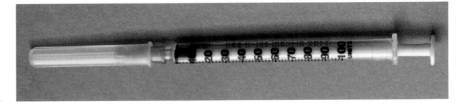

FIGURE 5-8

A 1-mL insulin syringe (for U 100 insulin). (© 2004 Lacey-Bordeaux Photography.)

Example

Order: 20 units NPH (unit 100) insulin every day subcutaneous.

Look at Figure 5-8. Note that there are four short lines between 10 units and 20 units. This indicates that each line is equal to 2 units on this syringe. Always check the markings on a syringe to be certain you understand what each line equals.

SELF TEST 7   1-mL Insulin Syringe

Use arrows on the insulin syringe in Figure 5-8 to indicate the following amounts. Check your answers at the end of this chapter.

22 units

34 units

50 units

Odd-numbered insulin doses should not be drawn up with the syringe in Figure 5-8. Another insulin syringe should be used to prepare these doses. Doses should be exact, not approximate.

LOW-DOSE INSULIN SYRINGE. The low-dose unit 100 insulin syringe with a 28-gauge, ½-inch needle (Fig. 5-9) has four short lines between 10 and 15. This indicates that each line is equal to 1 unit. The syringe is marked for 50 units, so any dose of insulin (unit 100) up to 50 units can be drawn up with this syringe.

SELF TEST 8   0.5-mL Insulin Syringe

Use arrows on the insulin syringe in Figure 5-9 to indicate the following amounts. Answers are given at the end of this chapter.

33 units

12 units

40 units

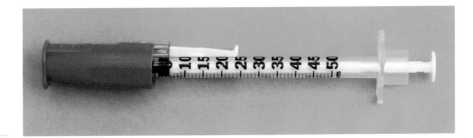

FIGURE 5-9

Low-dose insulin syringe for U 100 insulin. (© 2004 Lacey-Bordeaux Photography.)

Needles for Intramuscular and Subcutaneous Injections

Each of the four syringes discussed has a different injection needle.

Syringe	Gauge	Length, in.
3 mL	22	1½–3
1 mL	25	⅝–⅞
Unit 100 insulin	25–26	½–⅝
Unit 100 low-dose insulin	25–28	½–⅝

Gauge (g) indicates the diameter or width of the needle. *The higher the gauge number, the finer or smaller diameter the needle.* In the gauges just given, the low-dose insulin syringe has the needle with the smallest diameter (28 gauge) and, hence, is the finest needle in this group. A 16-gauge needle would be very wide and would have a wide opening. It is used to transfuse blood cells.

The *length* of the needle used depends on the route of injection. For deep intramuscular injections, a long needle is necessary. A short needle is used for subcutaneous injections.

The nurse determines what types of needle to use for adults and children depending on the route of administration, the size and condition of the patient, and the amount of adipose tissue present at the site (Fig. 5-10).

You have looked at medication orders, types of drug preparations, labels, systems of dosage, and measurement equipment. The next chapters will concentrate on solving dosage problems for oral and parenteral routes.

Needles usually used for **intradermal** injections are ⅜" to ⅝" (1 to 1.5 cm) long and are 25G. Such needles usually have short bevels.

Needles for **subcutaneous** injections are ⅝" to ⅞" (1.5 to 2 cm) long, have medium bevels, and are 25G to 23G.

Needles for **intramuscular** use are 1" to 3" (2.5 to 7.5 cm) long, have medium bevels, and are 23G to 18G.

Needles for **intravenous** use are 1" to 3" long, have long bevels, and are 25G to 14G.

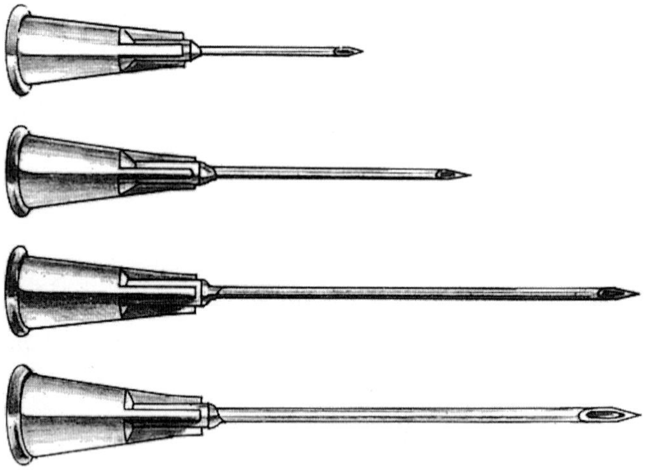

FIGURE 5-10

When choosing a needle, the nurse must consider the needle gauge, bevel, and length. Gauge refers to the inside diameter of the needle; the smaller the gauge, the larger the diameter. Bevel refers to the angle at which the needle tip is opened, and length is the distance from the tip to the hub of the needle.

PROFICIENCY TEST 1 **Drug Preparations and Equipment**

Name: _____

Complete these statements. Answers are given on page 395.

1. Elixirs may be contraindicated for patients with a history of _____

   or _____

2. The average dose of a fluidextract is _____

3. In giving medications parenterally, four common routes are _____ ,

   _____ , _____ , and _____

4. When a powder is reconstituted, what four facts must the nurse write on the label?

   a. _____

   b. _____

   c. _____

   d. _____

5. What route(s) require(s) aseptic technique in preparing and administering drugs?

   _____

6. An example of a drug listed as a magma is _____

7. What action must always be carried out before pouring an oral suspension?

   _____

8. List six drug preparations that can be administered topically.

   _____ _____

   _____ _____

   _____ _____

9. List two advantages in using transdermal medications.

   _____

   _____

10. Define an ointment. _____

    _____

11. List two practices that aid in pouring oral liquids accurately.

    a. _____

    b. _____

12. Define the following:

    a. Meniscus _____

    _____

    b. Needle gauge _____

    _____

(continued)

13. What factors determine the needle length chosen for an injection?

_____

_____

_____

14. List two rules for rounding off numbers.

a. _____

_____

b. _____

_____

15. What determines how dosage answers are rounded off?

_____

_____

_____

Answers

Self-Test 1 Terms

1. e	**4.** h	**6.** m	**8.** b	**10.** d	**12.** f
2. k	**5.** i	**7.** l	**9.** c	**11.** g	**13.** j
3. a					

Self-Test 2 Medicine Cup Measurements

1. Other equivalents are 2 tbsp, 1 oz, 8 drams, 30 mL.

2. No, a dram is slightly less than 5 mL.

3. Use the 2-dram line.

4. Fifteen milliliters is equal to 1 tbsp, ½ oz, and 4 drams.

5. **a.** Pour 2 tsp.

   b. 4 tsp × 5 mL = 20 mL; use the 20-mL line

   c. ½ oz. Use the line for ½ oz.

6. No, there is no line for 2 mL. Use a syringe to obtain the 2 mL and then pour the amount into a medicine cup.

Self-Test 3 3-mL Syringe Amounts

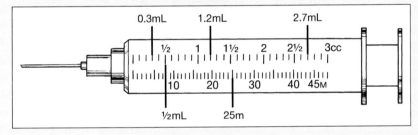

Self-Test 4 1-mL Syringe Amounts

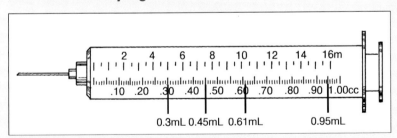

Self-Test 5 3-mL Syringe—Rounding Answers

a. 0.1 mL	✓	**e.** 0.2 mL	✓	**i.** 0.4 mL	✓
b. 1½ mL	✓	**f.** 8½ m	9 m	**j.** 0.65 mL	0.7 mL
c. 0.83 mL	0.8 mL	**g.** 1.7 mL	✓	**k.** 3 minims	✓
d. 0.98 m	1 minim	**h.** ½ mL	✓	**l.** 5.5 minims	6 minims

Self-Test 6 1-mL Syringe—Rounding Answers

a. 0.65 mL _____✓_____   **d.** 12.8 m _____✓_____   **g.** 0.758 mL __0.76 mL ·__

b. 12.5 m _____✓_____   **e.** 0.346 mL __0.35 mL__   **h.** 5 minims _____✓_____

c. 0.04 mL _____✓_____   **f.** 0.290 mL __0.29 mL__

Self-Test 7 1-mL Insulin Syringe

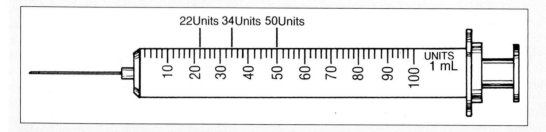

Self-Test 8 .5-mL Insulin Syringe

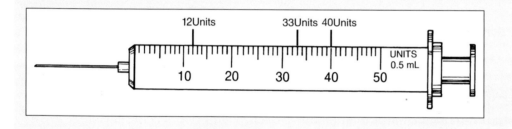

Calculation of Oral Medications—Solids and Liquids

Drugs for oral administration are prepared by pharmaceutical companies as solids (tablets, capsules) and liquids. When the dose ordered by the physician or health care provider differs from the supply, the nurse calculates the amount to be given. The problems are solved using a rule derived from ratio and proportion. All measurements need to be in the same system and the same unit or size (use smallest numbers).

In dosage calculations, three pieces of information are given:

1. The doctor's order

2. The quantity or strength of drug on hand

3. The solid or liquid form of supply drug (in which the drug comes)

The unknown is the amount of drug to administer, usually designated as X or x. These letters represent the above information:

D = doctor's order or desired dose

H = on hand or have

S = supply form

A = answer or amount of drug to give

▷ Proportion Expressed as Two Fractions

Using fractions, set up proportions so that like units are across from each other (the units and the numerator match and the units and denominators match). The first fraction is the known equivalent.

Example One tablet is equal to 50 mg would be written $\dfrac{1 \text{ tablet}}{50 \text{ mg}}$

The second fraction is the unknown and the desired dose. Example: x tablets is equal to 100 mg, and is written $\dfrac{\text{x tablets}}{100 \text{ mg}}$

The completed proportion looks like

$$\frac{S}{H} = \frac{x}{D} \qquad \frac{Supply}{Have} = \frac{x}{Desire}$$

In the previous example, it would look like: $\dfrac{1 \text{ tablet}}{50 \text{ mg}} = \dfrac{x \text{ tablets}}{100 \text{ mg}}$

Learning Aid

You can use the letter X or the letter A to denote the unknown amount. In this text, the letter X will be used with ratio/proportion problems and the letter A will be used when problems are solved using the formula method.

Next, solve for x. (Refer to Chapter 1, pages 14 to 17, to review solving proportions.) In our example, it would look like this:

1. $\dfrac{1 \text{ tablet}}{50 \text{ mg}} = \dfrac{x \text{ tablets}}{100 \text{ mg}}$

    $\dfrac{1 \text{ tablet}}{50 \text{ mg}} \diagdown \dfrac{x \text{ tablets}}{100 \text{ mg}}$

    $100 \times 1 = 50x$

Learning Aid

Always divide by the number that is multiplied by x.

2. $\dfrac{100 \times 1}{50} = \dfrac{50x}{50}$

3. $\dfrac{100}{50} = \dfrac{5\!\!\!/0\, x}{5\!\!\!/0}$

    $\dfrac{100}{50} = x$

Answer: 2 tablets = x

▶ Proportion Expressed as Two Ratios

A ratio using colons can be set up. Double colons separate the two ratios. The first ratio is the known equivalent; the second ratio is the desired dose and the unknown. The ratio must always follow the same sequence.

The ratio will look like

$\quad$ S : H : : x : D $\quad$ Supply : Have : : x : Desire

Using the previous example it would look like

$\quad$ 1 tablet : 50 mg : : x : 100 mg

Next, solve for x (Refer to Chapter 1, pages 14 to 17, to review solving ratios.)

1. 1 tablet : 50 mg : : x : 100 mg

2. $1 \times 100 = 50x$

3. $\dfrac{100}{50} = \dfrac{5\!\!\!/0\, x}{5\!\!\!/0}$

4. $\dfrac{100}{50} = x$

    Answer: 2 tablets = x

Formula Method

Both of these methods can be simplified by using the formula method. This is the formula derived from step 3:

$$\frac{D}{H} \times S = A \qquad \frac{Desire}{Have} \times Supply = Amount$$

The formula method eliminates the need to cross-multiply, which can be a possible source of error in calculation.

For the purpose of this book, the formula method, ratio method, and proportion method are shown side-by-side. The most important thing is for the nurse to understand thoroughly and use whichever method makes sense to him/her.

A fourth method used in dosage calculations is the dimensional analysis method. This is explained in Chapter 11.

The proficiency tests in this book show the answers with all four methods.

Oral Solids

Application of the Rule for Oral Solids

RULE	**FORMULA METHOD**

$$\frac{Desire}{Have} \times Supply = Amount\ or\ Answer$$

Learning Aid

Abbreviate the rule:

$$\frac{D}{H} \times S = A \qquad S:H::x:D \qquad \frac{S}{H} = \frac{x}{D}$$

RULE	**RATIO METHOD**

Supply : Have : : x : Desire

RULE	**PROPORTION METHOD**

$$\frac{Supply}{Have} = \frac{x}{Desire}$$

Example Order: Coreg 6.25 mg po bid

Supply: Read the label

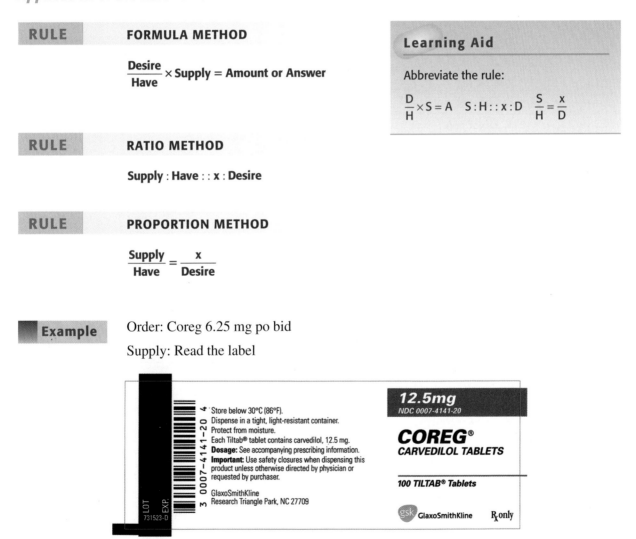

Used with permission of GlaxoSmithKline.

Desire: The desire is the order. In the example, desired is 6.25 mg.

Have: Have is the strength of the drug supplied in the container. In the example, the label indicates that each tablet contains 12.5 mg.

Supply: The supply is the unit form in which the drug comes. Coreg comes in tablet form. Because tablets and capsules are single entities, the stock for oral solid drugs is always one.

Amount: The amount is how much supply to give. For oral solids the answer will be the number of tablets or capsules to administer.

To solve any problem, first check that the order and the supply are in the same weight measure. If they are not, you must convert one or the other amount to its equivalent. In this example, no equivalent is needed; both the order and the supply are in milligrams.

Example   Desire: Coreg 6.25 mg po

Have: 12.5 mg

Supply: 1 tablet

RULE   **FORMULA METHOD**

$$\frac{D}{H} \times S = A$$

$$\frac{1\ \ 6.25\ mg}{2\ \ 12.5\ mg} \times 1\ tablet = A$$

½ tablet = A

Learning Aid

$$6.25\overline{)12.50}\ \ 2$$

RULE   **RATIO METHOD**

S : H : : x : D

1 tablet : 12.5 mg : : x : 6.25 mg

$6.25 \times 1 = 12.5x$

$$\frac{6.25}{12.5} = x$$

½ tablet = x

Learning Aid

Note that the ratio and proportion methods end with the same equation—in this case,

$$\frac{6.25}{12.5} = x$$

When illustrating these two methods, one combined final equation will be shown.

RULE   **PROPORTION METHOD**

$$\frac{S}{H} = \frac{x}{Desire}$$

$$\frac{1\ tablet}{12.5\ mg} \times \frac{x}{6.25\ mg}$$

$6.25 \times 1 = 12.5\ mg\ x$

$$\frac{6.25}{12.5} = x$$

½ tablet = x

Formula Method: Clearing Decimals

When the numerator and denominator in $\dfrac{D}{H}$ are decimals, add zeros to make the number of decimal places the same. Then drop the decimal points. This is a short arithmetic operation to replace long division:

$$\overset{\text{added}}{\underset{\downarrow}{\dfrac{0.5\underset{\frown}{0}\,\text{mg}}{0.25\,\text{mg}}}} \quad \dfrac{\text{numerator}}{\text{denominator or divisor}}$$

In division, the denominator is the divisor and must be cleared of decimal points before the arithmetic is carried out. The decimal point in the numerator is moved the same number of places. Refer to Chapter 1 for further help in division of decimals.

Example	Order: Lanoxin 0.125 mg po every day
	Supply: Read the label

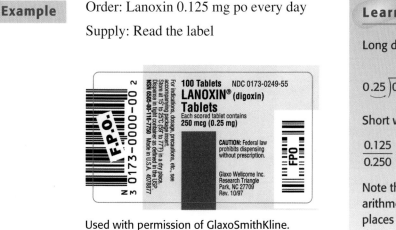

Used with permission of GlaxoSmithKline.

Learning Aid

Long division

$$0.25\,\overline{)\,0.125}\quad\overset{0.5}{}=\dfrac{5}{10}=\dfrac{1}{2}\,\text{tablet}$$

Short way

$$\dfrac{0.125}{0.250}=\dfrac{1}{2}\,\text{tablet}$$

Note that a zero was added. In short arithmetic when the number of decimal places is the same in the numerator and denominator, the decimal is dropped.

No equivalent is needed. It is stated on the label: 0.25 mg.

Formula Method

$$\dfrac{\overset{1}{0.1\underset{\frown}{2}5}\,\text{mg}}{\underset{2}{0.2\underset{\frown}{5}0}\,\text{mg}}\times 1\ \text{tablet}=\dfrac{1}{2}\ \text{tablet}$$

Ratio Method

1 tablet : 0.25 mg : : x : 0.125 mg

Proportion Method

$$\dfrac{1\ \text{tablet}}{0.25\ \text{mg}}\bowtie\dfrac{x}{0.125\ \text{mg}}$$

$$0.125\ \text{mg}=0.25x$$

$$\dfrac{\overset{1}{0.1\underset{\frown}{2}5}\,\text{mg}}{\underset{2}{0.2\underset{\frown}{5}0}\,\text{mg}}=x$$

$$\tfrac{1}{2}\ \text{tablet}=x$$

Example

Order: amoxicillin 1 g po q6h

Supply: 1 capsule equals 500 mg

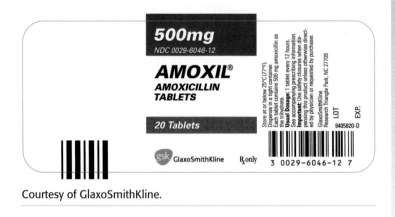

Courtesy of GlaxoSmithKline.

Equivalent: 1 g = 1000 mg

Formula Method

$$\frac{D}{H} \times S = A$$

$$\frac{\overset{2}{\cancel{1000}} \text{ mg}}{\underset{1}{\cancel{500}} \text{ mg}} \times 1 \text{ cap} = 2 \text{ caps}$$

Ratio Method

1 cap : 500 mg : : x : 1000 mg

Proportion Method

$$\frac{1}{500 \text{ mg}} \times \frac{x}{1000 \text{ mg}}$$

$$1000 = 500$$

$$\frac{1000}{500} = x$$

$$2 \text{ caps} = x$$

Example

Order: Synthroid 75 mcg po every day

Supply: Read the label

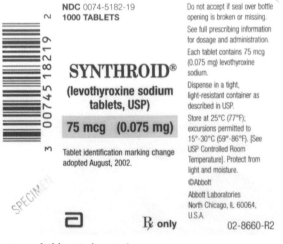

Courtesy of Abbott Laboratories.

Note that the label gives the equivalent measure:

75 mcg = 0.075 mg

Because the order and the supply are in the same weight measure, no calculation is necessary. Give 1 tablet.

Example

Order: Zyprexa 7.5 mg po every day

Supply: Read the label

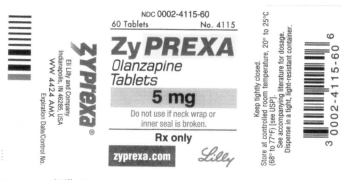

Courtesy of Lilly Co.

No equivalent is needed.

Formula Method

$$\frac{\overset{1.5}{\cancel{7.5}} \text{ mg}}{\underset{1}{\cancel{5}} \text{ mg}} \times 1 \text{ tablet} = 1\frac{1}{2} \text{ tablets}$$

Ratio Method

1 tablet : 5 mg :: x : 7.5 mg

Proportion Method

$$\frac{1 \text{ tablet}}{5 \text{ mg}} \times \frac{x}{7.5 \text{ mg}}$$

$$7.5 = 5x$$

$$\frac{7.5}{5} = x$$

$$1\frac{1}{2} \text{ tablets} = x$$

You can administer 1½ tablets because the supply is scored.

Example

Order: Lamictal 200 mg po every day

Supply: Read the label

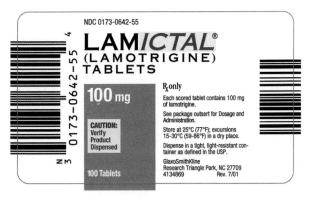

Courtesy of GlaxoSmithKline.

No equivalent is needed.

Formula Method

$$\frac{D}{H} \times S = A$$

$$\frac{\overset{2}{\cancel{200}} \text{ mg}}{\underset{1}{\cancel{100}} \text{ mg}} \times 1 \text{ tablet} = 2 \text{ tablets}$$

Ratio Method

$$S : H : : x : D$$

$$1 \text{ tablet} : 100 \text{ mg} : : x : 200 \text{ mg}$$

Proportion Method

$$\frac{S}{H} = \frac{x}{D}$$

$$\frac{1 \text{ tablet}}{100 \text{ mg}} \times \frac{x}{200 \text{ mg}}$$

$$200 = 100x$$

$$\frac{200}{100} = x$$

$$2 \text{ tablets} = x$$

Example

Order: furosemide 60 mg po every day

Supply: Read the label

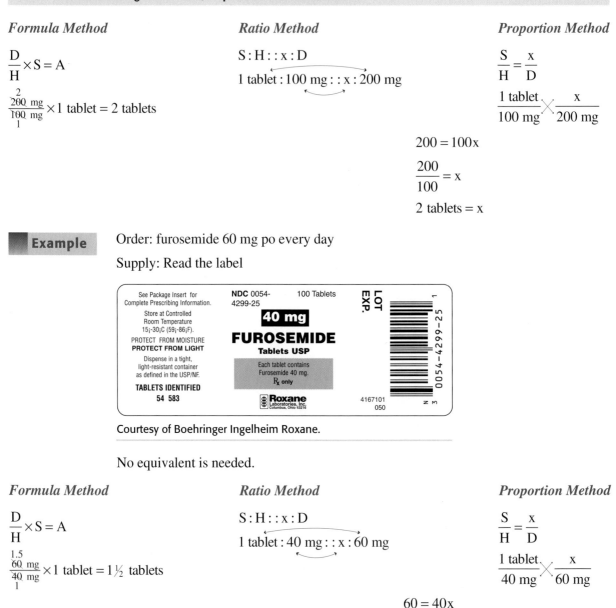

See Package Insert for Complete Prescribing Information.

Store at Controlled Room Temperature 15¡-30¡C (59¡-86¡F).

PROTECT FROM MOISTURE
PROTECT FROM LIGHT

Dispense in a tight, light-resistant container as defined in the USP/NF.

TABLETS IDENTIFIED 54 583

NDC 0054-4299-25   100 Tablets

LOT EXP.

40 mg

FUROSEMIDE

Tablets USP

Each tablet contains Furosemide 40 mg.

R$_x$ only

Roxane Laboratories, Inc. Columbus, Ohio 43216

4167101 050

0054-4299-25

Courtesy of Boehringer Ingelheim Roxane.

No equivalent is needed.

Formula Method

$$\frac{D}{H} \times S = A$$

$$\frac{\overset{1.5}{\cancel{60}} \text{ mg}}{\underset{1}{\cancel{40}} \text{ mg}} \times 1 \text{ tablet} = 1\tfrac{1}{2} \text{ tablets}$$

Ratio Method

$$S : H : : x : D$$

$$1 \text{ tablet} : 40 \text{ mg} : : x : 60 \text{ mg}$$

Proportion Method

$$\frac{S}{H} = \frac{x}{D}$$

$$\frac{1 \text{ tablet}}{40 \text{ mg}} \times \frac{x}{60 \text{ mg}}$$

$$60 = 40x$$

$$\frac{60}{40} = x$$

$$1\tfrac{1}{2} \text{ tablets} = x$$

Give 1½ tablets; tablets are scored.

Example

Order: Lexapro 20 mg po every day

Supply: Read the label

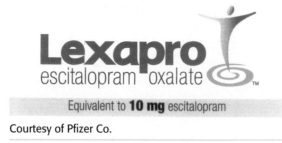

Lexapro
escitalopram oxalate ™

Equivalent to **10 mg** escitalopram

Courtesy of Pfizer Co.

Formula Method

$$\frac{D}{H} \times S = A$$

$$\frac{\overset{2}{\cancel{20}} \text{ mg}}{\underset{1}{\cancel{10}} \text{ mg}} \times 1 \text{ tablet} = 2 \text{ tablets}$$

Ratio Method

$$S : H : : x : D$$
$$1 \text{ tablet} : 10 \text{ mg} : : x : 20 \text{ mg}$$

Proportion Method

$$\frac{S}{H} = \frac{x}{D}$$
$$\frac{1 \text{ tablet}}{10 \text{ mg}} \times \frac{x}{20 \text{ mg}}$$

$$20 = 10x$$
$$\frac{20}{10} = x$$
$$2 \text{ tablets}$$

SELF-TEST 1   Oral Solids

Solve these practice problems. Answers are given at the end of the chapter. Remember the three methods:

Formula Method

$$\frac{D}{H} \times S = A$$

Ratio Method

$$S : H : : x : D$$

Proportion Method

$$\frac{S}{H} \times \frac{x}{D}$$

1. Order: Decadron 1.5 mg po bid
   Supply: tablets labeled 0.75 mg

2. Order: digoxin 0.25 mg po every day
   Supply: scored tablets labeled 0.5 mg

3. Order: ampicillin 0.5 g po q6h
   Supply: capsules labeled 250 mg

4. Order: prednisone 10 mg po tid
   Supply: tablets labeled 2.5 mg

5. Order: aspirin 650 mg po stat
   Supply: tablets labeled 325 mg

6. Order: cimetidine 0.8 g po at bedtime
   Supply: tablets labeled 400 mg

7. Order: Equanil 0.2 g po q4h
   Supply: scored tablets labeled 400 mg

8. Order: penicillin G potassium 200,000 units po q8h
   Supply: scored tablets labeled 400,000 units

9. Order: digoxin 0.5 mg po every day
   Supply: scored tablets labeled 0.25 mg

10. Order: Captopril 18.75 mg po tid
    Supply: scored tablets labeled 12.5 mg

11. Order: Allopurinol 600 mg po every day
    Supply: scored tablets labeled 300 mg

12. Order: Brethine 7.5 mg po bid
    Supply: scored tablets labeled 2.5 mg

(continued)

| SELF-TEST 1 | Oral Solids (Continued) |

13. Order: Captopril 6.25 mg po bid
   Supply: scored tablets labeled 25 mg

14. Order: Catapres 400 mcg po every day
   Supply: tablets labeled 0.2 mg

15. Order: Coumadin 7.5 mg po every day
   Supply: scored tablets labeled 5 mg

16. Order: Glyburide 0.625 mg every day
   Supply: scored tablets labeled 1.25 mg

17. Order: Naprosyn 0.5 g po every day
   Supply: scored tablets labeled 250 mg

18. Order: Hydrodiuril 37.5 mg po every day
   Supply: scored tablets labeled 25 mg

19. Order: Keflex 1 g po q6h
   Supply: capsules labeled 500 mg

20. Order: Baclofen 25 mg po tid
   Supply: scored tablets labeled 10 mg

Special Types of Oral Solid Orders

Drugs that contain a number of active ingredients are ordered by the number to be administered and do not require calculation. Over-the-counter (OTC) medications are often ordered by how many are to be administered.

Example   *EXAMPLE 1*

Vitamin B complex caplets 1 po every day

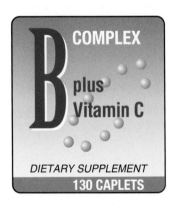

Interpret as: Give 1 caplet by mouth every day.

EXAMPLE 2

Aggrenox 25 mg/200 mg capsules 1 capsule po bid

NDC 0597-0001-60

Aggrenox®

(aspirin/extended-release dipyridamole)

25 mg/200 mg capsules

Rx only

60 capsules
Unit-of-use container

Boehringer
Ingelheim

Dosage: Read accompanying prescribing information.
Store at 25°C (77°F); excursions permitted to
15-30°C (59-86°F). [See USP Controlled Room
Temperature.] Protect from excessive moisture.
Mkd. by: Boehringer Ingelheim Pharmaceuticals, Inc.
Ridgefield, CT 06877 USA
Mfd. by: Boehringer Ingelheim Pharma GmbH & Co. KG
Biberach, Germany
Lic. from: Boehringer Ingelheim International GmbH
U.S. Pat. No. 6,015,577
© Copyright Boehringer Ingelheim International GmbH
2003, ALL RIGHTS RESERVED
Rev 1/30/03
43659/US/3

LOT   EXP

Courtesy of Boehringer Ingelheim Roxane.

Interpret as: Give 1 Aggrenox capsule by mouth twice a day.

Oral Liquids

Application of the Rule for Oral Liquids

Formula Method

$$\frac{\text{Desire}}{\text{Have}} \times \text{Supply} = \text{Amount}$$

Ratio Method

$$\text{Supply} : \text{Have} : : x : \text{Desire}$$

Proportion Method

$$\frac{\text{Supply}}{\text{Have}} = \frac{x}{\text{Desire}}$$

Example

Order: azithromycin oral susp 400 mg po
every day × 4 days

Supply: Read the label

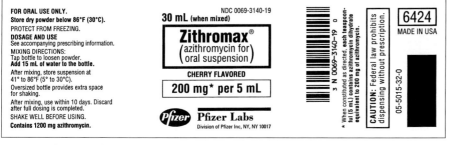

FOR ORAL USE ONLY.
Store dry powder below 86°F (30°C).
PROTECT FROM FREEZING.
DOSAGE AND USE
See accompanying prescribing information.
MIXING DIRECTIONS:
Tap bottle to loosen powder.
Add 15 mL of water to the bottle.
After mixing, store suspension at
41° to 86°F (5° to 30°C).
Oversized bottle provides extra space
for shaking.
After mixing, use within 10 days. Discard
after full dosing is completed.
SHAKE WELL BEFORE USING.
Contains 1200 mg azithromycin.

NDC 0069-3140-19
30 mL (when mixed)

Zithromax®
(azithromycin for
oral suspension)

CHERRY FLAVORED

200 mg* per 5 mL

Pfizer **Pfizer Labs**
Division of Pfizer Inc, NY, NY 10017

6424
MADE IN USA

* When constituted as directed, each teaspoon-
ful (5 mL) contains azithromycin dihydrate
equivalent to 200 mg of azithromycin.

CAUTION: Federal law prohibits
dispensing without prescription.

05-5015-32-0

Courtesy of Pfizer Labs.

Formula Method

$$\frac{\overset{2}{\cancel{400}} \text{ mg}}{\underset{1}{\cancel{200}} \text{ mg}} \times 5 \text{ mL} = 10 \text{ mL}$$

Ratio Method

5 mL : 200 mg : : x : 400 mg

Proportion Method

$$\frac{5 \text{ mL}}{200 \text{ mg}} \underset{\times}{} \frac{\text{x}}{400 \text{ mg}}$$

$$5 \times 400 = 200\text{x}$$

$$\frac{2000}{200} = \text{x}$$

$$10 \text{ mL} = \text{x}$$

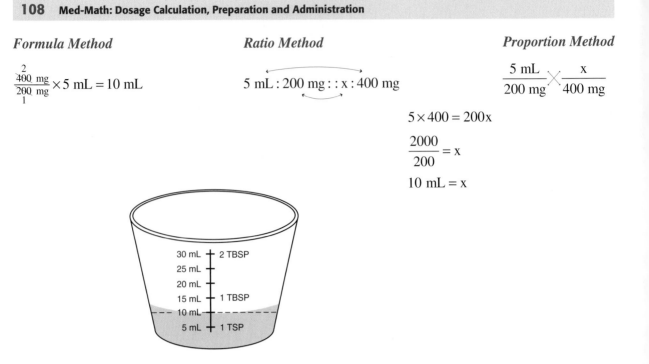

Administer 10 mL of Zithromax po every day for 4 days.

Before solving each problem, check to be certain that the order and your supply are in the same measure. If they are not, you must convert one or the other to its equivalent. Convert whichever one is easier for you to solve.

Example   Order: digoxin elixir 500 mcg × 1 dose

Supply: Read the label

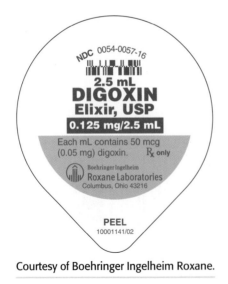

Courtesy of Boehringer Ingelheim Roxane.

Equivalent: 500 mcg = 0.5 mg

Formula Method

$$\frac{D}{H} \times S = A$$

$$\frac{\overset{4}{\cancel{0.5} \text{ mg}}}{\underset{1}{\cancel{0.125} \text{ mg}}} \times 2.5 \text{ mL} = 10 \text{ mL}$$

Ratio Method

$$S : H :: x : D$$

$$2.5 \text{ mL} : 0.125 \text{ mg} :: x : 0.5 \text{ mg}$$

Proportion Method

$$\frac{S}{H} = \frac{x}{D}$$

$$\frac{2.5 \text{ mL}}{0.125 \text{ mg}} \times \frac{x}{0.5 \text{ mg}}$$

$$2.5 \times 0.5 = 0.125 \text{ mg}$$

$$\frac{1.25}{0.125} = x$$

$$10 \text{ mL} = x$$

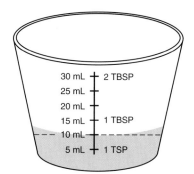

Administer 10 mL of Digoxin × 1 dose.

Learning Aid

Formula:
$$\begin{array}{r} 4. \\ 0.125 \overline{)0.500} \\ \underline{500} \\ 0 \end{array}$$

Ratio Proportion: $2.5 \times 0.5 = 1.25$

$$\begin{array}{r} 10. \\ 0.125 \overline{)1.250} \\ \underline{125} \\ 0 \end{array}$$

Example

Order: furosemide 34 mg po every day

Supply: Read the label

Learning Aid

Because the drug comes with a calibrated dropper, you are alerted that your answer will be a small amount.

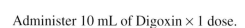

Courtesy of Boehringer Ingelheim Roxane.

No equivalent is needed.

Formula Method

$$\frac{D}{H} \times S = A$$

$$\frac{34 \text{ mg}}{10 \text{ mg}} \times 1 \text{ mL} = 3.4 \text{ mL}$$

$$10\overline{)34.0} \atop \begin{array}{r} 3.4 \\ \underline{30} \\ 40 \end{array}$$

Ratio Method

$$S : H :: x : D$$
$$1 \text{ mL} : 10 \text{ mg} :: x : 34 \text{ mg}$$

Proportion Method

$$\frac{S}{H} = \frac{x}{D}$$

$$\frac{1 \text{ mL}}{10 \text{ mg}} = \frac{x}{34 \text{ mg}}$$

$$34 = 10x$$

$$\frac{34}{10} = x$$

$$3.4 \text{ mL} = x$$

Use the calibrated dropper to administer 3.4 mL.

Example

Order: digoxin 0.375 mg po every day

Supply: Read the label

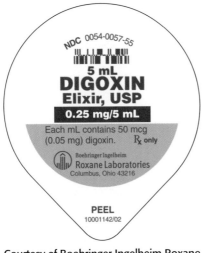

Courtesy of Boehringer Ingelheim Roxane.

No equivalent is needed.

Formula Method

$$\frac{D}{H} \times S = A$$

$$\frac{\overset{1.5}{0.375} \text{ mg}}{\underset{1}{0.25} \text{ mg}} \times 5 \text{ mL} = 1.5 \times 5 = 7.5 \text{ mL}$$

Ratio Method

$$S : H :: x : D$$
$$5 \text{ mL} : 0.25 \text{ mg} :: x : 0.375 \text{ mg}$$

Proportion Method

$$\frac{S}{H} = \frac{x}{D}$$

$$\frac{5 \text{ mL}}{0.25 \text{ mg}} = \frac{x}{0.375 \text{ mg}}$$

$$5 \times 0.375 = 0.25x$$

$$\frac{1.875}{0.25} = x$$

$$7.5 \text{ mL} = x$$

Use a needleless syringe to draw up 7.5 mL.

Learning Aid

Formula

$$0.25\overline{)0.375} = 1.5$$
$$\underline{25}$$
$$125$$

Ratio Proportion $5 \times 0.375 = 1.875$

$$0.25\overline{)1.875} = 7.5$$
$$\underline{175}$$
$$125$$
$$\underline{125}$$
$$0$$

Example

Order: amoxicillin oral suspension 500 mg po q8h

Supply: Read the label

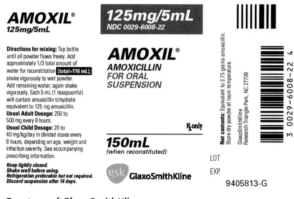

Courtesy of GlaxoSmithKline.

Formula Method

$$\frac{D}{H} \times S = A$$

$$\frac{\overset{4}{\cancel{500}}\ mg}{\underset{1}{\cancel{125}}\ mg} \times 5\ mL = 4 \times 5 = 20\ mL$$

Ratio Method

$$S : H : : x : D$$
$$5\ mL : 125\ mg : : x : 500\ mg$$

$$5 \times 500 = 125x$$
$$\frac{2500}{125} = x$$
$$20\ mL = x$$

Proportion Method

$$\frac{S}{H} = \frac{x}{D}$$
$$\frac{5\ mL}{125\ mg} \times \frac{x}{500\ mg}$$

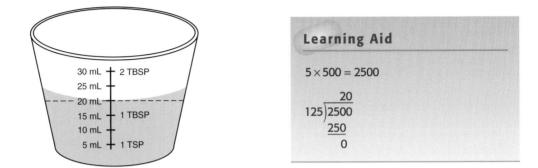

Administer 20 mL of Amoxil PO every 8 hours.

SELF-TEST 2 | Oral Liquids

Solve these oral liquid problems. Answers are given at the end of the chapter.

1. Order: erythromycin susp 0.75 g po qid
   Supply: liquid labeled 250 mg/mL

2. Order: ampicillin susp 500 mg po q8h
   Supply: liquid labeled 250 mg/5 mL

3. Order: Cephalexin in oral suspension 0.35 g po q6h
   Supply: liquid labeled 125 mg/5 mL

4. Order: cyclosporine 150 mg po stat and every day
   Supply: liquid labeled 100 mg/mL in a bottle with a calibrated dropper

5. Order: sulfisoxazole susp 300 mg po qid
   Supply: liquid labeled 0.5 g/5 mL

6. Order: digoxin 0.02 mg po every day
   Supply: pediatric elixir 0.05 mg/mL in a bottle with a dropper marked in tenths of a milliliter

7. Order: potassium chloride 30 mEq po every day
   Supply: liquid labeled 20 mEq/15 mL

8. Order: digoxin elixir 0.25 mg via nasogastric tube every day
   Supply: liquid labeled 0.25 mg/mL

9. Order: hydrocortisone cypionate oral susp 30 mg po q6h
   Supply: liquid labeled 10 mg/5 mL

10. Order: promethazine HCl syrup 12.5 mg po tid
    Supply: liquid labeled 6.25 mg/5 mL

11. Order: Vistaril 50 mg po qid
    Supply: syrup labeled 10 mg per 5 mL

12. Order: furosemide 40 mg po q12h
    Supply: liquid labeled 10 mg/mL

13. Order: potassium chloride 10 mEq po bid
    Supply: liquid labeled 20 mEq/30 mL

14. Order: Compazine 10 mg po tid
    Supply: syrup labeled 5 mg/5 mL

(continued)

SELF-TEST 2   **Oral Liquids (Continued)**

15. Order: phenobarbital 100 mg po hs
Supply: elixir labeled 20 mg/5 mL

16. Order: Tylenol gr 10 po q4h prn
Supply: elixir labeled 160 mg/5 mL

17. Order: Benadryl 25 mg po q4h
Supply: liquid labeled 12.5 mg/5 mL

18. Order: Thorazine 50 mg po tid
Supply: syrup labeled 10 mg/5 mL

19. Order: Docusate 100 mg po every day
Supply: syrup labeled 50 mg/15 mL

20. Order: codeine 0.06 g po q4–6h prn
Supply: liquid labeled 15 mg/5 mL

Special Types of Oral Liquid Orders

Some liquids, including OTC preparations and multivitamins, are ordered in the amount to be poured and administered. No calculation is required.

Example

EXAMPLE 1

Order: Robitussin syrup 2 tsp q4h prn po

Supply: liquid labeled Robitussin syrup

No calculation is needed. Pour 2 tsp and take every 4 hours by mouth as necessary.

EXAMPLE 2

Order: milk of magnesia 30 mL tonight po

Supply: liquid labeled milk of magnesia

No calculation is required. Pour 30 mL milk of magnesia and give tonight by mouth.

Mental Drill for Oral Solid and Liquid Problems

As you develop proficiency in solving problems, you will be able to calculate many answers without written work. This drill combines your knowledge of equivalents and dosage.

SELF-TEST 3 | Mental Drill Oral Solids

Solve the problems mentally and write only the amount to be given. Answers are given at the end of the chapter. Keep the rule in mind as you solve each problem.

Order	Supply (scored tablets)	Answer
1. 20 mg	10 mg	
2. 0.125 mg	0.25 mg	
3. 0.25 mg	0.125 mg	
4. 200,000 units	100,000 units	
5. 0.5 mg	0.25 mg	
6. 0.2 g	400 mg	
7. 1 g	1000 mg	
8. 0.1 g	100 mg	
9. 0.01 g	20 mg	
10. 650 mg	325 mg	
11. 500 mg	250 mg	
12. gr i	60 mg	
13. 50 mg	0.1 g	
14. 4 mg	2 mg	

SELF-TEST 4 | Mental Drill Oral Liquids

Order	Supply	Answer
1. 20 mg	10 mg/5 mL	
2. 10 mg	2 mg/5 mL	
3. 0.5 g	250 mg/5 mL	
4. 0.1 g	200 mg/10 mL	
5. 250 mg	0.1 g/6 mL	
6. 100 mg	50 mg/10 mL	
7. 12 mg	4 mg/5 mL	
8. 15 mg	30 mg/10 mL	
9. 15 mg	10 mg/4 mL	
10. 0.25 mg	0.5 mg/5 mL	

PROFICIENCY TEST 1 | **Calculation of Oral Doses**

Name: _____

For liquid answers, draw a line on the medicine cup indicating the amount you would pour.
Answers are given on page 396.

1. Order: KCl elixir 20 mEq po bid
Supply: liquid labeled 30 mEq/15 mL
Answer   _____

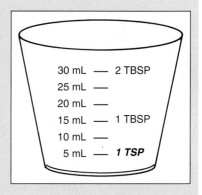

2. Order: Dilantin susp 150 mg po tid
Supply: liquid labeled 75 mg/7.5 mL
Answer   _____

3. Order: digoxin elixir 0.125 mg po every day
Supply: liquid labeled 0.25 mg/10 mL
Answer   _____

(continued)

PROFICIENCY TEST 1   **Calculation of Oral Doses (Continued)**

4. Order: Dilantin oral susp 375 mg po tid
   Supply: liquid labeled 125 mg/5 mL
   Answer   _____

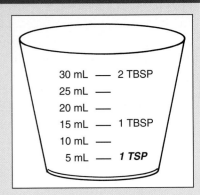

5. Order: Famotidine 40 mg
   Supply: suspension labeled 20 mg/2.5 mL
   Answer   _____

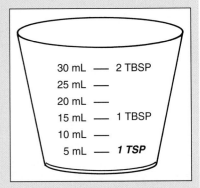

6. Order: digoxin 0.5 mg po every day
   Supply: tablets labeled 0.25 mg
   Answer   _____

7. Order: Lanoxin 100 mcg every day po
   Supply: 0.1-mg capsules
   Answer   _____

8. Order: Zyloprim 250 mg po every day
   Supply: scored tablets 100 mg
   Answer   _____

9. Order: ampicillin 0.5 g po q6h
   Supply: capsules labeled 250 mg
   Answer   _____

10. Order: Synthroid 0.3 mg po every day
    Supply: tablets labeled 300 mcg scored
    Answer   _____

PROFICIENCY TEST 2 | **Calculation of Oral Doses (Test 2)**

Name: _____

For liquid answers, draw a line on the medicine cup indicating the amount you would pour. Answers are given on page 400.

1. Order: ibuprofen 0.8 g po tid
   Supply: tablets labeled 400 mg
   Answer _____

2. Order: isoniazid 0.3 g po every day
   Supply: tablets labeled 300 mg
   Answer _____

3. Order: ethambutol HCl 600 mg po every day
   Supply: tablets scored and labeled 400 mg
   Answer _____

4. Order: acetaminophen 0.65 g po q4h
   Supply: tablets labeled 325 mg
   Answer _____

5. Order: ascorbic acid 250 mg po bid
   Supply: tablets scored and labeled 500 mg
   Answer _____

6. Order: nystatin oral susp 750,000 units po tid
   Supply: liquid labeled 100,000 units/mL
   Answer _____

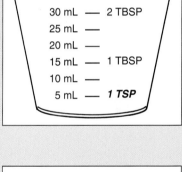

7. Order: oxacillin sodium 0.75 g po q6h
   Supply: liquid labeled 250 mg/5 mL
   Answer _____

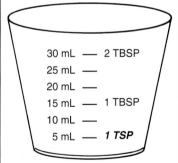

(continued)

8. Order: penicillin V potassium 500 mg po q6h
Supply: liquid labeled 250 mg/5 mL
Answer   _____

9. Order: Mylanta II 30 mL q4h prn
Supply: liquid labeled Mylanta II
Answer   _____

10. Order: theophylline 160 mg po q6h
Supply: liquid labeled 80 mg/15 mL
Answer   _____

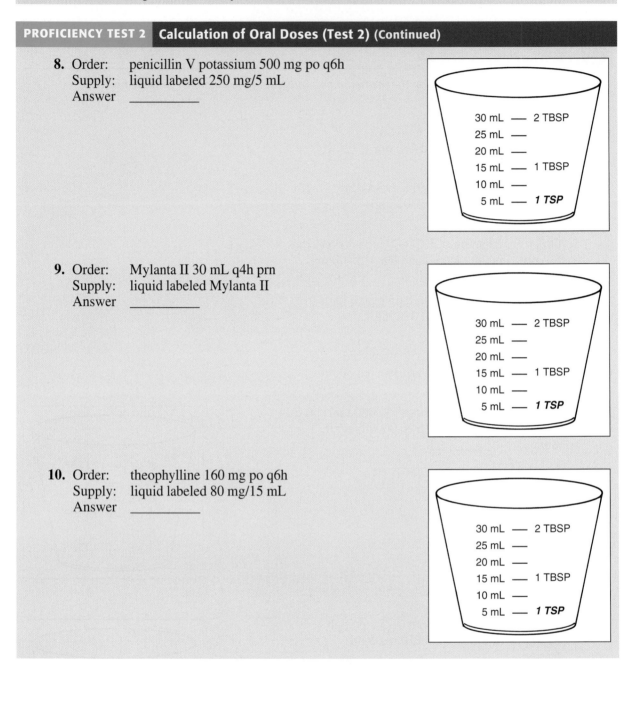

PROFICIENCY TEST 3 | **Calculation of Oral Doses (Test 3)**

Name: _____

Aim for 90% or better on this test. There are 20 questions and each is worth 5 points. Determine the amount to be given. If you have any difficulty, reread Chapter 6, which explains this information. Answers are given on page 404.

1. Order: potassium chloride 20 mEq po in juice bid
   Supply: liquid in a bottle labeled 30 mEq/15 mL

2. Order: syrup of tetracycline hydrochloride 80 mg po q6h
   Supply: liquid in a dropper bottle labeled 125 mg/5 mL

3. Order: propranolol 0.02 g po bid
   Supply: scored tablets labeled 10 mg

4. Order: ampicillin sodium 0.5 g po q6h
   Supply: capsules of 250 mg

5. Order: digoxin 0.5 mg po every day
   Supply: scored tablets of 0.25 mg

6. Order: prednisone 40 mg po every day
   Supply: liquid in a bottle labeled 5 mg/5 mL

7. Order: hydrochlorothiazide 75 mg po every day
   Supply: scored tablets 50 mg

8. Order: furosemide 40 mg po every day
   Supply: scored tablets of 80 mg

9. Order: digoxin 0.125 mg po
   Supply: liquid in a dropper bottle labeled 500 mcg/10 mL

10. Order: Dilantin susp 75 mg po tid
    Supply: liquid in a bottle labeled 50 mg/10 mL

11. Order: diazepam 5 mg po q4h prn
    Supply: scored tablets 2 mg

12. Order: Synthroid 0.15 mg po every day
    Supply: scored tablets 300 mcg

13. Order: Antabuse 375 mg po today
    Supply: scored tablets 250 mg

14. Order: ibuprofen 0.6 g po q4h prn
    Supply: film-coated tablets 300 mg

15. Order: chlorpheniramine maleate syr 1.5 mg po bid
    Supply: liquid in a bottle 1 mg/8 mL

16. Order: diphenhydramine maleate syrup 25 mg po q4h while awake
    Supply: liquid labeled 12.5 mg/5 mL

17. Order: simethicone liq 60 mg po in 1/2 glass H_2O
    Supply: liquid in a dropper bottle labeled 40 mg/0.6 mL

18. Order: chlorothiazide oral susp 0.5 g via NGT po every day
    Supply: liquid labeled 250 mg/5 mL

19. Order: meperidine HCl syrup 15 mg po q4h prn
    Supply: liquid labeled 50 mg/5 mL

20. Order: hydroxyzine susp 50 mg q6h po
    Supply: liquid labeled 25 mg/5 mL

Answers

Self-Test 1 Oral Solids

Formula Method	*Ratio Method*	*Proportion Method*
$\dfrac{D}{H} \times S = A$	$S : H : : x : D$	$\dfrac{S}{H} = \dfrac{x}{D}$

1. No equivalent needed

Formula Method

$$\dfrac{\overset{2}{\cancel{1.50}}\ \cancel{mg}}{\underset{1}{\cancel{0.75}}\ \cancel{mg}} \times 1\ \text{tablet} = 2\ \text{tablets}$$

Ratio Method

1 tablet : 0.75 mg : : x : 1.5 mg

Proportion Method

$$\dfrac{1\ \text{tablet}}{0.75\ \text{mg}} = \dfrac{x}{1.5\ \text{mg}}$$

$$1.5 = 0.75x$$

$$\dfrac{1.5}{0.75} = x$$

$$2\ \text{tablets} = x$$

Learning Aid

$$0.75\ \overline{)\,1.50\,}^{\ 2.}$$
$$\underline{1\ 50}$$
$$0$$

2. No equivalent necessary

Formula Method

$$\dfrac{\overset{1}{\cancel{0.25}}\ \cancel{mg}}{\underset{2}{\cancel{0.50}}\ \cancel{mg}} \times 1\ \text{tablet} = \dfrac{1}{2}\ \text{tablet}$$

Ratio Method

1 tablet : 0.5 mg : : x : 0.25 mg

Proportion Method

$$\dfrac{1\ \text{tablet}}{0.5\ \text{mg}} = \dfrac{x}{0.25\ \text{mg}}$$

$$0.25 = 0.5x$$

$$\dfrac{0.25}{0.5} = x$$

$$0.5\ \text{tablet} = x$$

Learning Aid

$$0.5\ \overline{)\,0.2.5\,}^{\ 0.5} \ \text{or}\ \dfrac{1}{2}$$
$$\underline{2\ 5}$$
$$0$$

3. Equivalent 0.5 g = 500 mg

Formula Method

$$\frac{\overset{2}{\cancel{500}} \text{ mg}}{\underset{1}{\cancel{250}} \text{ mg}} \times 1 \text{ capsule} = 2 \text{ capsules}$$

Ratio Method

1 capsule : 250 mg : : x : 500 mg

Proportion Method

$$\frac{1 \text{ capsule}}{250 \text{ mg}} = \frac{x}{500 \text{ mg}}$$

$$\frac{500}{250} = x$$

2 capsules = x

Learning Aid

$$250\overline{)500.}\ \ ^{2.}$$
$$\underline{500}$$
$$0$$

4. No equivalent necessary

Formula Method

$$\frac{\overset{4}{\cancel{10.0}} \text{ mg}}{\underset{1}{\cancel{2.5}} \text{ mg}} \times 1 \text{ tablet} = 4 \text{ tablets}$$

Ratio Method

1 tablet : 2.5 mg : : x : 10 mg

Proportion Method

$$\frac{1 \text{ tablet}}{2.5 \text{ mg}} = \frac{x}{10}$$

$$10 = 2.5x$$

$$\frac{10}{2.5} = x$$

4 tablets = x

Learning Aid

$$2.5\overline{)10.0}\ \ ^{4.}$$

5. No equivalent necessary

Formula Method

$$\frac{\overset{2}{\cancel{650}} \text{ mg}}{\underset{1}{\cancel{325}} \text{ mg}} \times 1 \text{ tablet} = 2 \text{ tablets}$$

Ratio Method

1 tablet : 325 mg : : x : 650 mg

Proportion Method

$$\frac{1 \text{ tablet}}{325 \text{ mg}} = \frac{x}{650 \text{ mg}}$$

$$650 = 325x$$

$$\frac{650}{325} = x$$

2 tablets = x

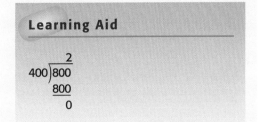

Learning Aid

$$325 \overline{\smash{)}650.} \quad \overset{2.}{}$$
$$\underline{650}$$
$$0$$

6. Equivalent 0.8 g = 800 mg

Formula Method

$$\frac{\overset{2}{\cancel{800}} \text{ mg}}{\underset{1}{\cancel{400}} \text{ mg}} \times 1 \text{ tablet} = 2 \text{ tablets}$$

Ratio Method

1 tablet : 400 mg : : x : 800 mg

Proportion Method

$$\frac{1 \text{ tablet}}{400 \text{ mg}} = \frac{x}{800 \text{ mg}}$$

$$800 = 400x$$

$$\frac{800}{400} = x$$

2 tablets = x

Learning Aid

$$400 \overline{\smash{)}800} \quad \overset{2}{}$$
$$\underline{800}$$
$$0$$

7. Equivalent 0.2 g = 200 mg

Formula Method

$$\frac{\overset{1}{\cancel{200}} \text{ mg}}{\underset{2}{\cancel{400}} \text{ mg}} \times 1 \text{ tablet} = \frac{1}{2} \text{ tablet}$$

Ratio Method

1 tablet : 400 mg : : x : 200 mg

Proportion Method

$$\frac{1 \text{ tablet}}{400 \text{ mg}} = \frac{x}{200 \text{ mg}}$$

$$200 = 400x$$

$$\frac{200}{400} = x$$

$$0.5 \text{ tablet} = x$$

> ### Learning Aid
>
> Move decimal point three places to the right.
>
> 0.200 = 200 mg
>
> Important! Do not invert the numbers in the answer. The answer is
>
> $\frac{1}{2}$ tablet, not 2 tablets.

8. No equivalent necessary

Formula Method

$$\frac{\overset{1}{\cancel{200{,}000}} \text{ units}}{\underset{2}{\cancel{400{,}000}} \text{ units}} \times 1 \text{ tablet} = \frac{1}{2} \text{ tablet}$$

Ratio Method

1 tablet : 400,000 units : : x : 200,000

Proportion Method

$$\frac{1 \text{ tablet}}{400{,}000 \text{ units}} = \frac{x}{200{,}000 \text{ units}}$$

$$200{,}000 = 400{,}000x$$

$$\frac{200{,}000}{400{,}000} = x$$

$$0.5 \text{ tablet} = x$$

> ### Learning Aid
>
>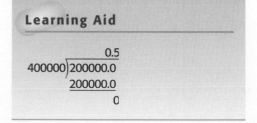

9. No equivalent necessary

Formula Method

$$\frac{\overset{2}{\cancel{0.50}}\ \text{mg}}{\underset{1}{\cancel{0.25}}\ \text{mg}} \times 1\ \text{tablet} = 2\ \text{tablets}$$

Ratio Method

1 tablet : 0.25 mg : : x : 0.5 mg

Proportion Method

$$\frac{1\ \text{tablet}}{0.25\ \text{mg}} = \frac{x}{0.5\ \text{mg}}$$

$$0.5 = 0.25x$$

$$\frac{0.50}{0.25} = x$$

$$2\ \text{tablets} = x$$

Learning Aid

$$0.25\overline{)0.50}\ \ \overset{2.}{}$$
$$\underline{50}$$
$$0$$

10. No equivalent necessary

Formula Method

$$\frac{\overset{1.5}{\cancel{18.75}}\ \text{mg}}{\underset{1}{\cancel{12.5}}\ \text{mg}} \times 1\ \text{tablet} = 1.5\ \text{tablets}$$

Ratio Method

1 tablet : 12.5 mg : : x : 18.75 mg

Proportion Method

$$\frac{1\ \text{tablet}}{12.5\ \text{mg}} = \frac{x}{18.75\ \text{mg}}$$

$$18.75 = 12.5x$$

$$\frac{18.75}{12.5} = x$$

$$1.5\ \text{tablets} = x$$

Learning Aid

$$12.5\overline{)18.75}\ \ \overset{1.5}{}$$
$$\underline{12\ 5}$$
$$6\ 25$$
$$\underline{6\ 25}$$
$$0$$

11. No equivalent needed

Formula Method

$$\frac{\overset{2}{\cancel{600}}\ \cancel{mg}}{\underset{1}{\cancel{300}}\ \cancel{mg}}\times 1 \text{ tablet} = 2 \text{ tablets}$$

Ratio Method

1 tablet : 300 mg : : x : 600 mg

Proportion Method

$$\frac{1 \text{ tablet}}{300 \text{ mg}} = \frac{x}{600 \text{ mg}}$$

$$600 = 300x$$

$$\frac{600}{300} = x$$

$$2 \text{ tablets} = x$$

Learning Aid

$$300\overline{)600}^{\;2}$$
$$\underline{600}$$
$$0$$

12. No equivalent needed.

Formula Method

$$\frac{\overset{3}{\cancel{7.5}}\ \cancel{mg}}{\underset{1}{\cancel{2.5}}\ \cancel{mg}}\times 1 \text{ tablet} = 3 \text{ tablets}$$

Ratio Method

1 tablet : 2.5 mg : : x : 7.5 mg

Proportion Method

$$\frac{1 \text{ tablet}}{2.5 \text{ mg}} = \frac{x}{7.5 \text{ mg}}$$

$$7.5 \text{ mg} = 2.5x$$

$$\frac{7.5}{2.5} = x$$

$$3 \text{ tablets} = x$$

Learning Aid

$$2.5\overline{)7.5}^{\;3}$$
$$\underline{7\ 5}$$

13. No equivalent needed

Formula Method

$$\frac{\overset{0.25}{\cancel{6.25}}\ \text{mg}}{\underset{1}{\cancel{25}}\ \text{mg}} \times 1\ \text{tablet} = 0.25\ \text{tablet}$$
(tablets can be quartered)

Ratio Method

1 tablet : 25 mg : : x : 6.25 mg

Proportion Method

$$\frac{1\ \text{tablet}}{25\ \text{mg}} = \frac{x}{6.25\ \text{mg}}$$

$$6.25\ \text{mg} = 25x$$

$$\frac{6.25}{25} = x$$

0.25 tablets or ¼ tablet

Learning Aid

$$25\overline{)6.25}$$ = 0.25
50
125
125
0

14. Equivalent: 0.2 mg = 200 mcg

Formula Method

$$\frac{\overset{2}{\cancel{400}}\ \text{mcg}}{\underset{1}{\cancel{200}}\ \text{mcg}} \times 1\ \text{tablet} = 2\ \text{tablets}$$

Ratio Method

1 tablet : 200 mcg : : x : 400 mcg

Proportion Method

$$\frac{1\ \text{tablet}}{200\ \text{mcg}} = \frac{x}{400\ \text{mcg}}$$

$$400 = 200x$$

$$\frac{400}{200} = x$$

2 tablets = x

Learning Aid

$$200\overline{)400}$$ = 2
400
0

15. No equivalent needed

Formula Method

$$\frac{\overset{1.5}{\cancel{7.5}} \text{ mg}}{\cancel{5} \text{ mg}} \times 1 \text{ tablet} = 1.5 \text{ tablets}$$

Ratio Method

1 tablet : 5 mg : : x : 7.5 mg

Proportion Method

$$\frac{1 \text{ tablet}}{5 \text{ mg}} = \frac{x}{7.5 \text{ mg}}$$

$$7.5 \text{ mg} = 5x$$

$$\frac{7.5}{5} = x$$

1.5 or 1½ tablets

Learning Aid

$$5\overline{)7.5} \;\; {}^{1.5}$$

```
      1.5
  5 ) 7.5
      5
      2 5
      2 5
        0
```

---

16. No equivalent needed

Formula Method

$$\frac{\overset{0.5}{\cancel{0.625}} \text{ mg}}{\cancel{1.25} \text{ mg}} \times 1 \text{ tablet} = 0.5 \text{ tablet}$$

Ratio Method

1 tablet : 1.25 mg : : x : 0.625 mg

Proportion Method

$$\frac{1 \text{ tablet}}{1.25 \text{ mg}} = \frac{x}{0.625 \text{ mg}}$$

$$0.625 = 1.25x$$

$$\frac{0.625}{1.25} = x$$

0.5 or ½ tablet = x

Learning Aid

```
          0.5
  1.25 ) 0.625
          625
            0
```

17. Equivalent: 0.5 g = 500 mg

Formula Method

$$\frac{\overset{2}{\cancel{500}} \text{ mg}}{\underset{1}{\cancel{250}} \text{ mg}} \times 1 \text{ tablet} = 2 \text{ tablets}$$

Ratio Method

1 tablet : 250 mg : : x : 500 mg

Proportion Method

$$\frac{1 \text{ tablet}}{250 \text{ mg}} = \frac{x}{500 \text{ mg}}$$

$$500 = 250x$$

$$\frac{500}{250} = x$$

2 tablets

> **Learning Aid**
>
> $$250\overline{)500} \quad \begin{array}{r} 2 \\ \underline{500} \\ 0 \end{array}$$

18. No equivalent needed

Formula Method

$$\frac{\overset{1.5}{\cancel{37.5}} \text{ mg}}{\underset{1}{\cancel{25}} \text{ mg}} \times 1 \text{ tablet} = 1.5 \text{ tablets}$$

Ratio Method

1 tablet : 25 mg : : x : 37.5 mg

Proportion Method

$$\frac{1 \text{ tablet}}{25 \text{ mg}} = \frac{x}{37.5 \text{ mg}}$$

$$37.5 = 25x$$

$$\frac{37.5}{25} = x$$

1.5 tablets or 1½ tablets

> **Learning Aid**
>
> $$25\overline{)37.5} \quad \begin{array}{r} 1.5 \\ \underline{25} \\ 125 \\ \underline{125} \\ 0 \end{array}$$

19. Equivalent: 1 g = 1000 mg

Formula Method

$$\frac{\overset{2}{\cancel{1000}}\text{ mg}}{\underset{1}{\cancel{500}}\text{ mg}}\times1 \text{ capsule} = 2 \text{ capsules}$$

Ratio Method

1 capsule : 500 mg : : x : 1000 mg

Proportion Method

$$\frac{1 \text{ capsule}}{500 \text{ mg}}=\frac{x}{1000 \text{ mg}}$$

$$1000 = 500x$$

$$\frac{1000}{500}=x$$

2 capsules

Learning Aid

$$\begin{array}{r} 2 \\ 500\overline{)1000} \\ \underline{1000} \\ 0 \end{array}$$

20. No equivalent needed

Formula Method

$$\frac{\overset{2.5}{\cancel{25}}\text{ mg}}{\underset{1}{\cancel{10}}\text{ mg}}\times1 \text{ tablet} = 2.5 \text{ tablets}$$

Ratio Method

1 tablet : 10 mg : : x : 25 mg

Proportion Method

$$\frac{1 \text{ tablet}}{10 \text{ mg}}=\frac{x}{25 \text{ mg}}$$

$$25 = 10x$$

$$\frac{25}{10}=x$$

2.5 tablets or 2½ tablets

Learning Aid

$$\begin{array}{r} 2.5 \\ 10\overline{)25.0} \\ \underline{20} \\ 50 \\ \underline{50} \\ 0 \end{array}$$

Self-Test 2 Oral Liquids

Formula Method

$$\frac{D}{H} \times S = A$$

Ratio Method

$$S : H : : x : D$$

Proportion Method

$$\frac{S}{H} = \frac{x}{D}$$

1. Equivalent 0.75 g = 750 mg

Formula Method

$$\frac{\overset{3}{750\ mg}}{\underset{1}{250\ mg}} \times 1\ mL = 3\ mL$$

Ratio Method

1 mL : 250 mg : : x : 750 mg

Proportion Method

$$\frac{1\ mL}{250\ mg} = \frac{x}{750\ mg}$$

$$750 = 250x$$

$$\frac{750}{250} = x$$

$$3\ mL = x$$

2. No equivalent necessary

Formula Method

$$\frac{\overset{2}{500\ mg}}{\underset{1}{250\ mg}} \times 5\ mL = 10\ mL$$

Ratio Method

5 mL : 250 mg : : x : 500 mg

Proportion Method

$$\frac{5\ mL}{250\ mg} = \frac{x}{500\ mg}$$

$$2500 = 250x$$

$$\frac{2500}{250} = x$$

$$10\ mL = x$$

3. Equivalent 0.35 g = 350 mg

Formula Method	*Ratio Method*	*Proportion Method*

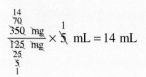

5 mL : 125 mg : : x : 350 mg

$$\frac{5 \text{ mL}}{125 \text{ mg}} = \frac{x}{350 \text{ mg}}$$

$$1750 = 125x$$

$$\frac{1750}{125} = x$$

$$14 \text{ mL} = x$$

> **Learning Aid**
>
> Alternate arithmetic
>
> $350 \times 5 = 1750$
>
> ```
>        14.
> 125)1750.
>     125
>     ---
>     500
>     500
>     ---
>       0
> ```

4. No equivalent necessary

Formula Method	*Ratio Method*	*Proportion Method*

$$\frac{\overset{3}{\cancel{150}} \text{ mg}}{\underset{2}{\cancel{100}} \text{ mg}} \times 1 \text{ mL} = \frac{3}{2} = 1.5 \text{ mL}$$

1 mL : 100 mg : : x : 150 mg

$$\frac{1 \text{ mL}}{100 \text{ mg}} = \frac{x}{150 \text{ mg}}$$

$$150 = 100x$$

$$\frac{150}{100} = x$$

$$1.5 \text{ mL} = x$$

> **Learning Aid**
>
> Alternate arithmetic
>
> ```
>         1.5
> 100)150.0
>     100
>     ---
>     500
>     500
>     ---
>       0
> ```

5. Equivalent: 0.5 g = 500 mg

Formula Method

$$\frac{300 \text{ mg}}{500 \text{ mg}} \times 5 \text{ mL} = \frac{3 \times 5}{5} = 3 \text{ mL}$$

Ratio Method

5 mL : 500 mg : : x : 300 mg

Proportion Method

$$\frac{5 \text{ mL}}{500 \text{ mg}} = \frac{x}{300 \text{ mg}}$$

$$1500 = 500x$$

$$\frac{1500}{500} = x$$

$$3 \text{ mL} = x$$

Learning Aid

$300 \times 5 = 1500$

$$\begin{array}{r} 3 \\ 500{\overline{\smash{\big)}\,1500}} \\ \underline{1500} \\ 0 \end{array}$$

6. No equivalent necessary

Formula Method

$$\frac{0.02 \text{ mg}}{0.05 \text{ mg}} \times 1 \text{ mL} = \frac{2}{5} = 0.4 \text{ mL}$$

Ratio Method

1 mL : 0.05 mg : : x : 0.02 mg

Proportion Method

$$\frac{1 \text{ mL}}{0.05 \text{ mg}} = \frac{x}{0.02 \text{ mg}}$$

$$0.02 = 0.05x$$

$$\frac{0.02}{0.05} = x$$

$$0.4 \text{ mL} = x$$

Learning Aid

$$\begin{array}{r} 0.4 \\ 0.05{\overline{\smash{\big)}\,0.020}} \\ \underline{20} \\ 0 \end{array}$$

7. No equivalent necessary

Formula Method

$$\frac{30 \ \cancel{mEq}}{20 \ \cancel{mEq}} \times 15 \ \text{mL} = \frac{3 \times 15}{2} = \frac{45}{2} = 22.5 \ \text{mL}$$

Ratio Method

15 mL : 20 mEq :: x : 30 mEq

Proportion Method

$$\frac{15 \ \text{mL}}{20 \ \text{mEq}} = \frac{x}{30 \ \text{mEq}}$$

$$15 \times 30 = 20x$$

$$\frac{450}{20} = x$$

$$22.5 \ \text{mL} = x$$

Learning Aid

$15 \times 30 = 450$

$$\begin{array}{r} 22.5 \\ \frac{45}{2} \overline{\smash)45.0} \\ \underline{4} \\ 5 \\ \underline{4} \\ 10 \end{array} \quad \text{or} \quad \begin{array}{r} 22.5 \\ \frac{450}{20} \overline{\smash)450.0} \\ \underline{40} \\ 50 \\ \underline{40} \\ 100 \end{array}$$

8. No equivalent necessary

Formula Method

$$\frac{0.25 \ \cancel{mg}}{0.25 \ \cancel{mg}} \times 1 \ \text{mL} = 1 \ \text{mL}$$

Ratio Method

1 mL : 0.25 mg :: x : 0.25 mg

Proportion Method

$$\frac{1 \ \text{mL}}{0.25 \ \text{mg}} = \frac{x}{0.25 \ \text{mg}}$$

$$0.25 = 0.25x$$

$$\frac{0.25}{0.25} = x$$

$$1 \ \text{mL} = x$$

9. No equivalent necessary

Formula Method

$$\frac{\overset{3}{\cancel{30}}\ \cancel{mg}}{\underset{1}{\cancel{10}}\ \cancel{mg}} \times 5\ mL = 15\ mL$$

Ratio Method

$$5\ mL : 10\ mg : : x : 30\ mg$$

Proportion Method

$$\frac{5\ mL}{10\ mg} = \frac{x}{30\ mg}$$

$$150 = 10x$$

$$\frac{150}{10} = x$$

$$15\ mL = x$$

Learning Aid

Alternate arithmetic

$30 \times 5 = 150$

```
       15.
  10)150.
     10
      50
      50
```

10. No equivalent necessary

Formula Method

$$\frac{\overset{10}{\cancel{12.5}}\ \cancel{mg}}{\underset{\underset{1}{1.25}}{\cancel{6.25}}\ \cancel{mg}} \times \overset{1}{\cancel{5}}\ mL = 10\ mL$$

Ratio Method

$$5\ mL : 6.25\ mg : : x : 12.5\ mg$$

Proportion Method

$$\frac{5\ mL}{6.25\ mg} = \frac{x}{12.5\ mg}$$

$$62.5 = 6.25x$$

$$\frac{62.5}{6.25} = x$$

$$10\ mL = x$$

Learning Aid

Alternate arithmetic

$12.5 \times 5 = 62.5$

```
          10.
  6.25)62.50
       62 5
          0
```

11. No equivalent necessary

Formula Method	*Ratio Method*	*Proportion Method*

$$\frac{\overset{5}{\cancel{50}} \text{ mg}}{\underset{1}{\cancel{10}} \text{ mg}} \times 5 \text{ mL} = 25 \text{ mL}$$

5 mL : 10 mg : : x : 50 mg

$$\frac{5 \text{ mL}}{10 \text{ mg}} = \frac{x}{50 \text{ mg}}$$

$$5 \times 50 = 10x$$

$$\frac{250}{10} = x$$

$$25 \text{ mL} = x$$

Learning Aid

$$5 \times 50 = 250$$

$$\begin{array}{r} 25 \\ 10\overline{)250} \\ \underline{20} \\ 50 \\ \underline{50} \\ 0 \end{array}$$

12. No equivalent necessary

Formula Method	*Ratio Method*	*Proportion Method*

$$\frac{\overset{4}{\cancel{40}} \text{ mg}}{\underset{1}{\cancel{10}} \text{ mg}} \times 1 \text{ mL} = 4 \text{ mL}$$

1 mL : 10 mg : : x : 40 mg

$$\frac{1 \text{ mL}}{10 \text{ mg}} = \frac{x}{40 \text{ mg}}$$

$$40 = 10x$$

$$\frac{40}{10} = x$$

$$4 \text{ mL} = x$$

Learning Aid

$$\begin{array}{r} 4 \\ 10\overline{)40} \\ \underline{40} \\ 0 \end{array}$$

13. No equivalent necessary

Formula Method

$$\frac{\overset{1}{\cancel{10}} \text{ mEq}}{\underset{2}{\cancel{20}} \text{ mEq}} \times 30 \text{ mL} = \frac{30}{2} = 15 \text{ mL}$$

Ratio Method

30 mL : 20 mEq : : x : 10 mEq

Proportion Method

$$\frac{30 \text{ mL}}{20 \text{ mEq}} = \frac{\text{x}}{10 \text{ mEq}}$$

$$30 \times 10 = 20x$$

$$\frac{300}{20} = x$$

$$15 \text{ mL} = x$$

Learning Aid

$30 \times 10 = 300$

$$20\overline{)300} \quad \begin{array}{r} 15 \\ \hline 20 \\ \hline 100 \\ 100 \\ \hline 0 \end{array}$$

14. No equivalent necessary

Formula Method

$$\frac{\overset{2}{\cancel{10}} \text{ mg}}{\underset{1}{\cancel{5}} \text{ mg}} \times 5 \text{ mL} = 10 \text{ mL}$$

Ratio Method

5 mL : 5 mg : : x : 10 mg

Proportion Method

$$\frac{5 \text{ mL}}{5 \text{ mg}} = \frac{\text{x}}{10 \text{ mg}}$$

$$10 \times 5 = 5x$$

$$\frac{50}{5} = x$$

$$10 \text{ mL} = x$$

Learning Aid

$10 \times 5 = 50$

$$5\overline{)50} \quad \begin{array}{r} 10 \\ \hline 5 \\ \hline 0 \end{array}$$

15. No equivalent necessary

Formula Method

$$\frac{\overset{5}{\cancel{100 \text{ mg}}}}{\underset{1}{\cancel{20 \text{ mg}}}} \times 5 \text{ mL} = 25 \text{ mL}$$

Ratio Method

5 mL : 20 mg : : x : 100 mg

Proportion Method

$$\frac{5 \text{ mL}}{20 \text{ mg}} = \frac{x}{100 \text{ mg}}$$

$$5 \times 100 = 20x$$

$$\frac{500}{20} = x$$

$$25 \text{ mL} = x$$

Learning Aid

$5 \times 100 = 500$

$$\begin{array}{r} 25 \\ 20\overline{)500} \\ \underline{40} \\ 100 \\ \underline{100} \end{array}$$

16. Equivalent: gr 10 = 650 mg

Formula Method

$$\frac{650 \text{ mg}}{160 \text{ mg}} \times 5 \text{ mL} = \frac{3250}{160} = 20.31 \text{ or } 20 \text{ mL}$$

Ratio Method

5 mL : 160 mg : : x : 650 mg

Proportion Method

$$\frac{5 \text{ mL}}{160 \text{ mg}} = \frac{x}{650 \text{ mg}}$$

$$650 \times 5 = 160x$$

$$\frac{3250}{160} = x$$

$$20.31 \text{ or } 20 \text{ mL}$$

Learning Aid

$650 \times 5 = 3250$

$$\begin{array}{r} 20.31 \\ 160\overline{)3250} \\ \underline{320} \\ 500 \\ \underline{480} \\ 200 \end{array}$$

17. No equivalent needed

Formula Method

$$\frac{\overset{2}{\cancel{25}} \text{ mg}}{\underset{1}{\cancel{12.5}} \text{ mg}} \times 5 \text{ mL} = 10 \text{ mL}$$

Ratio Method

$$5 \text{ mL} : 12.5 \text{ mg} :: x : 25 \text{ mg}$$

Proportion Method

$$\frac{5 \text{ mL}}{12.5 \text{ mg}} = \frac{x}{25 \text{ mg}}$$

$$5 \times 25 = 12.5x$$

$$\frac{125}{12.5} = x$$

$$10 \text{ mL} = x$$

Learning Aid

$$25 \times 5 = 125$$

$$12.5 \overline{)125.0} \begin{array}{r} 10 \\ \hline \end{array}$$
$$\underline{125}$$

18. No equivalent needed

Formula Method

$$\frac{\overset{5}{\cancel{50}} \text{ mg}}{\underset{1}{\cancel{10}} \text{ mg}} \times 5 \text{ mL} = 25 \text{ mL}$$

Ratio Method

$$5 \text{ mL} : 10 \text{ mg} :: x : 50 \text{ mg}$$

Proportion Method

$$\frac{5 \text{ mL}}{10 \text{ mg}} = \frac{x}{50 \text{ mg}}$$

$$5 \times 50 = 10x$$

$$\frac{250}{10} = x$$

$$25 \text{ mL} = x$$

Learning Aid

$$50 \times 5 = 250$$

$$10 \overline{)250} \begin{array}{r} 25 \\ \hline \end{array}$$
$$\underline{20}$$
$$50$$
$$\underline{50}$$
$$0$$

19. No equivalent needed

Formula Method

$$\frac{\overset{2}{\cancel{100}} \text{ mg}}{\underset{1}{\cancel{50}} \text{ mg}} \times 15 \text{ mL} = 30 \text{ mL}$$

Ratio Method

15 mL : 50 mg : : x : 100 mg

Proportion Method

$$\frac{15 \text{ mL}}{50 \text{ mg}} = \frac{\text{x}}{100 \text{ mg}}$$

$$15 \times 100 = 50x$$

$$\frac{1500}{50} = x$$

$$30 \text{ mL} = x$$

Learning Aid

$15 \times 100 = 1500$

$$\begin{array}{r} 30 \\ 50\overline{)1500} \\ \underline{150} \\ 0 \end{array}$$

20. Equivalent: 0.06 g = 60 mg

Formula Method

$$\frac{\overset{4}{\cancel{60}} \text{ mg}}{\underset{1}{\cancel{15}} \text{ mg}} \times 5 \text{ mL} = 20 \text{ mL}$$

Ratio Method

5 mL : 15 mg : : x : 60 mg

Proportion Method

$$\frac{5 \text{ mL}}{15 \text{ mg}} = \frac{\text{x}}{60 \text{ mg}}$$

$$5 \times 60 = 15x$$

$$\frac{300}{15} = x$$

$$20 \text{ mL} = x$$

Learning Aid

$60 \times 5 = 300$

$$\begin{array}{r} 20 \\ 15\overline{)300} \\ \underline{30} \\ 00 \end{array}$$

Self-Test 3 Mental Drill Oral Solids

1. 2 tablets	**5.** 2 tablets	**9.** ½ tablet	**13.** ½ tablet
2. ½ tablet	**6.** ½ tablet	**10.** 2 tablets	**14.** 2 tablets
3. 2 tablets	**7.** 1 tablet	**11.** 2 tablets	
4. 2 tablets	**8.** 1 tablet	**12.** 1 tablet	

Self-Test 4 Mental Drill Oral Liquids

1. 10 mL	**3.** 10 mL	**5.** 15 mL	**7.** 15 mL	**9.** 6 mL
2. 25 mL	**4.** 5 mL	**6.** 20 mL	**8.** 5 mL	**10.** 2.5 mL

Liquids for Injection

Liquid drugs for injection are prepared by pharmaceutical companies as sterile solutions, powders, or suspensions. Sterile techniques are used to prepare and administer them. As with oral medications, the nurse may be required to calculate the correct dosage.

RULE   **CALCULATING LIQUID INJECTIONS**

The rule used to solve liquid injection problems is the same as that for oral solids and liquids. ■

Formula Method

$$\frac{\text{Desire}}{\text{Have}} \times \text{Supply} = \text{Amount}$$

Ratio Method

$$\text{Supply} : \text{Have} :: \text{x} : \text{Desire}$$

Proportion Method

$$\frac{\text{Supply}}{\text{Have}} = \frac{\text{x}}{\text{Desire}}$$

Example   Order: Stelazine 1.5 mg IM q6h prn

Supply: Read the label

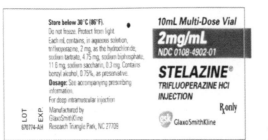

Courtesy of GlaxoSmithKline.

Desire is the order: 1.5 mg

Have is the strength of the drug supplied: 2 mg

Supply is the unit form of the drug: 1 mL

Amount or *Answer* is how much liquid to give by injection in mL. "x" is used in the ratio and proportion methods.

Formula Method	*Ratio Method*	*Proportion Method*

$$\frac{1.5 \text{ mg}}{2 \text{ mg}} \times 1 \text{ mL} = A$$

$$0.75 \text{ mL} = A$$

$$1 \text{ mL} : 2 \text{ mg} :: x : 1.5 \text{ mg}$$

$$\frac{1 \text{ mL}}{2 \text{ mg}} \times \frac{x}{1.5 \text{ mg}}$$

$$2x = 1.5$$

$$x = \frac{1.5}{2}$$

$$x = 0.75 \text{ mL}$$

Calculating Injection Problems

3-mL Syringe

The degree of accuracy in calculating injection answers depends on the syringe used. Figure 7-1 shows a 3-mL syringe marked in milliliters to the nearest tenth and in minims to the nearest whole number. *To calculate milliliter answers for this 3-mL syringe, the arithmetic is carried out to the hundredth place and the answer is rounded off to the nearest tenth.*

   1.25 mL becomes 1.3 mL

1-mL Precision Syringe

Figure 7-2 shows a 1-mL precision syringe marked in milliliters to the nearest hundredth and in minims to the nearest half-minim. *To calculate milliliters when the 1-mL syringe is used, the arithmetic is carried out to the thousandth place and the answer is rounded off to the nearest hundredth.*

   0.978 mL becomes 0.98 mL

> **Learning Aid**
>
> Rules for rounding off numbers can be reviewed in Chapter 1.

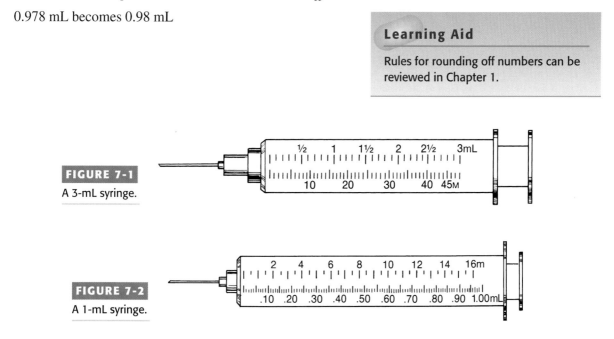

FIGURE 7-1
A 3-mL syringe.

FIGURE 7-2
A 1-mL syringe.

A syringe is provided for each of the examples that follow. Calculate milliliters to the degree of accuracy required by the syringe markings. *Calculation of minims is not provided because this is an apothecary measure.* Draw a line on the syringe indicating the answer for milliliters only. Minim (M or m) markings are still found on many syringes.

Example Order: Demerol HCl 75 mg IM q4h prn

Supply: Read the label.

ab 1 mL   NDC 0074-1179-31
                      LD-83

10 Carpuject®
sterile cartridge units
with Luer Lock

C II

DETECTO-SEAL® PAK Tamper Detection Package

Demerol®
meperidine
hydrochloride
injection, USP

Warning: May be habit forming.

50 mg/mL

Courtesy of Abbott Laboratories.

Formula Method

$$\frac{D}{H} \times S = A$$

$$\frac{\overset{3}{\cancel{75}} \text{ mg}}{\underset{2}{\cancel{50}} \text{ mg}} \times 1 \text{ mL} = \frac{3}{2} = 1.5 \text{ mL}$$

Ratio Method

$$1 \text{ mL} : 50 \text{ mg} :: x : 75 \text{ mg}$$

Proportion Method

$$\frac{1 \text{ mL}}{50 \text{ mg}} = \frac{x}{75 \text{ mg}}$$

$$\frac{75}{50} = x$$

$$1.5 \text{ mL} = x$$

Give 1.5 mL IM.

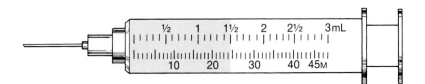

Example   Order: heparin sodium 1500 units subcutaneous bid
Supply: Read the label.

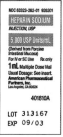

NDC 63323-262-01 926201
HEPARIN SODIUM
INJECTION, USP
5,000 USP Units/mL
(Derived from Porcine
Intestinal Mucosa)
For IV or SC Use   Rx only
1 mL Multiple Dose Vial
Usual Dosage: See insert.
**American Pharmaceutical
Partners, Inc.**
Los Angeles, CA 90024

401810A

LOT 313167
EXP 09/03

Formula Method

$$\frac{D}{H} \times S = A$$

$$\frac{\overset{3}{1500} \text{ units}}{\underset{5000}{10} \text{ units}} \times 1 \text{ mL} = \frac{3}{10} = 0.3 \text{ mL}$$

Give 0.3 mL.

Ratio Method

1 mL : 5000 units : : x : 1500 units

Proportion Method

$$\frac{1 \text{ mL}}{5000 \text{ units}} \times \frac{\text{x}}{1500 \text{ units}}$$

$$\frac{1500}{5000} = \text{x}$$

$$0.3 \text{ mL} = \text{x}$$

Learning Aid

$$\begin{array}{r} 3 0.3 \\ \hline 10\,)\overline{3.0} \end{array}$$

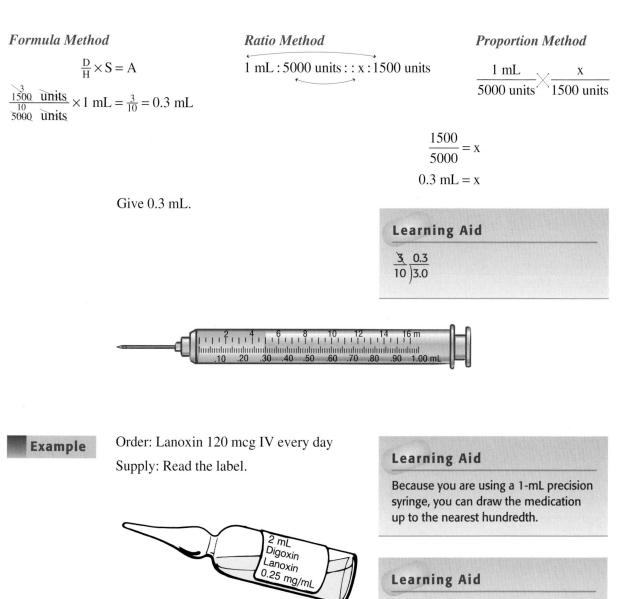

Example   Order: Lanoxin 120 mcg IV every day
Supply: Read the label.

2 mL
Digoxin
Lanoxin
0.25 mg/mL

Learning Aid

Because you are using a 1-mL precision syringe, you can draw the medication up to the nearest hundredth.

Learning Aid

0.25 mg = 250 mcg

Formula Method

$$\frac{D}{H} \times S = A$$

$$\frac{120 \text{ mcg}}{250 \text{ mcg}} \times 1 \text{ mL} = \frac{12}{25} \quad 25 \overline{\smash{)}12.00} \begin{array}{r} 0.48 \\ \underline{100} \\ 200 \\ \underline{200} \end{array}$$

Ratio Method

1 mL : 250 mcg : : x : 120 mcg

Proportion Method

$$\frac{1 \text{ mL}}{250 \text{ mcg}} \times \frac{x}{120 \text{ mcg}}$$

$$\frac{120}{250} = x$$

$$0.48 \text{ mL} = x$$

Give 0.48 mL IV.

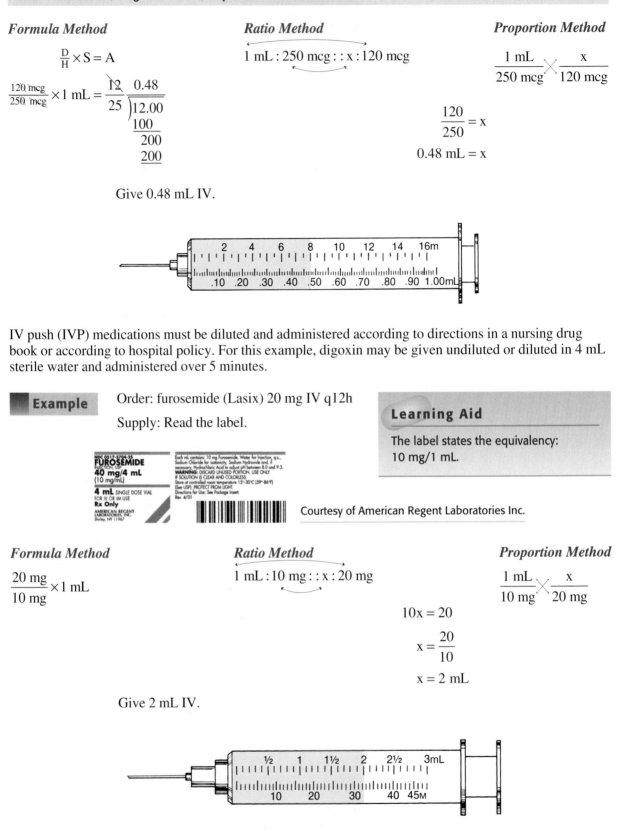

IV push (IVP) medications must be diluted and administered according to directions in a nursing drug book or according to hospital policy. For this example, digoxin may be given undiluted or diluted in 4 mL sterile water and administered over 5 minutes.

Example   Order: furosemide (Lasix) 20 mg IV q12h

Supply: Read the label.

Learning Aid

The label states the equivalency:
10 mg/1 mL.

NDC 0517-5704-25
FUROSEMIDE
INJECTION, USP
40 mg/4 mL
(10 mg/mL)
4 mL SINGLE DOSE VIAL
FOR IV OR IM USE
Rx Only
AMERICAN REGENT
LABORATORIES, INC.
Shirley, NY 11967

Each mL contains: 10 mg Furosemide, Water for Injection, q.s., Sodium Chloride for isotonicity, Sodium Hydroxide and, if necessary, Hydrochloric Acid to adjust pH between 8.0 and 9.3.
WARNING: DISCARD UNUSED PORTION. USE ONLY IF SOLUTION IS CLEAR AND COLORLESS.
Store at controlled room temperature 15°–30°C (59°–86°F) (See USP). PROTECT FROM LIGHT.
Directions for Use: See Package Insert.
Rev. 4/01

Courtesy of American Regent Laboratories Inc.

Formula Method

$$\frac{20 \text{ mg}}{10 \text{ mg}} \times 1 \text{ mL}$$

Ratio Method

1 mL : 10 mg : : x : 20 mg

Proportion Method

$$\frac{1 \text{ mL}}{10 \text{ mg}} \times \frac{x}{20 \text{ mg}}$$

$$10x = 20$$

$$x = \frac{20}{10}$$

$$x = 2 \text{ mL}$$

Give 2 mL IV.

Lasix IVP is given undiluted at a rate of 20 mg over 1 minute.

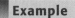 **Example**

Order: promethazine (Phenergan) 12.5 mg IV q4–6h prn

Supply: Read the label.

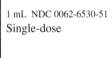

1 mL NDC 0062-6530-51
Single-dose

**Promethazine
Hydrochloride
Injection USP**

25 mg
(25 mg/mL)

FOR IV/IM USE

**Protect from Light
Prescription only**

Formula Method

$$\frac{12.5 \text{ mg}}{25 \text{ mg}} \times 1 \text{ mL} = A$$

$$0.5 \text{ mL} = A$$

Ratio Method

1 mL : 25 mg : : x : 12.5 mg

Proportion Method

$$\frac{1 \text{ mL}}{25 \text{ mg}} \times \frac{x}{12.5 \text{ mg}}$$

$$25x = 12.5 \text{ mg}$$

$$x = \frac{12.5}{25}$$

$$x = 0.5 \text{ mL}$$

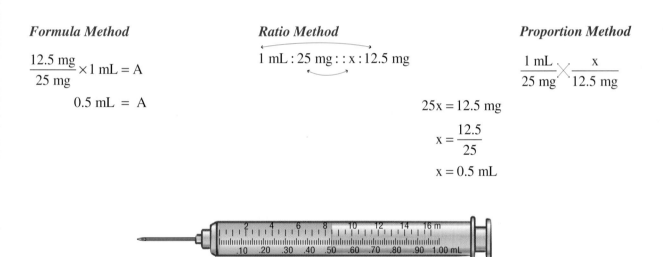

Promethazine IVP is given undiluted if less than 25 mg. Give each 25 mg over 1 minute.

SELF-TEST 1 | Calculation of Liquids for Injection

Practice calculations of injections from a liquid. Report your answer in milliliters; mark the syringe in milliliters. Answers are given at the end of the chapter.

1. Order: Cleocin 0.3 g IM q6h
      Supply: liquid in a vial labeled 300 mg/2 mL

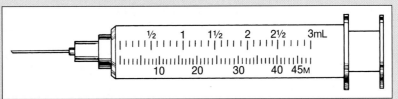

2. Order: morphine SO$_4$ 12 mg IV stat
      Supply: vial of liquid labeled 15 mg/mL

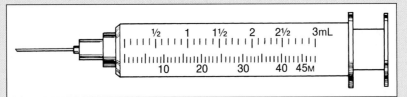

3. Order: vitamin B$_{12}$ 1 mg IM every day
      Supply: vial of liquid labeled 1000 mcg/mL

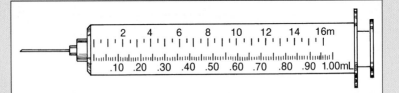

4. Order: gentamicin 9 mg IM q8h
      Supply: pediatric ampule labeled 20 mg/2 mL

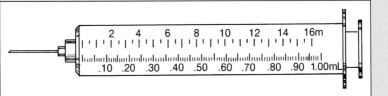

5. Order: digoxin 0.5 mg IV q6h × 3 doses
      Supply: vial labeled 0.25 mg/mL

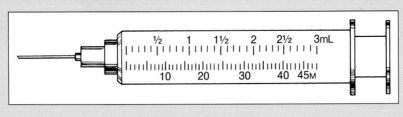

(continued)

6. Order: gentamicin 50 mg IM q8h
Supply: vial labeled 40 mg/mL

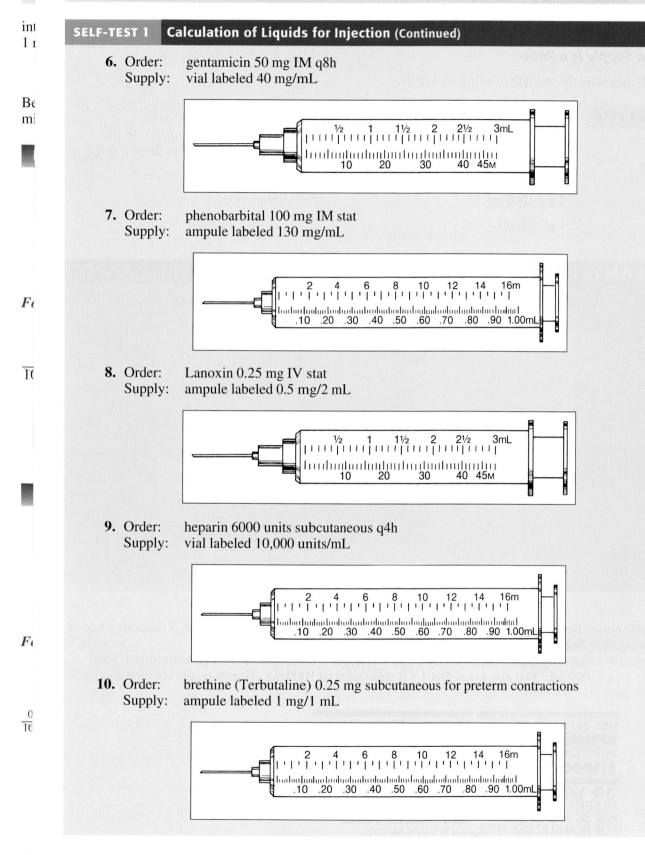

7. Order: phenobarbital 100 mg IM stat
Supply: ampule labeled 130 mg/mL

8. Order: Lanoxin 0.25 mg IV stat
Supply: ampule labeled 0.5 mg/2 mL

9. Order: heparin 6000 units subcutaneous q4h
Supply: vial labeled 10,000 units/mL

10. Order: brethine (Terbutaline) 0.25 mg subcutaneous for preterm contractions
Supply: ampule labeled 1 mg/1 mL

6. Order: scopolamine 0.5 mg subcutaneous stat
   Supply: vial labeled 0.4 mg/mL

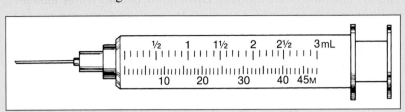

7. Order: NPH insulin 10 units and Humulin insulin 3 units subcutaneous every day 7 AM
   Supply: vials of NPH insulin U 100 and Humulin insulin U 100

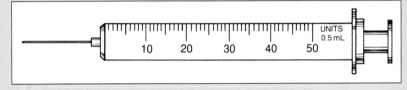

8. Order: add sodium bicarbonate 1.2 mEq to IV stat
   Supply: vial labeled infant 4.2% sodium bicarbonate 5 mEq (0.5 mEq/mL)

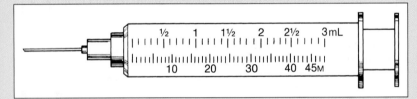

9. Order: dromostanolone proprionate 75 mg IM tiw
   Supply: vial labeled 50 mg/mL

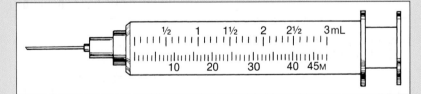

10. Order: adrenalin 500 mcg subcutaneous stat
   Supply: ampule of liquid labeled 1:1000

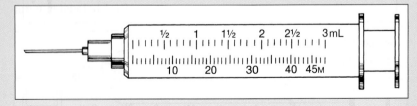

PROFICIENCY TEST 3 | **Calculations of Liquid Injections (Test 3)**

Name: _____

Aim for 90% or better on this test. There are 20 questions and each is worth 5 points. If you have any difficulty, reread and study Chapter 7, which explains this information. Assume you have only a 3-mL syringe. Answers are given on page 419.

1. Order: Lanoxin 0.25 mg IM every day
      Supply: ampule labeled 0.5 mg/2 mL

2. Order: diphenhydramine hydrochloride 40 mg IM stat
      Supply: ampule labeled 50 mg (2-mL size)

3. Order: morphine sulfate 8 mg IV q4h prn
      Supply: vial labeled 15 mg/mL

4. Order: Demerol hydrochloride 25 mg IM q4h prn
      Supply: vial labeled 100 mg/mL

5. Order: ascorbic acid 200 mg IM every day
      Supply: ampule labeled 500 mg/2 mL

6. Order: vitamin B_{12} 1500 mcg every day IM
      Supply: vial labeled 5000 mcg/mL

7. Order: atropine sulfate 0.6 mg IV at 7:30 AM
      Supply: vial labeled 0.4 mg/mL

8. Order: sodium amytal 0.1 g IM stat
      Supply: ampule 200 mg/3 mL

9. Order: hydromorphone HCl 1.5 mg IM q4h prn
      Supply: vial labeled 2 mg/mL

10. Order: penicillin G procaine 600,000 units IM q12h
      Supply: vial labeled 500,000 USP units/mL

11. Order: add nitroglycerin 200 mcg to IV stat
      Supply: vial labeled 0.8 mg/mL

12. Order: neostigmine methylsulfate 500 mcg subcutaneous
      Supply: ampule labeled 1:4000

13. Order: levorphanol tartrate 3 mg subcutaneous
      Supply: vial labeled 2 mg/mL

14. Order: epinephrine 0.4 mg subcutaneous stat
      Supply: ampule labeled 1:1000 (2-mL size)

15. Order: magnesium sulfate 500 mg IM
      Supply: ampule labeled 50% (2-mL size)

(continued)

PROFICIENCY TEST 3   **Calculations of Liquid Injections (Test 3) (Continued)**

16. Order: oxymorphone HCl 0.75 mg subcutaneous
   Supply: vial labeled 1.5 mg/mL

17. Order: add lidocaine 100 mg to IV stat
   Supply: ampule labeled 20%

18. Order: Lanoxin 0.125 mg IV 10 AM
   Supply: ampule labeled 0.25 mg/2 mL

19. Order: nalbuphine HCl 12 mg IM
   Supply: vial 10 mg/mL

20. Order: add 10 mEq KCl to IV
   Supply: vial 40 mEq/20 mL

PROFICIENCY TEST 4	Mental Drill in Liquids-for-Injection Problems

Name: _____

As you develop proficiency in solving problems, you will be able to calculate many answers without written work. This drill combines your knowledge of equivalents and dosages. Solve these problems mentally and write only the amount to give. Keep the rule in mind as you solve each problem. Answers are given on page 427.

Order	Supply	Give
1. 0.5 g IM	250 mg/mL	_____
2. 10 mEq IV	40 mEq/20 mL	_____
3. 0.5 mg IM	0.25 mg/mL	_____
4. 100 mg IM	0.2 g/2 mL	_____
5. 50 mg IM	100 mg = 1 mL	_____
6. 0.25 mg IM	0.5 mg/2 mL	_____
7. 0.3 mg subcutaneous	0.4 mg/mL	_____
8. 1 mg subcutaneous	1:1000 solution	_____
9. 1 g IV	5% solution	_____
10. 0.1 g IM	200 mg/5 mL	_____
11. 400,000 units IM	500,000 units/mL	_____
12. 0.5 mg IM	0.5 mg/2 mL	_____
13. 1 g IV	50% solution	_____
14. 75 mg IM	100 mg/2 mL	_____
15. 15 mg IM	1:100 solution	_____
16. 35 mg IM	100 mg/mL	_____
17. 0.6 mg subcutaneous	0.4 mg per mL	_____
18. 0.15 g IM	0.2 g/2 mL	_____

Name: _____

There are five questions and each is worth 20 points. Aim for 90% or better on this test. If you have any difficulty doing the problems, review and study Chapter 7. Answers are given on p. 427.

1. Order: Fortaz 250 mg IM q8h
   Supply: vial of powder labeled 1-g powder (refer to Fig. 7-13 on p. 171)

   a. Diluting fluid and number of milliliters:
   b. Solution and new supply:
   c. Rule and arithmetic:
   d. Amount to give:
   e. Write on label:
   f. Storage:

2. Order: ticarcillin disodium 1 g IM
   Supply: vial of powder labeled Ticar 1 g (Fig. 7-15)

   a. Diluting fluid and number of milliliters:
   b. Solution and new stock:
   c. Rule and arithmetic:
   d. Amount to give:
   e. Write on label:
   f. Storage:

FIGURE 7-15

Directions for use of ticarcillin disodium (Ticar). (Courtesy of GlaxoSmithKline.)

DIRECTIONS FOR USE
—1 Gm, 3 Gm and 6 Gm Standard Vials—
INTRAMUSCULAR USE: (Concentration of approximately 385 mg/ml).
For initial reconstitution use Sterile Water for Injection, USP, Sodium Chloride Injection, USP or 1% Lidocaine Hydrochloride solution* (without epinephrine).
Each gram of Ticarcillin should be reconstituted with 2 ml of Sterile Water for Injection, U.S.P., Sodium Chloride Injection, U.S.P. or 1% Lidocaine Hydrochloride solution* (without epinephrine) and **used promptly.** Each 2.6 ml of the resulting solution will then contain 1 Gm of Ticarcillin.
*[For full product information, refer to manufacturer's package insert for Lidocaine Hydrochloride.]
As with all intramuscular preparations, TICAR (Ticarcillin Disodium) should be injected well within the body of a relatively large muscle, using usual techniques and precautions.

3. Order: ampicillin sodium 300 mg IM q8h
   Supply: vial of 500 mg powder (Fig. 7-16)

   a. Diluting fluid and number of milliliters:
   b. Solution and new supply:
   c. Rule and arithmetic:
   d. Amount to give:
   e. Write on label:
   f. Storage:

4. Order: Mefoxin 300 mg IM q4h
   Supply: vial of powder 1 g (Fig. 7-17)

   a. Diluting fluid and number of milliliters:
   b. Solution and new supply:
   c. Rule and arithmetic:

(continued)

Intramuscular Use: 125 mg vial: Add 1 ml Sterile Water for Injection, USP, or Bacteriostatic Water for Injection, USP (TUBEX® Sterile Cartridge-Needle Unit) to give a final concentration of 125 mg per ml. For fractional doses, withdraw the ampicillin sodium solution as follows:

Dose	Withdraw
25 mg	0.2 ml
50 mg	0.4 ml
75 mg	0.6 ml
100 mg	0.8 ml
125 mg	1 ml

250 mg vial: Add 0.9 ml Sterile Water for Injection, USP, or Bacteriostatic Water for Injection, USP (TUBEX) to give a final concentration of 250 mg/ml. For fractional doses, withdraw the ampicillin sodium solution as follows:

Dose	Withdraw
125 mg	0.5 ml
150 mg	0.6 ml
175 mg	0.7 ml
200 mg	0.8 ml
225 mg	0.9 ml
250 mg	1 ml

For dilution of 500-mg, 1-gram, and 2-gram vials, dissolve contents of a vial with the amount of Sterile water for Injection, USP, or Bacteriostatic Water for Injection, USP, listed in the table below:

Label Claim	Recommended Amount of Diluent	Withdrawable Volume	Concentration in mg/ml
500 mg	1.8 ml	2.0 ml	250 mg
1.0 gram	3.4 ml	4.0 ml	250 mg
2.0 gram	6.8 ml	8.0 ml	250 mg

While the 1-gram and 2-gram vials are primarily for intravenous use, they may be administered intramuscularly when the 250-mg or 500-mg vials are unavailable. In such instances, dissolve in 3.4 or 6.8 ml Sterile Water for Injection, USP, or Bacteriostatic Water for Injection, USP, to give a final concentration of 250 mg/ml

The above solutions must be used within one hour after reconstitution.

FIGURE 7-16

Reconstitution directions for ampicillin sodium for IM or IV injection.

	— Preparation of Solution		
Strength	Amount of Diluent to be Added (mL) + +	Approximate Withdrawable Volume (mL)	Approximate Average Concentration (mg/mL)
1 gram Vial	2 (Intramuscular)	2.5	400
2 gram Vial	4 (Intramuscular)	5	400
1 gram Vial	10 (IV)	10.5	95
2 gram Vial	10 or 20 (IV)	11.1 or 21.0	180 or 95
1 gram Infusion Bottle	50 or 100 (IV)	50 or 100	20 or 10
2 gram Infusion Bottle	50 or 100 (IV)	50 or 100	40 or 20
10 gram Bulk	43 or 93 (IV)	49 or 98.5	200 or 100

+ +Shake to dissolve and let stand until clear.

Intramuscular
MEFOXIN, as constituted with Sterile Water for Injection, Bacteriostatic Water for Injection, or 0.5 percent or 1 percent lidocaine hydrochloride solution (without epinephrine), maintains satisfactory potency for 24 hours at room temperature, for one week under refrigeration (below 5 C), and for at least 30 weeks in the frozen state.

FIGURE 7-17

Directions to reconstitute Mefoxin (cefoxitin sodium). (Courtesy of Merck Co. Inc.)

    d. Amount to give:

    e. Write on label:

    f. Storage:

5. Order: cefazolin sodium 0.33 g IM q8h

       Supply: vial of powder labeled 1 g (see Fig. 7-8 on p. 166)

    a. Diluting fluid and number of milliliters:

    b. Solution and new supply:

    c. Rule and arithmetic:

    d. Amount to give:

    e. Write on label:

    f. Storage:

Answers

Self-Test 1 Calculation of Liquids for Injection

1. Equivalent: 0.3 g = 300 mg

Formula Method

$$\frac{\overset{1}{\cancel{300}\text{ mg}}}{\underset{1}{\cancel{300}\text{ mg}}} \times 2 \text{ mL} = 2 \text{ mL}$$

Ratio Method

2 mL : 300 mg : : x : 300 mg

Proportion Method

$$\frac{2 \text{ mL}}{300 \text{ mg}} = \frac{x}{300 \text{ mg}}$$

$$\frac{600}{300} = x$$

$$2 \text{ mL} = x$$

Give 2 mL IM.

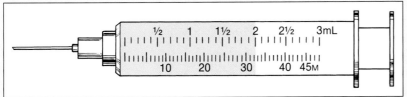

2. *Formula Method*

$$\frac{\overset{4}{\cancel{12}\text{ mg}}}{\underset{5}{\cancel{15}\text{ mg}}} \times 1 \text{ mL} = \frac{4}{5} \overset{0.8}{\cancel{)4.0}}$$

Ratio Method

1 mL : 15 mg : : x : 12 mg

Proportion Method

$$\frac{1 \text{ mL}}{15 \text{ mg}} = \frac{x}{12 \text{ mg}}$$

$$\frac{12}{15} = x$$

$$0.8 \text{ mL} = x$$

Give 0.8 mL IV. Follow directions for dilution and rate of administration.

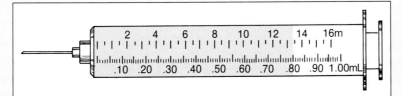

3. Equivalent: 1 mg = 1000 mcg

Formula Method

$$\frac{\overset{1}{\cancel{1000}\text{ mcg}}}{\underset{1}{\cancel{1000}\text{ mcg}}} \times 1 \text{ mL} = 1 \text{ mL}$$

Ratio Method

1 mL : 1000 mcg : : x : 1000 mcg

Proportion Method

$$\frac{1 \text{ mL}}{1000 \text{ mcg}} = \frac{x}{1000 \text{ mcg}}$$

$$\frac{1000}{1000} = x$$

$$1 \text{ mL} = x$$

Give 1 mL IM (see next page).

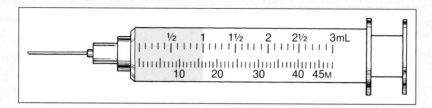

4. *Formula Method*

$$\frac{9 \ \cancel{mg}}{20 \ \cancel{mg}} \times 2 \ mL = \frac{18}{20} \begin{array}{r} 0.9 \\ \overline{)18.0} \\ \underline{18.0} \end{array}$$

Ratio Method

2 mL : 20 mg : : x : 9 mg

Proportion Method

$$\frac{2 \ mL}{20 \ mg} = \frac{x}{9 \ mg}$$

$$\frac{18}{20} = x$$

$$0.9 \ mL = x$$

Give 0.9 mL IM using a 1-mL precision syringe.

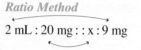

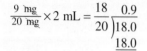

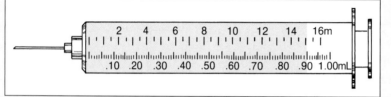

5. *Formula Method*

$$\frac{\overset{2}{\cancel{0.50}} \ mg}{\underset{1}{\cancel{0.25}} \ mg} \times 1 \ mL = 2 \ mL$$

Ratio Method

1 mL : 0.25 mg : : x : 0.5 mg

Proportion Method

$$\frac{1 \ mL}{0.25 \ mg} = \frac{x}{0.5 \ mg}$$

$$\frac{0.5}{0.25} = x$$

$$2 \ mL = x$$

Give 2 mL IM. Follow dilution and administration guidelines.

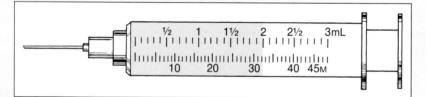

6. *Formula Method*

$$\frac{50 \ \cancel{mg}}{40 \ \cancel{mg}} \times 1 \ mL = \frac{5}{4} \begin{array}{r} 1.25 \\ \overline{)5.00} \\ \underline{4} \\ 10 \\ \underline{8} \\ 20 \\ \underline{20} \end{array}$$

Ratio Method

1 mL : 40 mg : : x : 50 mg

Proportion Method

$$\frac{1 \ mL}{40 \ mg} = \frac{x}{50 \ mg}$$

$$\frac{50}{40} = x$$

$$1.25 \ mL = x$$

Give 1.3 mL IM (see next page).

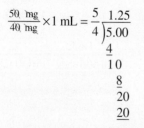
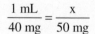
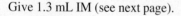
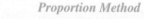

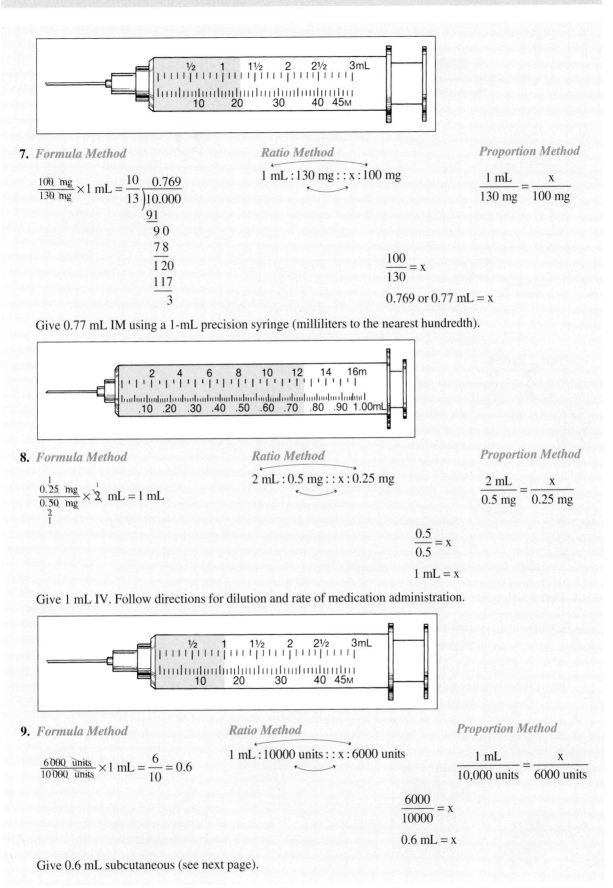

7. *Formula Method*

$$\frac{100 \text{ mg}}{130 \text{ mg}} \times 1 \text{ mL} = \frac{10}{13} \overline{)10.000} \; 0.769$$

$$\underline{9\,1}$$
$$\quad 9\,0$$
$$\quad \underline{7\,8}$$
$$\quad 1\,20$$
$$\quad \underline{1\,17}$$
$$\quad\quad 3$$

Ratio Method

1 mL : 130 mg : : x : 100 mg

Proportion Method

$$\frac{1 \text{ mL}}{130 \text{ mg}} = \frac{x}{100 \text{ mg}}$$

$$\frac{100}{130} = x$$

0.769 or 0.77 mL = x

Give 0.77 mL IM using a 1-mL precision syringe (milliliters to the nearest hundredth).

8. *Formula Method*

$$\frac{\overset{1}{0.25} \text{ mg}}{\underset{2}{0.50} \text{ mg}} \times \overset{1}{2} \text{ mL} = 1 \text{ mL}$$

Ratio Method

2 mL : 0.5 mg : : x : 0.25 mg

Proportion Method

$$\frac{2 \text{ mL}}{0.5 \text{ mg}} = \frac{x}{0.25 \text{ mg}}$$

$$\frac{0.5}{0.5} = x$$

1 mL = x

Give 1 mL IV. Follow directions for dilution and rate of medication administration.

9. *Formula Method*

$$\frac{6000 \text{ units}}{10\,000 \text{ units}} \times 1 \text{ mL} = \frac{6}{10} = 0.6$$

Ratio Method

1 mL : 10000 units : : x : 6000 units

Proportion Method

$$\frac{1 \text{ mL}}{10,000 \text{ units}} = \frac{x}{6000 \text{ units}}$$

$$\frac{6000}{10000} = x$$

0.6 mL = x

Give 0.6 mL subcutaneous (see next page).

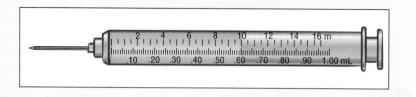

10. *Formula Method*

$$\frac{0.25 \text{ mg}}{1 \text{ mg}} \times 1 \text{ mL}$$

0.25 mL

Ratio Method

1 mL : 1 mg : : x : 0.25 mg

Proportion Method

$$\frac{1 \text{ mL}}{1 \text{ mg}} = \frac{x}{0.25 \text{ mg}}$$

0.25 mL = x

Give 0.25 mL subcutaneous.

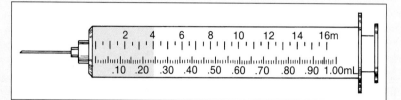

Self-Test 2 Ratios

RATIO	? g per ? mL	? g = ? mL	? g/? mL
1:20	1 g per 20 mL	1 g = 20 mL	1 g/20 mL
2:15	2 g per 15 mL	2 g = 15 mL	2 g/15 mL
1:500	1 g per 500 mL	1 g = 500 mL	1 g/500 mL
2:2000	2 g per 2000 mL	2 g = 2000 mL	2 g/2000 mL
1:4	1 g per 4 mL	1 g = 4 mL	1 g/4 mL
2:25	2 g per 25 mL	2 g = 25 mL	2 g/25 mL
4:50	4 g per 50 mL	4 g = 50 mL	4 g/50 mL
1:100	1 g per 100 mL	1 g = 100 mL	1 g/100 mL
3:75	3 g per 75 mL	3 g = 75 mL	3 g/75 mL
5:1000	5 g per 1000 mL	5 g = 1000 mL	5 g/1000 mL

Self-Test 3 Using Ratios with Liquids for Injection

1. Equivalent: 1:2000 means

   1 g in 2000 mL

   1 g = 1000 mg

Hence, the solution is 1000 mg/2000 mL.

Formula Method

$$\frac{D}{H} \times S = A$$

$$\frac{0.5 \text{ mg}}{1000 \text{ mg}} \times \overset{2}{2000} \text{ mL} = 0.5$$

$$\frac{\times \ 2}{1.0}$$

Ratio Method

2000 mL : 1000 mg : : x : 0.5 mg

Proportion Method

$$\frac{2000 \text{ mL}}{1000 \text{ mg}} = \frac{x}{0.5 \text{ mg}}$$

$$\frac{1000}{1000} = x$$

1 mL = x (see next page)

Give 1 mL subcutaneous.

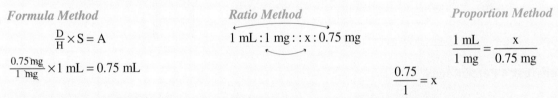

2. Equivalent: 1:5000 means

  1 g in 5000 mL

  1 g = 1000 mg

Hence, the solution is 1000 mg/5000 mL.

Formula Method

$\frac{D}{H} \times S = A$

$\frac{1\,mg}{1000\,mg} \times 5000\,mL = 5\,mL$

Ratio Method

5000 mL : 1000 mg : : x : 1 mg

Proportion Method

$\frac{5000\,mL}{1000\,mg} = \frac{x}{1\,mg}$

$\frac{5000}{1000} = x$

5 mL = x

Add 5 mL to IV. (This is correct because route is IV not IM).

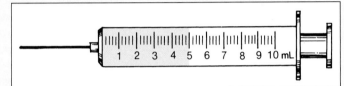

3. Equivalent: 1:1000 means

  1 g in 1000 mL

  1 g = 1000 mg

Hence, the solution is 1000 mg/1000 mL or 1 mg/mL.

Formula Method

$\frac{D}{H} \times S = A$

$\frac{0.75\,mg}{1\,mg} \times 1\,mL = 0.75\,mL$

Ratio Method

1 mL : 1 mg : : x : 0.75 mg

Proportion Method

$\frac{1\,mL}{1\,mg} = \frac{x}{0.75\,mg}$

$\frac{0.75}{1} = x$

0.75 mL = x

You have a 1-mL syringe marked in hundredths. Draw up 0.75 mL. Do not round off.

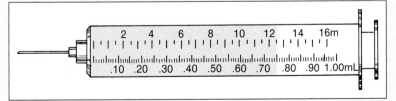

4. Equivalent: 1:1000 means

  1 g in 1000 mL

  1 g = 1000 mg

Hence, the solution is 1000 mg/1000 mL.

Formula Method

$$\frac{0.5\,\cancel{mg}}{1000\,\cancel{mg}} \times 1000\,mL$$

0.5 mL

Ratio Method

1000 mL : 1000 mg : : x : 0.5 mg

Proportion Method

$$\frac{1000\,mL}{1000\,mg} = \frac{x}{0.5\,mg}$$

$$\frac{500}{1000} = x$$

$$0.5\,mL = x$$

Give 0.5 mL subcutaneous.

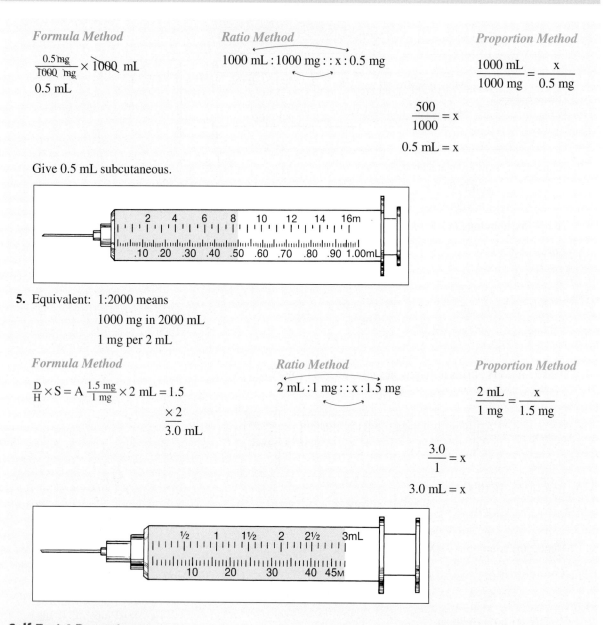

5. Equivalent: 1:2000 means

1000 mg in 2000 mL

1 mg per 2 mL

Formula Method

$$\frac{D}{H} \times S = A \quad \frac{1.5\,mg}{1\,mg} \times 2\,mL = 1.5$$

$$\begin{array}{r} \times 2 \\ \hline 3.0\,mL \end{array}$$

Ratio Method

2 mL : 1 mg : : x : 1.5 mg

Proportion Method

$$\frac{2\,mL}{1\,mg} = \frac{x}{1.5\,mg}$$

$$\frac{3.0}{1} = x$$

$$3.0\,mL = x$$

Self-Test 4 Percentages

PERCENTAGE	? g per 100 mL	? g = 100 mL	? g/100 mL
0.9%	0.9 g per 100 mL	0.9 g = 100 mL	0.9 g/100 mL
10%	10 g per 100 mL	10 g = 100 mL	10 g/100 mL
0.45%	0.45 g per 100 mL	0.45 g = 100 mL	0.45 g/100 mL
50%	50 g per 100 mL	50 g = 100 mL	50 g/100 mL
0.33%	0.33 g per 100 mL	0.33 g = 100 mL	0.33 g/100 mL
5%	5 g per 100 mL	5 g = 100 mL	5 g/100 mL
30%	30 g per 100 mL	30 g = 100 mL	30 g/100 mL
1.5%	1.5 g per 100 mL	1.5 g = 100 mL	1.5 g/100 mL
1%	1 g per 100 mL	1 g = 100 mL	1 g/100 mL
20%	20 g per 100 mL	20 g = 100 mL	20 g/100 mL

Self-Test 5 Using Percentages with Liquids for Injection

1. Equivalent: 1% 1 g in 100 mL

1 g = 1000 mg

Hence, the solution is 1000 mg/100 mL.

Formula Method

$$\frac{\overset{1}{\cancel{5}}\ \text{mg}}{\underset{\underset{2}{10}}{\cancel{1000}}\ \text{mg}} \times \overset{1}{\cancel{100}}\ \text{mL} = \frac{1}{2}\ \text{mL or } 0.5$$

Ratio Method

100 mL : 1000 mg : : x : 5 mg

Proportion Method

$$\frac{100\ \text{mL}}{1000\ \text{mg}} = \frac{x}{5\ \text{mg}}$$

$$\frac{500}{1000} = x$$

$$0.5\ \text{mL} = x$$

Give 0.5 mL subcutaneous.

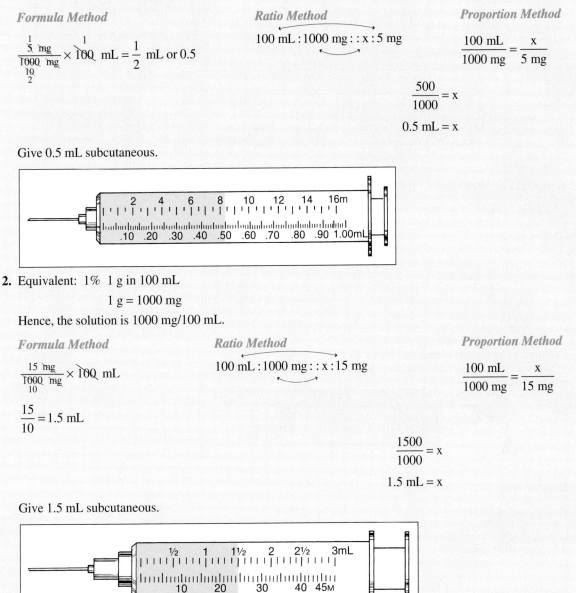

2. Equivalent: 1% 1 g in 100 mL

1 g = 1000 mg

Hence, the solution is 1000 mg/100 mL.

Formula Method

$$\frac{15\ \text{mg}}{\underset{10}{\cancel{1000}}\ \text{mg}} \times \overset{}{\cancel{100}}\ \text{mL}$$

$$\frac{15}{10} = 1.5\ \text{mL}$$

Ratio Method

100 mL : 1000 mg : : x : 15 mg

Proportion Method

$$\frac{100\ \text{mL}}{1000\ \text{mg}} = \frac{x}{15\ \text{mg}}$$

$$\frac{1500}{1000} = x$$

$$1.5\ \text{mL} = x$$

Give 1.5 mL subcutaneous.

3. Equivalent: 1% 1 g in 100 mL

1 g = 1000 mg

Hence, the solution is 1000 mg/100 mL.

Formula Method

$$\frac{3\,\text{mg}}{\underset{10}{\cancel{1000}}\,\text{mg}} \times \overset{1}{\cancel{100}}\ \text{mL} = \frac{3}{10} = 0.3\ \text{mL}$$

Ratio Method

$$100\ \text{mL} : 1000\ \text{mg} :: x : 3\ \text{mg}$$

Proportion Method

$$\frac{100\ \text{mL}}{1000\ \text{mg}} = \frac{x}{3\ \text{mg}}$$

$$\frac{300}{1000} = x$$

$$0.3\ \text{mL} = x$$

Give 0.3 mL subcutaneous.

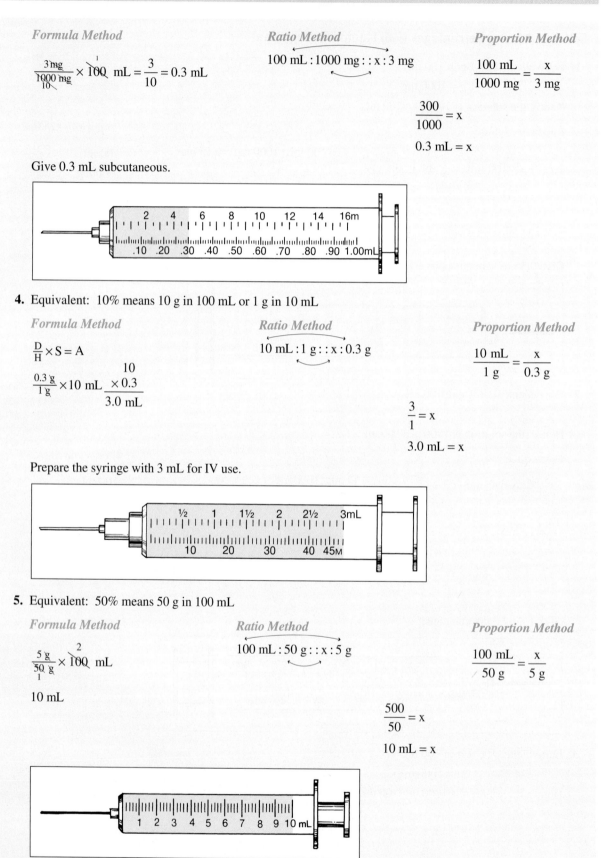

4. Equivalent: 10% means 10 g in 100 mL or 1 g in 10 mL

Formula Method

$$\frac{D}{H} \times S = A$$

$$\frac{0.3\,\text{g}}{1\,\text{g}} \times 10\ \text{mL} \quad \begin{array}{r} 10 \\ \times 0.3 \\ \hline 3.0\ \text{mL} \end{array}$$

Ratio Method

$$10\ \text{mL} : 1\ \text{g} :: x : 0.3\ \text{g}$$

Proportion Method

$$\frac{10\ \text{mL}}{1\ \text{g}} = \frac{x}{0.3\ \text{g}}$$

$$\frac{3}{1} = x$$

$$3.0\ \text{mL} = x$$

Prepare the syringe with 3 mL for IV use.

5. Equivalent: 50% means 50 g in 100 mL

Formula Method

$$\frac{5\,\text{g}}{\underset{1}{50}\,\text{g}} \times \overset{2}{\cancel{100}}\ \text{mL}$$

10 mL

Ratio Method

$$100\ \text{mL} : 50\ \text{g} :: x : 5\ \text{g}$$

Proportion Method

$$\frac{100\ \text{mL}}{50\ \text{g}} = \frac{x}{5\ \text{g}}$$

$$\frac{500}{50} = x$$

$$10\ \text{mL} = x$$

Self-Test 6 Insulin Calculations

1.

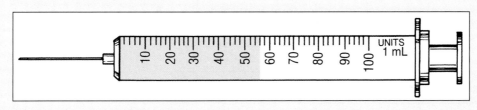

2.

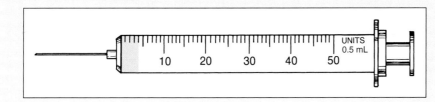

3.

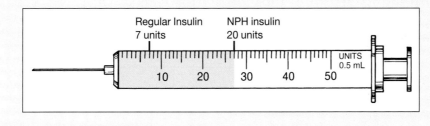

4.

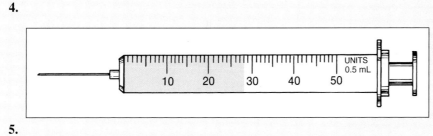

5.

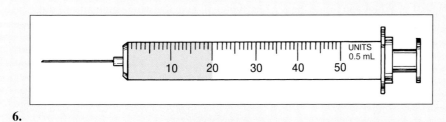

6.

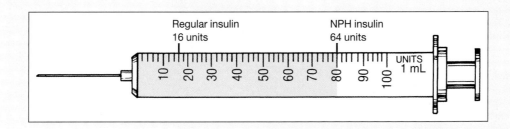

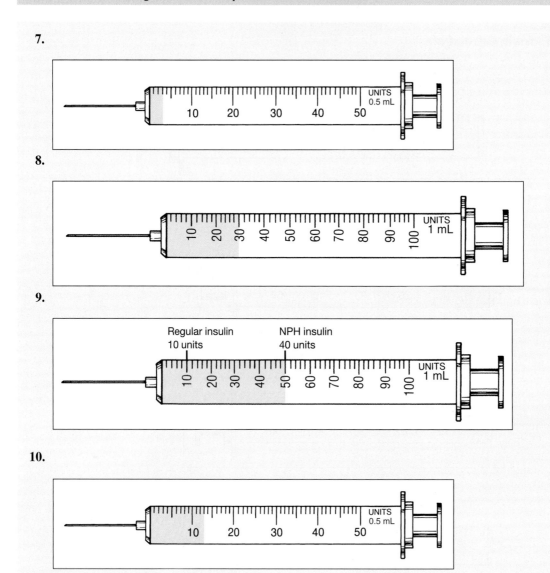

7.

8.

9.

Regular insulin
10 units

NPH insulin
40 units

10.

Self-Test 7 Injections from Powders

1. You want 1 g. The supply is 1 g. When you dilute the powder, you will give the whole amount of fluid, *whatever the amount is*. The manufacturer states it will be 3.6 mL/1 g. If you solve the arithmetic you have

Formula Method

$$\frac{D}{H} \times S = A$$

Ratio Method

1 mL : 280 mg : : x mL : 1000 mg

$$\frac{1000}{280} = x$$

Proportion Method

$$\frac{1 \text{ mL}}{280 \text{ mg}} = \frac{x}{1000 \text{ mg}}$$

$$\frac{1000 \text{ mg}}{280 \text{ mg}} \times 1 \text{ mL} = \frac{100}{28} \quad 28 \overline{)100.00} \quad = 3.6 \text{ mL} = x$$

$$\begin{array}{r} 3.57 \\ 28\overline{)100.00} \\ \underline{84} \\ 160 \\ \underline{140} \\ 200 \\ \underline{196} \end{array}$$

    a. 3 mL sterile water for injection

    b. 1 g in 3.6 mL; 280 mg/mL

    c. Not necessary

    d. Give 3.6 mL in two syringes.

    e. Discard the vial; it is empty.

    f. Discard the vial in appropriate receptacle.

2. a. 1.8 mL sterile water for injection

    b. 250 mg/mL

Formula Method	*Ratio Method*	*Proportion Method*
c. $\dfrac{D}{H} \times S = A$	1 mL : 250 mg : : x mL : 250 mg	$\dfrac{1 \text{ mL}}{250 \text{ mg}} = \dfrac{x}{250 \text{ mg}}$
$\dfrac{250 \text{ mg}}{250 \text{ mg}} \times 1$		$\dfrac{250}{250} = x$
		1 mL = x

    d. Give 1 mL IM.

    e. Nothing! Read the last line: "The above solutions must be used within 1 hour after reconstitution." You must discard the remaining fluid!

    f. None

3. a. Choose 500 mg powder. (Can you see why?)

    b. Add 2 mL sterile water for injection.

    c. 225 mg/mL

    d. Not necessary: You want 225 mg; you made 225 mg/mL.

    e. Give 1 mL IM.

    f. 225 mg/mL, date, time, initials

    g. Refrigerate; stable for 96 hours

4. a. 3.0 mL sterile water for injection

    b. 280 mg/mL

Formula Method	*Ratio Method*	*Proportion Method*
c. $\dfrac{D}{H} \times S = A$	1 mL : 280 mg : : x mL : 500 mg	$\dfrac{1 \text{ mL}}{280 \text{ mg}} = \dfrac{x}{500 \text{ mg}}$
$\dfrac{500 \text{ mg}}{280 \text{ mg}} \times 1 \text{ mL} = \dfrac{50}{28} \; \begin{array}{r} 1.78 \\ \overline{)50.00} \\ \underline{28} \\ 220 \\ \underline{196} \\ 240 \\ \underline{224} \\ 16 \end{array}$		$\dfrac{500}{280} = x$ 1.78 or 1.8 mL = x

    d. Give 1.8 mL IM.

    e. 280 mg/mL, date, time, initials

    f. Refrigerate; stable for 7 days

5. a. Add 2 mL sterile water for injection.

    b. 400 mg/mL

Formula Method

c. $\dfrac{D}{H} \times S = A$

$\dfrac{\overset{1}{\cancel{200}} \text{ mg}}{\underset{2}{\cancel{400}} \text{ mg}} \times 1 \text{ mL} = \dfrac{1}{2} \text{ mL or } 0.5 \text{ mL}$

Ratio Method

1 mL : 400 mg : : x mL : 200 mg

Proportion Method

$\dfrac{1 \text{ mL}}{400 \text{ mg}} = \dfrac{x}{200 \text{ mg}}$

$\dfrac{200}{400} = x$

$0.5 \text{ mL} = x$

d. Give ½ mL (0.5 mL).

e. 400 mg/mL, date, time, initials

f. Refrigerate; stable for 1 week

6. a. 3.0 mL sterile water for injection

b. 280 mg/mL

c. Give 0.3 mL IM (3-mL syringe) or 0.32 mL (1-mL precision syringe).

d. 280 mg/mL, date, time, initials

7. a. 2 mL sterile water for injection

b. 225 mg/mL

c. 2 mL IM

d. 225 mg/mL, date, time, initials

8. a. 1.8 mL sterile water for injection

b. 250 mg/mL

c. 1.6 mL

d. 250 mg/mL, date, time, initials

9. a. 3 mL sterile water for injection

b. 280 mg/mL

c. 1.8 mL

d. 280 mg/mL, date, time, initials

10. a. 2 mL sterile water for injection

b. 400 mg/mL

c. 1.3 mL IM

d. 400 mg/mL, date, time, initials

CHAPTER

8

Calculation of Basic IV Drip Rates

Administration of parenteral fluids and medications by the IV route is common medical practice and is a specialty within nursing and health care. Texts such as *Plumer's Principles and Practice of Intravenous Therapy* (Lippincott, 2001) present detailed and extensive information. This chapter presents basic knowledge—types of fluids, equipment, calculation of drip rates, and recording intake. Chapter 9 presents rules and calculations for special types of IV orders.

▶ Types of Intravenous Fluids

Intravenous fluids are packaged in sterile plastic bags or glass bottles. The nurse selects the IV fluid ordered and prepares the solution. Care is essential. An error in choosing the correct IV may result in serious fluid and electrolyte imbalance.

The written order for an IV may differ from the printed supply label. Always seek expert advice when in doubt about which solution to use.

Common abbreviations for IV fluids are D, dextrose; W, water; and NS, normal (or isotonic) saline. Often, a percent of these is indicated. For example, D5W means 5% dextrose in water; 0.9%NS means 0.9% saline in water.

Example	Written Order	Supply Label
	1000 mL D5W	1000 mL D5%W
	500 mL D5S	500 mL D5%0.9NS
	250 mL D5½NS	250 mL D5%0.45NS
	500 mL D5⅓NS	500 mL D5%0.33NS
	500 mL NS	500 mL 0.9%NS
	1000 mL ½NS	1000 mL 0.45%NS

▶ Kinds of Intravenous Drip Factors

IV fluids are administered through infusion sets that consist of plastic tubing attached at one end to the IV bag and at the other end to a needle or catheter inserted into a blood vessel. The top of the infusion set contains a chamber. Sets that contain a needle in the chamber are called *microdrip* because the drops are small. To deliver 1 mL fluid to the patient, 60 drops must fall (60 gtt = 1 mL). All microdrip sets deliver 60 gtt/mL.

Infusion sets that do not have a needle in the chamber are called *macrodrip* (Fig. 8-1). Macrodrip amounts per milliliter differ according to the manufacturer.

For example, Baxter-Travenol macrodrip sets deliver 10 gtt/mL; Abbott sets deliver 15 gtts/mL. The package label will state the drops per milliliter (gtt/mL). You need to know this information to calculate IV drip rates.

The tubing for these sets includes a clamp that the nurse can open or close to regulate the drip rate; a second hand on a watch or clock is used to count the drops per minute (Fig. 8-2).

Infusion Pumps

Electric infusion pumps also are used to deliver IV fluid. Some are easy to operate; others are more elaborate. The nurse enters two pieces of information: the total number of milliliters to be infused and the number of milliliters per hour. Pumps used in specialty units also allow the nurse to input the name of the medication, and the pump automatically calculates the rate in mg, mcg, etc., as well as mL/h. Figure 8-3 shows a photo of the face of an infusion pump. IV tubing is connected to the pump. If an order reads "500 mL D5W IV. Run 50 mL/hr," the nurse would press Volume for Infusion, 500; Rate for Infusion, 50; and On. The pump would automatically deliver 50 mL/hr over a 10-hour period.

IV pumps can also run IVPB. If an order reads "Ampicillin 2 g IVPB in 100 mL NS over 1 hour," the nurse would press Secondary Volume, 100; Secondary Rate, 100; and On. The pump would interrupt the main IV to administer the IVPB over 1 hour, then resume the primary flow.

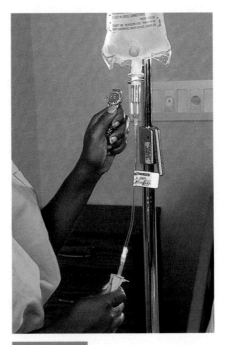

FIGURE 8-2

Timing the IV drip rate. (© B. Proud.) (With permission From Taylor, C., Lillis, C., & LeMone, P. [2004]. *Photo atlas of medication administration.* Philadelphia: Lippincott Williams & Wilkins, p. 46.)

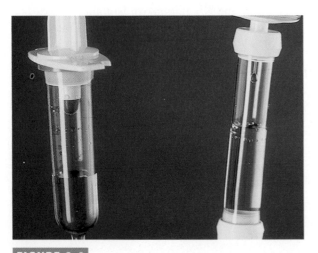

FIGURE 8-1

Drip chambers for macrodrip and microdrip IV tubing.

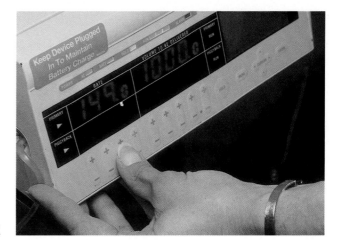

FIGURE 8-3

IV rate is programmed into the infusion pump in mL/hr.

Labeling IVs

Every IV must be identified so that any professional can check what fluid is infusing and the drip rate. The following information is a typical order:

Patient name, room, bed number, and date

Order: 500 mL D5W½NS. Run 50 mL/hr.

Label			
Patient	*James Latham*	Room	*1411B*
Date, Time	*6/26, 1000A*	Rate	*50 gtt/min*
Order	*500 mL D5W1/2NS*	Run	*50 mL/hr*
Time	*10 A–8 P*	Initials	*CB*

Note that the physician orders 50 mL/hr. Because the IV fluid amount is 500 mL, it will take 10 hours to complete; the time is 10 AM to 8 PM (10 hours). Using microdrip tubing, 50 mL/hr = 50 gtt/min, the rate set by the nurse. In the next section we study how to calculate IV drip rates. Our goal is to deliver the amount of fluid ordered in the time ordered with a continuous and even drip rate.

Calculating Basic IV Drip Rates

Routine IV orders contain the number of milliliters of fluid and the time of administration:

Example	250 mL D5W IV at 250 mL/hr	Fluid amount: 250 mL	Time: 1 hour
	1000 mL Ringer's lactate IV 8 AM–8 PM	Fluid amount: 1000 mL	Time: 12 hours
	500 mL D5½NS with 20 mEq KCl IV to run 75 mL/hr on a pump	Fluid amount: 500 mL	Time: 75 mL/hour

The equipment used by the nurse determines the drip factor and the calculations needed. With an infusion pump, calculations are in mL/hr because *the pump is set in mL/hr.* IV drips set in gtt/min depend on whether microdrip or macrodrip tubing is used.

RULE

> Problems in IV calculations are solved in two steps. Step 1 is used to solve problems requiring an infusion pump and to simplify the arithmetic needed for microdrip and macrodrip. Step 2 solves micro- and macrodrip problems. ■

Step 1. $\dfrac{\text{Total number of milliliters ordered}}{\text{number of hours to run}} = \text{number of mL/hr}$

Step 2. $\dfrac{\text{Number of milliliters per hour} \times \text{tubing drip factor (TF)}}{\text{number of minutes}} = \text{drops per minute}$

Learning Aid

Step 1. $\dfrac{\#\ \text{mL}}{\#\ \text{hr}} = \text{mL/hr}$

Step 2. $\dfrac{\text{mL/hr} \times \text{TF}}{\#\ \text{min}} = \text{gtt/min}$

Note that in Step 2, mL/hr is the answer from Step 1.

Note: Often the terms *drop factor, drip factor,* or *gtt factor* are used instead of *tubing drip factor.* We use *TF* in this text to mean all these terms.

Learning Aid

Remember the abbreviation "gtt" is "drop."

Explanation

Step 1. $\dfrac{\#\ \text{mL}}{\#\ \text{hr}} = \text{mL/hr}$

mL: The physician or healthcare provider will indicate the number of milliliters to be infused in the order.

hr: The number of hours to run depends on the way the order is written. For example, if the order is written

q8h = 8 hours at a time

10 AM–4 PM = 6 hours

mL/hr = the answer to step 1

Step 2. $\dfrac{\#\ \text{mL/hr} \times \text{TF}}{\#\ \text{min}} = \text{gtt/min}$

mL/hr: the answer from Step 1

TF: tubing drip factor is either microdrip (60 gtt = 1 mL) or macrodrip

Depending on the manufacturer, macrodrip could be 10 gtt = 1 mL, 15 gtt = 1 mL, or 20 gtt = 1 mL.

min: Number of minutes is always 60 for this problem. In step 1 you found mL/hr, but you need gtt/min because there are 60 minutes in an hour, divide by 60.

gtt/min: The drip factor calculated to deliver an even flow of fluid over a specified time. The nurse regulates the drip rate using a second hand on a watch or a clock. If the drip rate is calculated to be 80 gtt/min, the nurse opens the clamp and regulates the drip until there are 20 gtt in 15 seconds. This provides 80 gtt/min.

In the problems requiring calculation in this text, the drip factor will be given to you. In the clinical area, you must read the package label to identify the gtt/mL.

Application of the Rule

Example

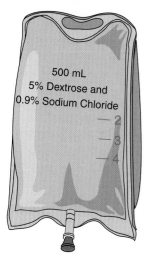

Order: 1000 mL Ringer's lactate IV 8 AM–8 PM

Available: an infusion pump

Logic: 8 AM to 8 PM is 12 hours for the IV to run. The infusion pump regulates the rate in milliliters per hour. Only step 1 is necessary.

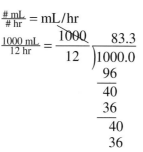

$$\frac{\# \, mL}{\# \, hr} = mL/hr$$

$$\frac{1000 \, mL}{12 \, hr} = \frac{1000}{12}$$

$$\begin{array}{r} 83.3 \\ 12 \, \overline{)1000.0} \\ \underline{96} \\ 40 \\ \underline{36} \\ 40 \\ 36 \end{array}$$

> **Learning Aid**
>
> Carry out arithmetic one decimal place and round off the answer to the nearest whole number.

Label the IV.

Set the pump as follows:

Total # mL: 1000

mL/hr: 83

Example

Order: 500 mL D5NS IV 12 NOON–4 PM

Available: microdrip at 60 gtt/mL; macrodrip at 20 gtt/mL

Logic: The IV will run 4 hours. Because no pump is available, the nurse must choose the drip factor; two steps are necessary. Solve for both drip factors and choose one.

Step 1. $\frac{\# \, mL}{\# \, hr} = mL/hr$

$$\frac{500}{4} \quad \begin{array}{r} 125. \\ \overline{)500.} \end{array} = 125 \, mL/hr$$

> **Learning Aid**
>
> Note that the answer to Step 1 is 125 mL/hr.
>
> The answer to Step 2 is 125 gtt/min for microdrip. See next page.

Step 2. $\frac{\# \, mL/hr \times TF}{\# \, min} = gtt/min$

Macrodrip

$$\frac{125 \times \overset{1}{20}}{\underset{3}{60}} = \frac{125}{3} \quad \begin{array}{r} 41.6 \\ 3 \, \overline{)125.0} \\ \underline{12} \\ 5 \\ \underline{3} \\ 20 \end{array}$$

Macrodrip at 42 gtt/min

Microdrip

$$\frac{125 \times \overset{1}{\cancel{60}}}{\underset{1}{\cancel{60}}} = 125 \text{ gtt/min}$$

Microdrip at 125 gtt/min

Logic: Answers are macrodrip at 42 gtt/min and microdrip at 125 gtt/min. Choose one. (See the explanation for choosing the infusion set, after this discussion.)

Label the IV.

Set the drip rate.

Example

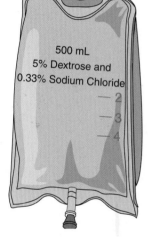

500 mL
5% Dextrose and
0.33% Sodium Chloride

Order: 500 mL D5⅓NS IV KVO for 24°

Available: microdrip at 60 gtt/mL; macrodrip 10 gtt/mL

Logic: Because no pump is available, choose the IV set. This is a two-step problem. The IV will run 24 hours.

Step 1. $\frac{\# \text{ mL}}{\# \text{ hr}} = \text{mL/hr}$

$$\frac{500}{24} \overset{20.8}{\overline{\smash{\big)}500.0}} = 21 \text{ mL/hr}$$
$$\underline{48}$$
$$200$$
$$\underline{192}$$

Step 2. $\frac{\text{mL/hr} \times \text{TF}}{\# \text{ min}} = \text{gtt/min}$

Logic: The answer from step 1 is 21 mL/hr. The number of minutes is 60. Work out the problem for micro- and macrodrip and make a nursing judgment about which tube to use.

Macrodrip

$$\frac{21 \times \cancel{10}}{\cancel{60}} = \frac{21}{6} \overset{3.5}{\overline{\smash{\big)}21.0}}$$
$$\underline{18}$$
$$30$$
$$\underline{30}$$

Macrodrip at 4 gtt/min

Microdrip

$$\frac{21 \times \cancel{60}}{\cancel{60}} = 21 \text{ gtt/min}$$

Logic: A 4-gtt/min macrodrip is too slow. Choose microdrip. (See the explanation on p. 206 for choosing the infusion set.)

Label the IV.

Select a microdrip infusion set.

Set the drip rate at 21 gtt/min.

SELF-TEST 1 | **Calculation of Drip Factors**

Calculate the drip factor for the following IV orders given in milliliters per hour or number of hours. Answers are given at the end of the chapter.

1. Order: 150 mL D5W0.33NS IV q8h
   Available: infusion pump

2. Order: 250 mL D5W; run at 25 mL/hr
   Available: infusion pump

3. Order: 1000 mL D5NS; run 100 mL/hr
   Available: macrodrip (20 gtt/mL); microdrip (60 gtt/mL)

4. Order: 180 mL D5 1/3 NS 12 NOON–6 PM
   Available: macrodrip (10 gtt/mL); microdrip (60 gtt/mL)

5. Order: 1000 mL D5W0.45NS IV 4 PM–12 MIDNIGHT
   Available: macrodrip (15 gtt/mL); microdrip (60 gtt/mL)

6. Order: 250 mL D5W IV q8h
   Available: infusion pump

7. Order: 500 mL NS IV over 2 h
   Available: infusion pump

8. Order: 1000 mL D5NS IV 4 AM–4 PM
   Available: macrodrip (15 gtt/mL); microdrip (60 gtt/mL)

9. Order: 1000 mL D5W0.45 NS IV; run 150 mL/hr
   Available: macrodrip (10 gtt/mL); microdrip (60 gtt/mL)

10. Order: 150 mL 0.9 NS IV; over 1 h
    Available: macrodrip (20 gtt/mL); microdrip (60 gtt/mL)

Determining Hours an IV Will Run

It is helpful for the nurse to calculate approximately how long an IV will last so that the next IV can be prepared or new orders written. The rule is simple:

$$\frac{\text{number of milliliters ordered}}{\text{number of milliliters per hour}} = \text{number of hours to run}$$

Learning Aid

$$\frac{\#\ mL}{\#\ mL/hr} = \#\ hr$$

Example

Order: 500 mL NS IV; run 75 mL/hr

Rule: $\frac{\#\ mL}{\#\ mL/hr} = hr$

$$\frac{500\ mL}{75\ mL/hr} = 75\overline{)500.00}$$

6.67
450
50 0
45 0
5 00

The IV will last approximately 6.7 hours.

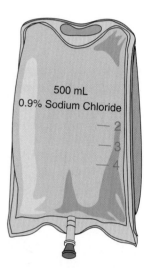

500 mL
0.9% Sodium Chloride

Example

Order: 1000 mL D5½ NS IV 8 AM–8 PM

No math necessary; 8 AM–8 PM = 12 hours

The IV will last 12 hours.

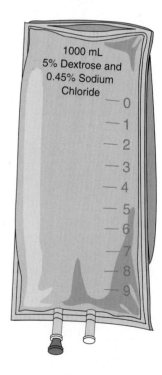

1000 mL
5% Dextrose and
0.45% Sodium
Chloride

Example

Order: aminophylline 500 mg in 250 mL D5W IV at 50 mL/hr

Rule: $\frac{\#\ mL}{\#\ mL/hr} = \#\ hr$

$\frac{250\ mL}{50\ mL} = 5\ hr$

The IV will last 5 hours.

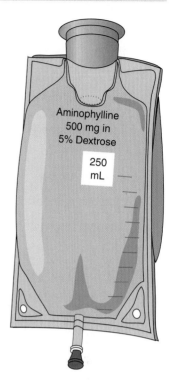

Aminophylline
500 mg in
5% Dextrose

250
mL

SELF-TEST 2 **IV Infusions—Hours**

Calculate the hours that the following IV orders will run. Answers are given at the end of this chapter.

 1. Order: 250 mL D5½ NS IV at 30 mL/hr

 2. Order: Ringer's lactate 500 mL IV; run 60 mL/hr

 3. Order: 1000 mL D5NS IV 4 PM–2 AM

 4. Order: 1000 mL D5W IV KVO 24 hours

 5. Order: 500 mL D51/2NS at 70 mL/hr

 6. Order: 500 mL D5W IV at 50 mL/hr

 7. Order: LR 1000 mL IV 10 hours

 8. Order: 250 mL NS IV at 100 mL/hr

 9. Order: 1000 mL NS IV 12 NOON–6 PM

10. Order: 500 mL NS IV over 5 hours

Choosing the Infusion Set

Experience will enable you to judge which IV tubing to use. Clinically you will be guided in making a choice. There is no problem when an electric infusion pump is used. The pump will deliver the amount programmed. There are specialized pumps in neonatal and intensive care units that can deliver 1 mL/hr and specialized syringe pumps that can deliver less than 1 mL/hr.

Some guidelines may be helpful when an IV pump is not available.

Use Microdrip When

- The IV is to be administered over a long period
- A small amount of fluid is to be infused
- The macrodrops per minute are too few (Why? IV fluid flows by gravity. Blood flowing in the vein exerts a pressure. If the IV is too slow, blood pressure may force blood into the tube where it clots. The IV will stop.)

Use Macrodrip When

- A large amount of fluid is ordered in a short time
- The microdrips per minute are too many and counting the drip rate becomes too difficult

Need for Continuous Observation

Many factors may interfere with the drip rate. Do not assume that once an IV is started it will continue to flow at the rate it was set. Check the IV frequently; IVs flow by gravity. As the amount of fluid decreases in the IV bag, pressure changes occur that may affect the rate. The patient's movements may kink the tube and shut off the flow, or the movements may change the position of the needle or catheter in the vein. The needle may be forced against the side of the blood vessel thereby changing the flow, or it may be forced out of the vessel, allowing fluid to enter the tissues (infiltration). Signs of possible infiltration are swelling, pain, coolness, or pallor at the insertion site.

Infusion pumps have an alarm system that beeps to alert the nurse when the rate cannot be maintained or when the infusion is about to be completed.

▶ Adding Medications to IVs

When a continuous IV order includes a medication, add the medication to the IV and determine the rate of flow. In some institutions, the pharmacist adds the medications; in others, nurses add the medication.

Medications Ordered Over Several Hours

Example   Order: 1000 mL D5W with 20 mEq KCl IV 10 AM–10 PM

Available: vial of KCl 40 mEq/20 mL, microdrip (60 gtt/min), macrodrip (20 gtt/min)

Formula Method

Logic: $\frac{D}{H} \times S = A$

$$\frac{\overset{1}{\cancel{20}\ mEq}}{\underset{\underset{1}{2}}{\cancel{40}\ mEq}} \times \overset{10}{\cancel{20}}\ mL = 10\ mL$$

Ratio Method

20 mL : 40 mEq : : x mL : 20 mEq

Proportion Method

$$\frac{20mL}{40mEq} \diagup\!\!\!\!\times\!\!\!\!\diagdown \frac{x}{20mEq}$$

$$\frac{400}{40} = x$$

$$10mL = x$$

Add 10 mL KCl to the IV bag.

Use two steps to solve the drip factor.

Choose the tubing. The IV will run 12 hours.

Step 1. $\frac{\#\text{ mL}}{\#\text{ hr}} = \text{mL/hr}$

$\frac{1000}{12} = 83\text{ mL/hr}$

Step 2. $\frac{\#\text{mL/hr} \times \text{TF}}{\#\text{min}} = \text{gtt/min}$

For macrodrip: $\frac{83 \times \overset{1}{20}}{\underset{3}{60}} = 28\text{ gtt/min}$

For microdrip: mL/hr = gtt/min; hence, 83 gtt/min

Choose either drip rate.

Label the IV.

Example

Order: 5 milliunits penicillin G potassium in 1000 mL D5W IV q8h

Available: macrodrip (10 gtt/mL), microdrip (60 gtt/mL)

Logic: Milliunits means million units. The order is for 5 million units of penicillin G potassium. Penicillin comes in 5-milliunit vials of powder. Directions say that the drug must be reconstituted with a minimum of 100 mL. The order states to add 5 milliunits to 1000 mL. The order is safe because you are adding 5 milliunits to 1000 mL. Use a 10-mL syringe to remove fluid aseptically from the 1000-mL bag of D5W and inject it into the powder to make a solution. Withdraw the solution and inject it into the bag. You now have 1000 mL D5W with the medication added. The IV will run 8 hours.

Two steps are needed:

Step 1. $\frac{\#\text{ mL}}{\#\text{ hr}} = \text{mL/hr}$

$\frac{\cancel{1000}}{8} \quad 125 \overline{)1000.} = 125\text{ mL/hr}$

Step 2. $\frac{\#\text{mL/hr} \times \text{TF}}{\#\text{min}} = \text{gtt/min}$

Macrodrip: $\frac{125 \times 10}{60} = \frac{\cancel{125}}{6} \quad \frac{20.8}{6\overline{)125.0}} = 21\text{ gtt/min}$

Microdrip = 125 gtt/min; macrodrip = 21 gtt/min

Choose one.

Label the IV.

Example

Order: aminophylline 250 mg in 250 mL D5W IV; run at 50 mL/hr

Available: ampule of aminophylline labeled 1 g in 10 mL; Buretrol that delivers 60 gtt/mL (microdrip). See Figure 8-4.

Logic: The ampule of aminophylline has 1 g in 10 mL. This is equivalent to 1000 mg in 10 mL. You want 250 mg.

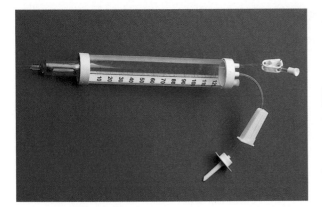

FIGURE 8-4

A Buretrol is an IV delivery system with tubing and a chamber that can hold 150 mL delivered as microdrip (1 mL = 60 drops). (This device is sometimes called a Volutrol.) The top of the Buretrol has a port so that a reservoir of fluid can be added. The Buretrol is a volume control because no more than 150 mL can be infused at one time.

Formula Method

$$\frac{D}{H} \times S = A$$

$$\frac{\overset{1}{\cancel{250}}}{\underset{4}{\cancel{1000}}} \times 10 = \frac{\overset{1}{\cancel{10}}}{4} \quad \begin{array}{r} 2.5 \text{ mL} \\ 4\overline{)10.0} \end{array}$$

Ratio Method

$$10 \text{ mL} : 1000 \text{ mg} : : x \text{ mL} : 250 \text{ mg}$$

Proportion Method

$$\frac{10 \text{ mL}}{1000 \text{ mg}} \times \frac{x}{250 \text{ mg}}$$

$$\frac{2500}{1000} = x$$

$$2.5 \text{ mL} = x$$

Draw up 2.5 mL and inject it into 250 mL D5W. You have 250 mg aminophylline in 250 mL D5W. Label the bag.

You want 50 mL/hr, and you have a Buretrol 60 gtt/mL.

$$\frac{\text{mL/hr} \times \text{TF}}{60} = \frac{50 \times 60}{60} = 50 \text{ gtt/min}$$

Label the IV: Rate, 50 mL/hr

Learning Aid

The Buretrol is microdrip. No calculation is needed.

mL/hr = gtt/min

SELF-TEST 3 | **IV Infusion Rates**

Calculate how much medication is needed (if applicable) and the infusion rate. Answers are given at the end of the chapter.

1. Order: 500 mL D5W IV with vitamin C 500 mg at 60 mL/hr
   Available: ampule of vitamin C labeled 500 mg/2 mL; microdrip tubing at 60 gtt/mL

2. Order: 250 mg hydrocortisone sodium succinate in 1000 mL D5W 8 AM–12 MIDNIGHT
   Available: vial of hydrocortisone sodium succinate labeled 250 mg with a 2-mL diluent; microdrip tubing

3. Order: aminophylline 250 mg in 250 mL D5W IV; run 50 mL/hr
   Available: infusion pump, vial of aminophylline labeled 500 mg/10 mL

4. Order: 250 mL D5½ NS with KCl 10 mEq IV 12 NOON–6 PM
   Available: microdrip tubing, vial of potassium chloride labeled 20 mEq/10 mL

Medications for Intermittent Intravenous Administration

Some IV medications are not administered continuously but only intermittently, such as q4h, q6h, or q8h. This route is termed *intravenous piggyback* or IVPB (Fig. 8-5).

Most of these drugs are prepared in powder form. The manufacturer specifies the type and amount of diluent needed to reconstitute the drug, which is connected by IV tubing to the main IV line.

The health care provider may write a detailed order: vancomycin 0.5 g IVPB in 100 mL D5W over 1 hr. More often the health care provider will write only the drug, route, and time interval, relying on the nurse to research the manufacturer's directions for the amount and type of diluent and the time for the infusion to run (e.g., Order: cefazolin 1 g IVPB q6h).

Explanation

The rule to solve IVPB problems is similar to the IV rule:

$$\frac{\# \text{ mL} \times \text{TF}}{\# \text{ min}} = \text{gtt/min}$$

mL: The type and amount of diluent will be stated on the label or in the package insert. Nurses' drug references and the *Physicians Drug Reference* also contain this information.

TF: The tubing for IVPB is called a secondary administration set and has a macrodrip factor. It is shorter than main line IV tubing. In the clinical setting, check the label for the tubing drip factor.

min: The manufacturer may or may not indicate the number of minutes needed for the IVPB medication to be infused. When the number is not given, a general rule to follow for adults is to allow 30 minutes for every 50 mL solution.

Example	Order: cefazolin 1 g IVPB q6h

Supply: package insert for IVPB dilution of cefazolin sodium. Reconstitute with 50 to 100 mL of sodium chloride injection or other solution listed under administration. Other solutions listed include D5W, D10W, D5LR, and D5NS.

Let's use 50 mL D5W. It is the most common IVPB diluent and we have 50-mL bags. No time for infusion is given in the directions for "piggyback" vials. Use 30 minutes for 50 mL.

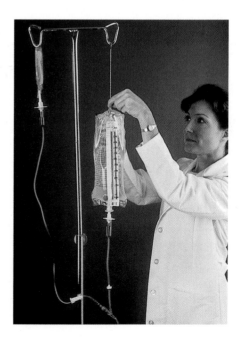

FIGURE 8-5

Photo of a primary IV line (*right*) and an IVPB (or secondary) line (*left*). Fluid flows continuously through the primary line into the patient's vein. At timed intervals, medication placed in an intravenous piggyback bag (IVPB) is attached by tubing to the primary IV for delivery to the patient. The primary fluid is lowered and the IVPB fluid flows. After the IVPB has infused, the primary fluid begins infusing again. An IV infusion pump may also be used, and medication in the IVPB is infused through the pump.

$$\frac{\#\,mL \times TF}{\#\,min} = gtt/min$$

$\#\,mL = 50\ mL\ D5W$

$TF = 10\ gtt/mL$ (For a secondary asministration, no set time for administration is given. Follow the general adult rule of 30 minutes for every 50 mL.

$\#\,min = 30$

$$\frac{50 \times 10}{30} = 16.6 = 17\ gtt/min$$

You are ready to prepare the IVPB. You have a vial of powder labeled 1 g. You need the whole amount. You have a 50-mL bag of D5W. You need the whole amount. Use a reconstitution device to mix the powder and the diluent. A reconstitution device is a sterile implement containing two needles that connects the vial and the 50-mL bag. It enables the nurse to dilute the powder and place it in the IV bag without using a syringe (Fig. 8-6). Some manufacturers now enclose this device with the IV bag. Once the powder is reconstituted, label the IV bag.

Medication Added	
Patient *Tom Smith*	Room *1503*
Date *cefazolin 1 g*	Flow Rate *17 gtt/min*
Base solution *50 mL D5W*	Initials *RT*
Time to Run *12 NOON–12:30 PM*	Date *6/14*

Note that the Time to Run is 12 NOON to 12:30 PM. Why? The order was q6h (6 AM–12 NOON, 6 PM–12 MIDNIGHT) and the time of infusion was 30 minutes.

It is time-consuming to look through package inserts for directions. Drug references such as *Lippincott's Nursing Drug Guide* provide concise information.

Example   Order: vancomycin 1 g IVPB 7 AM

Supply: 500 mg powder

Package insert directions: 250 mL (1 g)/D5W

Run over 2 hours (1 g). Refrigerate for 7 days.

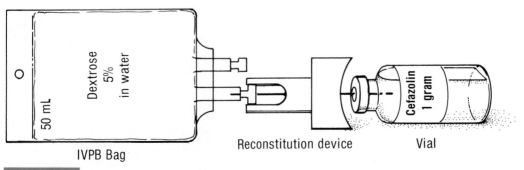

IVPB Bag   Reconstitution device   Vial

FIGURE 8-6

Reconstitution device. The IVPB bag is squeezed, forcing fluid into the vial of powder, which is then diluted. The three parts are turned to a vertical position—vial up, IVPB bag down. The IVPB bag is squeezed and released. This creates a negative pressure, allowing the diluted medication to flow into the IVPB bag.

Rule: $\frac{\#mL \times TF}{\#min} = gtt/min$

$$\frac{250 \times 10}{120} = \frac{250}{12} \overline{)250.0}^{20.8} = 21$$

Use a reconstitution device to add 1 g vancomycin (two vials of 500 mg) to 250 mL D5W. Label the IV. Set the rate at 21 gtt/min. The IVPB will run 2 hours.

SELF-TEST 4   IVPB Drip Factors

Solve these drip factors for IVPB problems. Answers are given at the end of this chapter.

1. Order: acyclovir 500 mg IVPB q8h
   Supply: 500 mg powder
   Package directions: 100 mL/D5W. Infuse 1 hour/once a day
   Available: macrodrip tubing at 10 gtt/mL

2. Order: ceftazidime 1 g IVPB q12h
   Supply: 1 g powder
   Package directions: 50 mL (1 g)/D5W. Infuse in 15–30 minutes/store for 7 days
                              (REFRIGERATED)
   Available: macrodrip tubing at 10 gtt/mL

3. Order: cefotaxime 1 g IVPB q6h
   Supply: 1 g powder
   Package directions: 50 mL (1 g)/D5W. Infuse in 15–30 minutes/store for 5 days
                              (REFRIGERATED)
   Available: macrodrip tubing at 10 gtt/mL

4. Order: Ampicillin 500 mg IV q6h
   Supply: 2 g in 5 mL
   Package directions: 50 mL (500 mg)/D5W. Infuse in 15–30 minutes
   Available: microdrip tubing at 60 gtt/mL

5. Order: tobromycin 50 mg IV q8h
   Supply: 80 mg in 2 mL
   Package directions: 100 mL (50 mg)/D5W. Infuse in 60 minutes
   Available: macrodrip tubing at 15 gtt/mL

6. Order: ticarcillin 500 mg IV q6h
   Supply: 1 g in 5 mL
   Package directions: 50 mL (500 mg)/D5W. Infuse in 30 minutes
   Available: macrodrip tubing at 15 gtt/mL

Admixture IVs

The institutional pharmacy may reconstitute and prepare IVPB solutions in a sterile environment using a laminar flow hood. This procedure saves nursing time: Drugs are prepared, labeled, and screened for incompatibilities. However, the nurse is not relieved of responsibility. Check the diluent and volume with guidelines. Check the dose and the expiration date of the reconstituted solution. Note whether the admixture should be refrigerated before use or whether it can remain at room temperature until hung. The nurse must calculate the drip rate and record this information on the IVPB label before hanging the bag.

Changing the Intravenous Drip Rate

Setting the drip rate for an IV does not relieve the nurse of the responsibility to check the IV frequently. Many factors can interfere with the flow—kinking of the tube, movement of the client, the effect of gravity, or placement of the needle or catheter. If a discrepancy in flow exists, it may be necessary to recalculate the IV drip.

Example

As you make rounds, you check a client's IV. The label reads:

1000 mL D5W IV to run 8 AM–4 PM *8 hours*

The tubing is macrodrip (10 gtt/mL). Rate is set at 20 gtt/min.

It is now 1 PM. You note that there is 600 mL left in the IV. Should you change the drip?

Logic: **Step 1.** Calculate how many milliliters per hour.

$$\frac{1000}{8} = 125 \text{ mL/hr}$$

Step 2. It is now 1 PM. Therefore 5 hours have elapsed since the IV was started.

125 ml/hr
$\times 5$
625 mL should have been delivered.

Step 3. Because there are 600 mL left in the IV, only 400 mL were delivered.

625 mL should have been delivered
− 400 mL were delivered
225 mL behind

1000 mL
5% Dextrose
—0 —1 —2 —3 —4 —5 —6 —7 —8 —9

Conclusion: The nurse will have to make a judgment about whether to increase the IV drip on the basis of an assessment of the client's status. It may be necessary to consult with the physician or healthcare provider.

Recording Intake

An accurate account must be kept of parenteral intake as well as liquids taken orally and/or enterally (eg, tube feedings). Each institution will provide a flow sheet to record fluid input over a period of time specified. Usually when an IVPB is infusing, the primary IV stops infusing. After the IVPB is completed, the primary IV flow rate begins again. (Refer to Fig. 8-5.)

SELF-TEST 5 **Fluid Intake**

Answer the following questions regarding fluid intake. Answers are given at the end of this chapter.

1. A total of 900 mL of an IV solution is to infuse at 100 mL/hr. If it is 9 AM when the infusion starts, at what time will it be completed?

2. A patient is receiving an antibiotic IVPB in 75 mL q6h to run over 1 hour plus a maintenance IV of 125 mL/hr. What is the 24-hour intake parenterally?

3. An IV of 1000 mL D5NS is infusing at 10 microdrips per minute. What is the parenteral intake for 8 hours?

4. A doctor orders 500 mL aminophylline 0.5 g to infuse at 50 mL/hr. How many mg will the patient receive each hour?

5. A total of 20,000 units of heparin is added to 500 mL D5W, and the order is to infuse IV at 30 mL/hr. How many hours will the IV run?

6. A patient is receiving an antibiotic IVPB in 50 mL q8h to run over 1 hour plus a maintenance IV of 100 mL/hr. What is the 24-hour intake parenterally?

7. A total of 500 mL of an IV solution is to infuse at 50 mL/hr. If it is 6 AM when the infusion starts, at what time is it completed?

8. IV of D5W 1000 mL is infusing at 125 mL/hr. How many hours will the IV run?

9. A patient is receiving an antibiotic IVPB in 250 mL q6h. What is the 24-hour intake parenterally?

10. A physician orders 100 units regular insulin in 100 mL to infuse at 10 mL/hr. How many units will the patient receive each hour?

Solve these problems related to intravenous and IVPB drip rates. Aim for a high degree of accuracy. Answers are given at the end of the chapter. Review material that you find difficult.

1. Order: 1500 mL D5W 8 AM–8 PM
   Available: macrodrip tubing (10 gtt/mL)
   What is the drip rate?

2. Order: 250 mL D5 ½ NS IV KVO (give over 12 hours)
   Available: microdrip tubing
   What is the drip rate?

3. Order: 150 mL D5 ⅓ NS IV; run 20 mL/hr
   Available: infusion pump
   a. What is the drip rate?
   b. How long will the IV last?

4. Order: 1000 mL D5NS with 15 mEq KCl IV; run 100 mL/hr
   Available: macrotubing (20 gtt/mL) and microdrip
   a. How many hours will this run?
   b. How many milliliters of KCl will you add to the IV if KCl comes in a vial labeled 40 mEq/20 mL?
   c. What tubing will you use?
   d. What are the gtt/min?

5. Order: aminophylline 1 g in 500 mL D5W IV at 75 mL/hr
   Available: vial of aminophylline 1 g in 10 mL; infusion pump
   a. How many mL of aminophylline should be added to the IV?
   b. How will you set the drip rate?

6. Order: amikacin 0.4 g IVPB q8h
   Supply: 2-mL vial labeled 250 mg/mL
   Package directions: 100 mL/D5W 30 minutes
   Available: macrodrip tubing 10 gtt/mL
   a. How many mL of amikacin should be added to the IV?
   b. What are the gtt/min?

7. Order: 500 mL D5 1/2 NS IV q8h
   Available: microdrip tubing
   What are the gtt/min?

8. Order: 1000 mL D5W IV q24h
   Available: macrodrip tubing (15 gtt/mL)
   What is the drip rate?

9. Order: Heparin 25,000 units in 250 mL NS at 20 mL/hr
   How long will the IV last?

10. Order: 500 mL NS over 4 h
    Available: macrodrip tubing (20 gtt/mL)
    What is the drip rate?

IV Problems

Solve these problems related to drip rates. Answers are given at the end of this chapter.

1. Order: aqueous penicillin G 1 milliunits in 100 mL D5W IVPB q6h over 40 minutes
(macrodrip tubing at 10 gtt/mL)
   Supply: vial labeled 5 million units of powder. Directions say to inject 18 mL sterile water
for injection to yield 20 mL solution. Reconstituted solution is stable for 1 week.
   a. How would you prepare the penicillin?
   b. What solution will you make?
   c. What amount of penicillin solution should be placed into the bag of 100 mL D5W?
   d. What is the drip factor for the IVPB?

2. A total of 1000 mL of an IV solution is to infuse at 100 mL/hr. If the infusion starts at 8 AM, at what time will it be completed?

3. Order: gentamicin 60 mg IVPB in 50 mL D5W over 30 minutes using macrodrip
(20 gtt/mL)
   Supply: vial of gentamicin 40 mg/mL; 50-mL bag of D5W; order is correct
   a. How many mL of gentamicin will you add to the 50-mL bag of D5W?
   b. What is the drip factor for the IVPB?

4. Calculate the drip factor for 1500 mL D5 1/2 NS to run 12 hours by macrodrip (10 gtt/mL).

5. Intralipid, 500 mL q6h, is ordered for a patient together with a primary IV that is infusing at 80 mL/hr. Calculate the 24-hour parenteral intake. (Total will be amount of lipids plus primary IV amount.)

6. Order: 1000 mL D5W with 20 mEq KCl and 500 mg vitamin C at 60 mL/hr. No infusion
pump is available.

   a. Approximately how many hours will the IV run?
   b. Which tubing will you choose—macrodrip at 10 gtt/mL or microdrip at 60 gtt/mL?
   c. What are the drops per minute for the tubing that you choose?

Name: _____

There are 10 questions related to IV and IVPB calculations. If you have any difficulty doing these problems, review the material in Chapter 8 that explains this information. Answers are given on page 429.

1. Order: 1000 mL D5NS; run 150 mL/hr IV
   Supply: IV bag of 1000 mL D5NS

   a. Approximately how many hours will the IV run?
   b. Which tubing will you choose—macrodrip (10 gtt/mL) or microdrip (60 gtt/mL)?
   c. What will be the drip rate?

2. Order: 100 mL Ringer's solution 12 NOON–6 PM IV

   a. What size tubing will you use?
   b. What are the gtt/min?

3. Order: 150 mL NS IV over 3 hours
   Supply: bag of 250 mL normal saline for IV and macrotubing, 15 gtt/mL; microtubing, 60 gtt/mL

   a. What would you do to obtain 150 mL NS?
   b. What IV tubing would you use?
   c. What are the gtt/min?

4. Order: 500 mL D5W IVKVO. Solve for 24 hours. An infusion pump is available. What should be the setting on the infusion pump?

5. Order: doxycycline 100 mg IVPB qd
   Supply: 100 mg powder
   Package directions: 250 mL/D5W to infuse over 1 hour; macrodrip tubing 10 gtt/mL

   a. State the amount and type of IV fluid you will use and the time for infusion you will use.
   b. What are the gtt/min?

6. Order: aminophylline 500 mg in 250 mL D5W to run 8 hours IV
   Available: vial of aminophylline labeled 1 g in 10 mL; microdrip tubing
   a. How much aminophylline is needed?
   b. What is the drip rate?

7. A patient is receiving a primary IV at the rate of 125 mL/hr. The doctor orders cefoxitin 1 g in 75 mL D5W q6h to run over 1 hour
   Calculate the 24-hour parenteral intake.

8. Order: 1000 mL D5 1/2 NS to run at 90 mL/hr; infusion pump available

   a. What will be the pump setting?
   b. Approximately how long will the IV run?

9. A doctor orders 500 mL aminophylline 0.5 g to infuse at 50 mL/hr. How many milligrams will the patient receive each hour?

10. Order: Bactrim 5 mL IVPB q6h
    Supply: vial of 5 mL; one 5-mL vial per 75 mL D5W run over 60 to 90 minutes.
    The main IV line is connected to an infusion pump. What will you do? Refer to Figure 8-4 on p. 208.

    a. State the type and amount of IV fluid you would use and the time for infusion.
    b. How would you program the infusion pump?

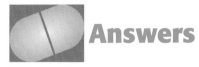

Answers

Self-Test 1 Calculation of Drip Factors

1. Logic: This is a continuous IV of 150 mL every 8 hours. There is a pump available. You only need step 1. It will run 8 hours.

$$\frac{\#\,mL}{\#\,hr} = mL/hr \qquad \frac{150\ mL}{8} \quad \begin{array}{r} 18.7\ mL/hr \\ 8\overline{)150.0} \\ \underline{8} \\ 70 \\ \underline{64} \\ 6\,0 \\ \underline{5\,6} \end{array}$$

Label the IV. Set the pump: total # mL = 150; mL/hr = 19.

2. Logic: This is a continuous IV. A pump is available. The order states mL/hr. There is no calculation needed. Label the IV. Set the pump as follows: total # mL = 250; mL/hr = 25.

3. Logic: The order gives 100 mL/hr; mL/hr = gtt/min microdrip, so you know the microdrip is 100 gtt/min. Work out the macrodrip factor and choose the tubing. You need step 2.

Macrodrip

Step 2. $\frac{mL/hr \times TF}{\#\,min} = gtt/min$

$$\frac{100 \times \overset{1}{\cancel{20}}}{\underset{3}{\cancel{60}}} = \frac{100}{3} = 33.3$$

Macrodrip at 33 gtt/min

Microdrip at 100 gtt/min

Either drip rate could be used. Label the IV.

4. Logic: This is a small volume over several hours; use microdrip. Macrodrip would be too slow (5 gtt/min).

Step 1. $\frac{\#\,mL}{\#\,hr} = mL/hr \qquad \frac{\overset{30}{\cancel{180}}}{\underset{1}{\cancel{6}}} = 30\ mL/hr$

Step 2. $\frac{mL/hr \times TF}{\#\,min} = gtt/min$

Microdrip is 30 gtt/min because mL/hr = gtt/min.

5. Logic: This is a large volume over several hours; use macrodrip. Solve using two steps and decide.

Step 1. $\frac{\#\,mL}{\#\,hr} = mL/hr \qquad \frac{\overset{125}{\cancel{1000}}}{\underset{1}{\cancel{8}}} = 125\ mL/hr$

Step 2. $\frac{mL/hr \times TF}{\#\,min} = gtt/min$

You know microdrip will be 125 gtt/min because mL/hr = gtt/min.

Macrodrip

$$\frac{125 \times \overset{1}{\cancel{15}}}{\underset{4}{\cancel{60}}} = \frac{\cancel{125}}{4} \quad \begin{array}{r} 31.2 \\ 4\overline{)125.0} \\ \underline{12} \\ 5 \\ \underline{4} \\ 1\,0 \\ \underline{8} \end{array}$$

Macrodrip at 31 gtt/min

Microdrip at 125 gtt/min

Use macrodrip.

Label the IV.

6. Logic: This is a continuous IV of 250 mL every 8 hours. There is a pump available. You only need step 1. It will run 8 hours.

$$\frac{\#\,mL}{\#\,hr} = mL/hr \qquad \frac{250\ mL}{8} \quad \begin{array}{r} 31.2\ mL/hr \\ 8\overline{)250.0} \\ \underline{24} \\ 10 \\ \underline{8} \\ 2.0 \end{array}$$

Label the IV. Set the pump: total # mL = 250; mL/hr = 31.

7. Logic: This is a continuous IV of 500 mL over 2 hours. There is a pump available. You only need step 1

It will run 2 hours.

$$\frac{\#\,mL}{\#\,hr} = mL/hr \qquad \frac{500\ mL}{2} \quad \begin{array}{r} 250.0\ mL/hr \\ 2\overline{)500.0} \\ \underline{4} \\ 10 \\ \underline{10} \\ 0 \end{array}$$

Label the IV. Set the pump: total # mL = 500; mL/hr = 250.

8. Logic: This is a large volume over several hours; use macrodrip. Solve using two steps.

Step 1. $\dfrac{\# \text{ mL}}{\# \text{ hr}} = \text{mL/hr}$

$$\begin{array}{r} 83.3 \text{ mL} \\ 12 \overline{)1000.0} \\ \underline{96} \\ 40 \\ \underline{36} \\ 40 \end{array}$$

Step 2. $\dfrac{\# \text{ mL/hr} \times \text{TF}}{\# \text{ min}} = \text{gtt/min}$

$$\dfrac{83 \times \overset{1}{\cancel{15}}}{\underset{4}{\cancel{60}}} = \dfrac{83}{4} \quad \begin{array}{r} 20.7 \\ 4 \overline{)83.0} \\ \underline{8} \\ 3 \\ \underline{0} \\ 3\,0 \end{array}$$

Macrodrip at 21 gtt/min, microdrip at 83 gtt/min
Label the IV.

9. Logic: This is a large volume at a fast rate. Use macrodrip. Solve using step 2 only.

$$\dfrac{\# \text{ mL/hr} \times \text{TF}}{\# \text{ min}} = \text{gtt/min}$$

$$\dfrac{150 \times \overset{1}{\cancel{10}}}{\underset{6}{\cancel{60}}} = \dfrac{150}{6} \quad \begin{array}{r} 25.0 \text{ gtt/min} \\ 6 \overline{)150.0} \\ \underline{12} \\ 30 \\ \underline{30} \\ 0 \end{array}$$

Macrodrip at 25 gtt/min, microdrip at 150 gtt/min
Label the IV.

10. Logic: This is a large volume over a short time. Use macrodrip tubing. The rate is 150 mL/hr (150 mL over 1 hour). Use step 2 only.

$$\dfrac{\# \text{ mL/hr} \times \text{TF}}{\# \text{ min}} = \text{gtt/min}$$

$$\dfrac{150 \times \overset{1}{\cancel{20}}}{\underset{3}{\cancel{60}}} = \dfrac{150}{3} \quad \begin{array}{r} 50 \text{ gtt/min} \\ 3 \overline{)150.0} \\ \underline{15} \\ 0 \end{array}$$

Macrodrip at 50 gtt/min, microdrip at 150 gtt/min
Label the IV.

Self-Test 2 IV Infusions—Hours

1. 8.3 hours approximately
2. 8.3 hours approximately
3. 10 hours (no math)
4. 24 hours (no math)
5. 7.1 hours approximately
6. 10 hours (no math)
7. 10 hours (no math)
8. 2.5 hours
9. 6 hours (no math)
10. 5 hours (no math)

Self-Test 3 IV Infusion Rates

1. Logic: You want vitamin C 500 mg and the supply is 500 mg in 2 mL. Use a syringe to add the 2 mL to 500 mL D5W. You have microdrip available. The IV is to run at 60 mL/hr. Remember mL/hr = gtt/min for microdrip. No math necessary. Set the microdrip at 60 gtt/min. Label the IV.

2. Logic: You want 250 mg hydrocortisone sodium succinate, and it comes 250 mg with a 2-mL diluent. Use a syringe to reconstitute the hydrocortisone with 2 mL diluent and add it to the IV. 8 AM–12 MIDNIGHT is 16 hours. Solve using two steps.

Step 1. $\dfrac{\# \text{ mL}}{\# \text{ hr}} = \text{mL/hr}$

$$\dfrac{1000}{16} \quad \begin{array}{r} 62.5 \\ 16 \overline{)1000.0} \\ \underline{96} \\ 40 \\ \underline{32} \\ 8\,0 \\ \underline{8\,0} \end{array} = 63 \text{ mL/hr}$$

Step 2. mL/hr = gtt/min for microdrip. No math for microdrip. Microdrip = 63 gtt/min.
Label the IV.

3. Logic: You want 250 mg aminophylline. Supply is 500 mg/10 mL.

Formula Method

$\frac{D}{H} \times S = A$ $\frac{250 \text{ mg}}{500 \text{ mg}} \times 10 \text{ mL} = 5 \text{ mL}$

Ratio Method

10mL : 500 mg :: x mL : 250 mg

Proportion Method

$\frac{10 \text{ mL}}{500 \text{ mg}} = \frac{x}{250 \text{ mg}}$

$\frac{2500}{500} = x$

$5 = x$

Add 5 mL aminophylline to 250 mL D5W. Order is 50 mL/hr. You have an infusion pump. No math. Set the pump as follows: total # mL = 250; mL/hr = 50.

4. Logic: You want KCl 10 mEq. Supply is 20 mEq/10 mL.

Formula Method

$\frac{D}{H} \times S = A$ $\frac{10 \text{ mEq}}{20 \text{ mEq}} \times 10 \text{ mL} = 5 \text{ mL}$

Ratio Method

10 mL : 10 mEq :: x mL : 20 mEq

Proportion Method

$\frac{10 \text{ mL}}{20 \text{ mEq}} = \frac{x}{10 \text{ mEq}}$

$\frac{100}{20} = x$

$5 \text{ mL} = x$

Add 5 mL KCl to 250 mL D5W½NS. 12 NOON–6 PM is 6 hours. One step is needed because you have microdrip tubing.

$\frac{\# \text{ mL}}{\# \text{ hr}} = \text{mL/hr}$ $\frac{250}{6}$ $6 \overline{)250.0}$ = 42 mL/hr   41.6

$\underline{24}$

10

$\underline{6}$

4 0

$\underline{3\ 6}$

mL/hr = gtt/min microdrip

Set the microdrip at 42 gtt/min.

Label the IV.

Self-Test 4 IVPB Drip Factors

1. Logic: acyclovir comes in 500 mg powder. Use a reconstitution device to add the powder to 100 mL D5W; # min = 60; TF = 10 gtt/mL for IVPB.

   Rule: $\frac{\text{\# mL} \times \text{TF}}{\text{\# min}} = \text{gtt/min}$

   $$\frac{100 \times 10}{60} = \frac{100}{6} \quad 6\overline{)100.0}\,{}^{16.6} = 17 \text{ gtt/min}$$

   Label the IVPB.

   Set the rate at 17 gtt/min.

2. Logic: ceftazidime comes in a 1-g powder

   Use a reconstitution device to add the powder to 50 mL D5W; # min, 30; TF, 10 gtt/mL for IVPB

   Rule: $\frac{\text{\# mL} \times \text{TF}}{\text{\# min}} = \text{gtt/min}$

   $$\frac{50 \times 10}{30} = \frac{50}{3} = 16.6 = 17 \text{ gtt/min}$$

   Label the IVPB.

   Set the rate at 17 gtt/min.

3. Logic: cefotaxime comes as a 1-g powder

   Use a reconstitution device to add the powder to 50 mL D5W; # min, 30; TF, 10 gtt/mL for IVPB

   Rule: $\frac{\text{\# mL} \times \text{TF}}{\text{\# min}} = \text{gtt/min}$

   $$\frac{50 \times 10}{30} = 16.6 = 17\text{gtt/min}$$

   Label the IVPB

   Set the rate at 17 gtt/min.

4. Logic: ampicillin comes as a 2-g powder.

   Reconstitute in 4.5 mL diluent = total volume 5 mL (2 g = 5 mL, 2000 mg = 5 mL)

   Formula Method

   $\frac{500 \text{ mg}}{2000 \text{ mg}} \times 5 \text{ mL} = 1.25 \text{ mL}$

   Ratio Method

   5 mL : 2000 mg : : x mL : 500 mg

   Proportion Method

   $\frac{5 \text{ mL}}{2000 \text{ mg}} = \frac{\text{x}}{500 \text{ mg}}$

   $\frac{2500}{2000} = \text{x}$

   $1.25 \text{ mL} = \text{x}$

   Add 1.25 mL to 50 mL D5W. Total min = 30; TF = 60 gtt/mL.

   $\frac{\text{\# mL} \times \text{TF}}{\text{\# min}} = \text{gtt/min}$

   $$\frac{50 \times \overset{2}{60}}{\underset{1}{30}} = 100 \text{ gtt/min}$$

   Label the IVPB.

   Set the rate at 100 gtt/min.

5. Logic: tobramycin comes as 80-mg. Reconstitute in 2 mL diluent = 2 mL (80 mg = 2 mL)

Formula Method

$\dfrac{50 \text{ mg}}{80 \text{ mg}} \times 2 \text{ mL} = 1.25 \text{ mL}$

Ratio Method

2 mL : 80 mg : : x mL : 50 mg

Proportion Method

$\dfrac{2 \text{ mL}}{80 \text{ mg}} = \dfrac{x}{50 \text{ mg}}$

$\dfrac{100}{80} = x$

$1.25 \text{ mL} = x$

Add 1.25 mL to 100 mL D5W.

Total # min = 60; TF = 15 gtt/mL

$\dfrac{\# \text{ mL} \times \text{TF}}{\# \text{ min}} = \text{gtt/min}$

$\dfrac{100 \times \overset{1}{\cancel{15}}}{\underset{4}{\cancel{60}}} = 25 \text{ gtt/min}$

Label the IVPB.

Set the rate at 50 gtt/min.

6. Logic: ticarcillin comes as a 1-g powder. Reconstitute in 4.5 mL of diluent = 5 mL (1 g or 1000 mg = 5 mL)

Formula Method

$\dfrac{500 \text{ mg}}{1000 \text{ mg}} \times 5 \text{ mL} = 2.5 \text{ mL}$

Ratio Method

5 mL : 1000 mg : : x mL : 500 mg

Proportion Method

$\dfrac{5 \text{ mL}}{1000 \text{ mg}} = \dfrac{x}{500 \text{ mg}}$

$\dfrac{2500}{1000} = x$

$2.5 \text{ mL} = x$

Add 2.5 mL to 50 mL D5W.

Total min, 30; TF, 15 gtt/mL

$\dfrac{\# \text{ mL} \times \text{TF}}{\# \text{ min}} = \text{gtt/min}$

$\dfrac{50 \times \overset{1}{\cancel{15}}}{\underset{2}{\cancel{30}}} = 25 \text{ gtt/min}$

Self-Test 5 Fluid Intake

1. Logic: 900 mL at 100 mL/hr = 9 hours to run. If the IV starts at 9 AM, + 9 hours = 6 PM.

2. Logic: IVPB is 75 mL q6h or four times in 24 hours

   75
   × 4
   300 mL

   The patient is receiving 125 mL for 20 hours (24 hours − 4 hours that the IVPB is running).

   125
   × 20
   000
   250
   2500 mL

   2500 mL
   + 300 mL
   2800 mL in 24 hours

3. Logic: IV is infusing at 10 microdrips/min. It takes 60 microdrips to make 1 mL., so 1 mL in 6 min, 10 mL in 60 min.

   10 mL in 60 min (1 hr)
   $\times$ 8 hr
   _____
   80 mL in 8 hr

4. Logic: The IV is 0.5 g or 500 mg in 500 mL. This is equal to 1 mg/mL. The patient receives 50 mL/hr, so the patient receives 50 mg each hour.

5. Logic: The IV is infusing at 30 mL/hr and the solution is 500 mL.

$$\frac{500 \text{ mL}}{30 \text{ mL/hr}} = \frac{50}{3} = 16.6 \text{ hours (approximately)}$$

6. Logic: IVPB 50 mL q8h or three times in 24 hours

   50
   $\times$ 3
   _____
   150 mL

   The patient is receiving 100 mL for 21 hours (24 hours − 3 hours that the IVPB is running).

   100
   $\times$ 21
   _____
   100
   + 200
   _____
   2100 mL

   2100 mL
   + 150 mL
   _____
   2250 mL in 24 hours

7. Logic: 500 mL at 50 mL/hr = 10 hours to run. If the IV starts at 6 AM + 10 hours = 4 PM.

8. Logic: The IV is infusing at 125 mL/hr and the solution is 1000 mL.

$$\frac{1000 \text{ mL}}{125 \text{ mL/hr}} = 8 \text{ hours}$$

9. Logic: IVPB is 250 mL q6h or four times in 24 hours

   250
   $\times$ 4
   _____
   1000 mL in 24 hours

10. Logic: The IV is 100 units in 100 mL or 1 unit/mL. The patient receives 10 mL/hr so the patient receives 10 units/hr.

Self-Test 6 IV Drip Rates

1. $\frac{\text{\# mL}}{\text{\# hr}} = \text{mL/hr}$

$$\frac{1500}{12} \quad 12\overline{)1500.} = 125 \text{ mL/hr}$$

   125.
   12
   ___
   30
   24
   ___
   60
   60

Macrodrip

$$\frac{\# mL/hr \times TF}{\# min} = gtt/min \qquad \frac{125 \times 10}{60} = \frac{125}{6} \quad \begin{array}{r} 20.8 \\ 6 \overline{)125.0} \\ \underline{12} \\ 5\,0 \\ \underline{4\,8} \end{array}$$

$= 21$ gtt/min

2. $\frac{\# mL}{\# hr} = mL/hr \qquad \frac{250}{12} \quad \begin{array}{r} 20.8 \\ 12 \overline{)250.0} = 21 \text{ ml/hr} \\ \underline{24} \\ 10\,0 \\ \underline{9\,6} \end{array}$

    \# mL/hr $\times$ TF = gtt/min 21 $\times$ 60 = 21 gtt/min

    You could also say mL/hr = gtt/min microdrip, so 21 mL/hr = 21 gtt/min.

3. $\frac{150 \text{ mL}}{20 \text{ mL/hr}} = \frac{15}{2} \quad \begin{array}{r} 7.5 \text{ hr} \\ 2 \overline{)15.0 \text{ hr}} \end{array}$

    a. The drip rate is 20 mL/hr. No math is necessary. Set the infusion pump.

    b. The IV will last approximately 7½ hours.

4. **a.** $\frac{\overset{10}{1000} \text{ mL}}{100 \text{ mL/hr}} = 10 \text{ hr}$

    b.

Formula Method	*Ratio Method*	*Proportion Method*
$\frac{D}{H} \times S = A$	20 mL : 40 mEq : : x mL : 15 mEq	$\frac{20 \text{ mL}}{40 \text{ mEq}} = \frac{x}{15 \text{ mEq}}$
$\frac{15 \text{ mEq}}{\underset{2}{40} \text{ mEq}} \times \overset{1}{20} \text{ mL} = \frac{15}{2} = 7.5 \text{ mL}$		$\frac{300}{40} = 7.5 \text{ mL}$

    c. Microdrip

    Order states to run at 100 mL/hr. mL/hr = gtt/min microdrip, so microdrip at 100 gtt/min.

    Macrodrip

    $\frac{100 \times \overset{1}{20}}{\underset{3}{60}} = \frac{100}{3} = 33 \text{ gtt/min}$

    Choose either tubing.

    d. 33 gtt/min macrodrip: 100 gtt/min microdrip

5. **a.** You desire 1 g. Aminophylline comes 1 g in 10 mL. Add 10 mL to the IV of 500 mL D5W and label.

    b. You have an infusion pump; there is no math.

    Set the pump:

    total \# mL = 500; mL/hr = 75

6. $0.4 \text{ g} = 400 \text{ mg}$

| *Formula Method* | *Ratio Method* | *Proportion Method* |

$\frac{D}{H} \times S = A$

$1 \text{ mL} : 250 \text{ mg} :: x \text{ mL} : 400 \text{ mg}$

$\dfrac{\overset{8}{400} \text{ mg}}{\underset{5}{250} \text{ mg}} \times 1 \text{ mL}$

$\dfrac{1 \text{ mL}}{250 \text{ mg}} = \dfrac{x}{400 \text{ mg}}$

$\frac{400}{250} = x$

1.6 mL

$\dfrac{\cancel{8}}{5} \overset{1.6 \text{ mL}}{\big) 8.0}$

Add 1.6 mL amikacin to 100 mL D5W.

TF = 10 gtt/mL for IVPB. Total min, 30

$\dfrac{\# \text{ mL} \times \text{TF}}{\# \text{ min}} = \text{gtt/min}$

$\dfrac{100 \text{ mL} \times \cancel{10}}{\cancel{30}} = \dfrac{100}{3} = 33.3$

$= 33 \text{ gtt/min}$

Label the IV.

Set the rate at 33 gtt/min.

7. $\dfrac{\# \text{ mL}}{\# \text{ hr}} = \text{mL/hr}$ $\dfrac{500}{8}$ $\overset{62.5}{\big) 500.0} = 63 \text{ mL/hr}$

$\dfrac{48}{20}$

$\dfrac{16}{4\,0}$

$\underline{4\,0}$

You are using microdrip tubing, so mL/hr = gtt/min. Set the rate at 63 gtt/min.

8. $\dfrac{\# \text{ mL}}{\# \text{ hr}} = \text{mL/hr}$ $\dfrac{1000}{24}$ $\overset{41.6}{\big) 1000.0} = 42 \text{ mL/hr}$

$\dfrac{96}{40}$

$\dfrac{24}{16\,0}$

$\dfrac{\# \text{ mL/hr} \times \text{TF}}{\# \text{ min}} = \text{gtt/min}$ $\dfrac{42 \times \overset{1}{\cancel{15}}}{\underset{4}{\cancel{60}}} = 11 \text{ gtt/min}$

9. $\dfrac{250 \text{ mL}}{20 \text{ mL/hr}} = \dfrac{250}{20}$ $\overset{12.5}{\big) 250.0}$

$\dfrac{20}{50}$

$\dfrac{40}{10\,0}$

The IV will last 12.5 hours.

10. $\dfrac{\#\ mL}{\#\ hr} = mL/hr$ $\quad \dfrac{\cancel{500}}{4}\ \ \begin{array}{r} 125 \\ \overline{)500} \\ \underline{4} \\ 10 \\ \underline{8} \\ 20 \end{array} = 125\ mL/hr$

$\dfrac{\#\ mL/hr \times TF}{\#\ min} = gtt/min \qquad \dfrac{125 \times \overset{1}{\cancel{20}}}{\underset{3}{\cancel{60}}} = \dfrac{125}{3} = 42\ gtt/min$

Self-Test 7 IV Problems

1. **a.** Add 18 mL sterile water for injection to the vial of 5 million units.

   b. Solution is 5 milliunits/20 mL.

   c. You want 1 milliunit.

Formula Method

$\dfrac{D}{H} \times S = A$

$\dfrac{1\ milliunit}{5\ milliunit} \times \overset{4}{\cancel{20}}\ mL = 4\ mL$

Ratio Method

20 mL : 5 milliunits : : x mL : 1 milliunit

Proportion Method

$\dfrac{20\ mL}{5\ milliunits} = \dfrac{x}{1}$

$\dfrac{20}{5} = 4\ mL$

   d. $\dfrac{\#\ mL \times TF}{\#\ min} = gtt/min \qquad \dfrac{\overset{25}{\cancel{100}}\ mL \times \cancel{10}}{\underset{1}{\cancel{40}}} = 25\ gtt/min$

2. Logic: 1000 mL is infusing at 100 mL/hr, so the IV will take

   $\dfrac{\overset{10}{\cancel{1000}}}{\underset{1}{\cancel{100}}} = 10$ hours to complete.

   If it starts at 8 AM, it should finish 10 hours later at 6 PM.

3. **a.**

Formula Method

$\dfrac{D}{S} \times S = A$

$\dfrac{\overset{3}{\cancel{60}}\ mg}{\underset{2}{\cancel{40}}\ mg} \times 1\ mL$

$\dfrac{3}{2} = 1.5\ mL$

Ratio Method

1 mL : 40 mg : : x mL : 60 mg

Proportion Method

$\dfrac{1\ mL}{40\ mg} = \dfrac{x\ mL}{60\ mg}$

$\dfrac{60}{40} = x$

1.5 mL

   Add 1.5 mL gentamicin.

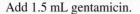

b. $\dfrac{\# \text{ mL} \times \text{TF}}{\# \text{ min}} = \text{gtt/min}$

$$\dfrac{50 \text{ mL} \times 20}{30} = \dfrac{100}{3} \quad \begin{array}{r} 33.3 \\ 3\overline{)100.00} \end{array} = 33 \text{ gtt/min}$$

4. Step 1. $\dfrac{\# \text{ mL}}{\# \text{ hr}} = \text{mL/hr}$

$$\dfrac{1500}{12} \quad \begin{array}{r} 125. \\ 12\overline{)1500.} \\ \underline{12} \\ 30 \\ \underline{24} \\ 60 \\ \underline{60} \end{array} = 125 \text{ mL/hr}$$

Step 2. $\dfrac{\# \text{ mL/hr} \times \text{TF}}{60} = \text{gtt/min}$

$$\dfrac{125 \times 10}{60} = \dfrac{125}{6} \quad \begin{array}{r} 20.8 \\ 6\overline{)125.0} \\ \underline{12} \\ 5\,0 \\ \underline{4\,8} \end{array} = 21 \text{ gtt/min}$$

5. Logic: Intralipid 500 mL q6h means the patient is receiving 500 mL four times every 24 hours

$$\begin{array}{r} 500 \\ \times\ 4 \\ \hline 2000 \text{ mL} \end{array}$$

The IV is infusing 80 mL/hr. There are 24 hours in a day, so

$$\begin{array}{r} 24 \\ \times\ 80 \\ \hline 1920 \end{array}$$

Adding these we have
$$\begin{array}{r} 2000 \text{ mL} \\ +1920 \text{ mL} \\ \hline 3920 \text{ mL} \end{array}$$

6. a. You have 1000 mL running at 60 mL/hr, therefore

$$\begin{array}{r} 16.6 \\ 60\overline{)1000.0} \\ \underline{60} \\ 400 \\ \underline{360} \\ 40\,0 \end{array} = \text{approximtely } 16\,\tfrac{1}{2} \text{ hours}$$

b. Logic: If you want 60 mL/hr and use microdrip tubing, the drip factor will be 60 gtt/min:

$$\frac{\#\ mL \times TF}{60} = \frac{60 \times 60}{60} = 60 \text{ gtt/min}$$

If you use macrodrip tubing you have $\frac{60 \times 10}{60} = 10$ gtt/min.

Because the IV will run over 16 hours, choose *microdrip tubing*.

c. The drip factor will be 60 gtt/min. *Note:* It is not incorrect to choose the macrodrip at 10 gtt/min. However, because the IV will run so many hours, a good flow might help to keep the IV running.

Special Types of Intravenous Calculations

In Chapter 8 we studied rules and calculations for microdrip and macrodrip factors, the use of the infusion pump, and IVPB orders. In this chapter we consider rules and calculations for orders written in units, milliunits, milligrams, and micrograms; how to calculate the safety of doses based on kilograms of body weight and body surface area (BSA); and how orders for patient-controlled analgesia (PCA) are handled.

The dosage calculations in this chapter are medications that are mixed in IV fluids and delivered as continuous infusions. The medications must be administered via infusion pumps to ensure a correct rate and accuracy of dose (Fig. 9-1). In most hospital settings, the medications and IV solutions are prepared by the pharmacy.

▶ Medications Ordered in Units/hr or mg/hr

Patient medications may be administered as continuous IVs. Solutions for these medications are standardized to decrease the possibility of error. Check guidelines to verify dose, dilution, and rate. If any doubts exist, consult with the prescribing physician.

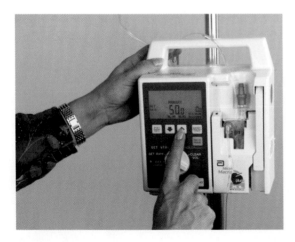

FIGURE 9-1

Infusion pump. (With permission from Evans-Smith, P. [2005]. *Taylor's clinical nursing skills.* Philadelphia: Lippincott Williams & Wilkins.)

Units/hr—Rule and Calculation

The order will indicate the amount of drug to be added to IV fluid and the flow rate in units per hour.

| Example | Order: heparin sodium 40,000 units in 1000 mL D5W IV, infuse 800 units/hr on a pump |

Logic: We know the solution and the amount to administer. Because a pump will be used, the answer will be in mL/hr.

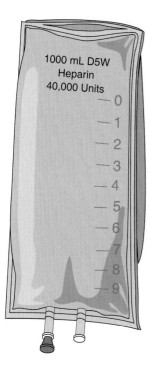

Learning Aid

An explanation of infusion pumps is given in Chapter 8.

Formula Method

Rule: $\frac{D}{H} \times S = A$

$$\frac{\overset{20}{\cancel{800 \text{ units/hr}}}}{\underset{\underset{1}{40}}{\cancel{40,000 \text{ units}}}} \times \cancel{1000} \text{ mL} =$$

20 mL/hr on a pump

Note that units cancel out and the answer is mL/hr.

How many hours will the IV run?

Rule: $\frac{\# \text{ mL}}{\# \text{ mL/hr}}$

$\frac{1000 \text{ mL}}{20 \text{ mL/hr}} = 50$ hours

Note: Most hospitals require changing the IV fluids every 24 hours.

Ratio Method

1000 mL : 40000 units : : x mL : 800 units

Proportion Method

$$\frac{x \text{ mL}}{800 \text{ units}} \times \frac{1000 \text{ mL}}{40000 \text{ units}}$$

$40,000x = 800000$

$$x = \frac{800000}{40000}$$

$x = 20$ mL/hr

Learning Aid

Desire = 800 units/hr

Have = 40,000 units

Supply = 1000 mL D5W

Example   Order: heparin sodium 1100 units/hr IV

Supply: infusion pump, standard solution of 25,000 units in 250 mL D5W

Learning Aid

Standard solutions are prepared by the pharmacy.

Learning Aid

Units cancel and the answer is mL/hr, the setting for the infusion pump.

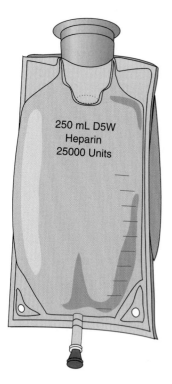

250 mL D5W
Heparin
25000 Units

Formula Method

Rule: $\frac{D}{H} \times S = A$

$\frac{1100 \text{ units/hr} \times 250 \text{ mL}}{\underset{1}{\overset{100}{\cancel{25,000 \text{ units}}}}} =$

11 mL/hr on a pump

Ratio Method

$\overset{\frown}{250 \text{ mL} : 25000 \text{ units} :: x \text{ mL} : 1100 \text{ units}}$

Proportion Method

$\frac{x \text{ mL}}{1100 \text{ units}} \times \frac{250 \text{ mL}}{25000 \text{ unit}}$

$x \text{ mL} = \frac{275000}{25000}$

$x = 11 \text{ mL/hr}$

How many hours will the IV run?

Rule: $\frac{\# \text{ mL}}{\# \text{ mL/hr}}$

$\frac{250 \text{ mL}}{11 \text{ mL/hr}} = 22.75 \text{ or } 23 \text{ hours}$

Example Order: regular insulin 10 units/hr IV

Available: infusion pump, standard solution of 125 units regular insulin in 250 mL NS

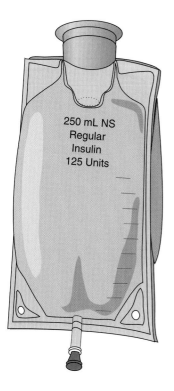

250 mL NS
Regular
Insulin
125 Units

Formula Method

Rule: $\frac{D}{H} \times S = A$

$\frac{10 \text{ units}}{125 \text{ units}} \times 250 \text{ mL}$

= 20 mL/hr on a pump

Ratio Method

250 mL : 125 units : : x mL : 10 units

Proportion Method

$\frac{x \text{ mL}}{10} \times \frac{2500}{125}$

$x \text{ mL} = \frac{2500}{125 \text{ units}}$

$x = 20 \text{ mL/hr}$

How many hours will the IV run?

Rule: $\frac{\# \text{ mL}}{\# \text{ mL/hr}}$

$\frac{250 \text{ mL}}{20 \text{ mL/hr}} = 12.5$ or approximately 13 hours

mg/hr; g/hr—Rule and Calculation

The order will indicate the amount of drug to be added to the IV fluid and the amount to administer.

There are five steps in solving mcg/min:

1. Reduce the number in the standard solution.
2. Change mg to mcg.
3. Reduce the number in the solution to mcg/1 mL.
4. Substitute 60 gtt for the mL.
5. Use the formula, ratio, or proportion method to solve for mL/hr.

Example

Order: dopamine 400 mcg/min IV

Supply: infusion pump, standard solution 400 mg in 250 mL D5W

Step 1. Reduce the numbers in the standard solution.

$$\frac{\overset{8}{\cancel{400}} \text{ mg}}{\underset{5}{\cancel{250}} \text{ mL}} = 8 \text{ mg} / 5 \text{ mL}$$

Step 2. Change mg to mcg.

8 mg = 8000 mcg
Solution is 8000 mcg/5 mL.

Step 3. Reduce number in solution to mcg/1 mL.

$$\frac{\overset{1600}{\cancel{8000}} \text{ mcg}}{\underset{1}{\cancel{5}} \text{ mL}} = 1600 \text{ mcg/mL}$$

Step 4. Substitute 60 gtt for the mL. 1600 mcg/60 gtt

Step 5. $\frac{D}{H} \times S = A$

250 mL D5W
Dopamine
400 mg

Learning Aid

D = order: 400 mcg/min

H = 1600 mcg

S = 60 gtt

Formula Method

$$\frac{\overset{1}{\cancel{400}} \text{ mcg /min}}{\underset{4}{\underset{1}{\cancel{1600}}} \text{ mcg}} \times \overset{15}{\cancel{60}} \text{ gtt} = 15 \text{ gtt microdrop}$$
$$\text{or } 15 \text{ mL/hr}$$

Ratio Method

$$60 : 1600 :: x \text{ mL} : 400$$

Proportion Method

$$\frac{x \text{ mL}}{400 \text{ mg}} \times \frac{60 \text{ gtt}}{1600 \text{ mg}}$$

$$1600x = 24000$$

$$x = \frac{24000}{1600}$$

$$x = 15 \text{ mL/hr}$$

To set the infusion pump, you must input

- Total # mL ordered

- mL/hr to run

Set the pump: total # mL = 250
(standard solutions); mL/hr = 15

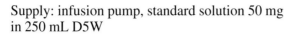

Learning Aid

When using an infusion pump,
gtt/min = mL/hr. The pump can be set
only in mL/hr.

Example

Order: aramine 60 mcg/min IV

Supply: infusion pump, standard solution 50 mg
in 250 mL D5W

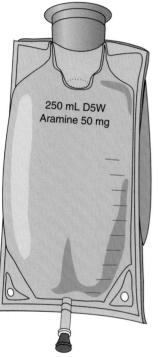

250 mL D5W
Aramine 50 mg

Step 1. Reduce the number in the standard solution.

$$\frac{\overset{1}{\cancel{50}} \text{ mg}}{\underset{5}{\cancel{250}} \text{ mL}} = 1 \text{ mg/5 mL}$$

Step 2. Change mg to mcg.

1 mg = 1000 mcg
Solution is 1000 mcg/5 mL.

Step 3. Reduce number in solution.

$$\frac{\overset{200}{\cancel{1000}} \text{ mcg}}{\underset{1}{\cancel{5}} \text{ mL}} = 200 \text{ mcg/mL}$$

Step 4. Substitute 60 gtt for the mL.

200 mcg/60 gtt

Step 5. $\frac{D}{H} \times S = A$

Learning Aid

1 mL = 60 gtt microdrip

Learning Aid

D = the order: 60 mcg/min

H = 200 mcg

S = 60 gtt

Formula Method

$$\frac{\overset{3}{\cancel{60} \text{ mcg/min}}}{\underset{1}{\cancel{200} \text{ mcg}}} \times \cancel{60} \text{ gtt} =$$

18 gtt/min = 18 mL/hr

Ratio Method

$$60 : 200 :: x \text{ mL} : 60 \text{ mg}$$

Proportion Method

$$\frac{x \text{ mL}}{60 \text{ mg}} \times \frac{60 \text{ gtt}}{200 \text{ mcg}}$$

$$200x = 3600$$

$$x = \frac{3600}{200}$$

$$x = 18 \text{mL/hr}$$

Set the pump: total # mL = 250 (standard solutions); mL/hr = 18

mcg/kg/min—Rule and Calculation

Example   Order: dopamine 2 mcg/kg/min

Supply: infusion pump, standard solution 200 mg in 250 mL D5W; client weighs 176 lb

Note that this order is somewhat different. We are to give 2 mcg/kg body weight. First we must weigh the patient, convert pounds to kilograms if the scale is not in kilograms, then multiply the number of kilograms by 2 mcg. Once we have determined this answer, we follow the steps given earlier.

The patient weighs 176 lb.

$$\frac{176 \text{ lb}}{2.2} \qquad \frac{80}{176.0} = 80 \text{ kg}$$

250 mL D5W
Dopamine
200 mg

> **Learning Aid**
>
> To convert lb to kg, divide by 2.2.

$$\begin{array}{r} 80 \text{ kg} \\ \times\ 2 \text{ mcg} \\ \hline 160 \text{ mcg} \end{array}$$ The order now is 160 mcg/min.

1. Reduce the number in the standard solution.

$$\frac{\overset{4}{200 \text{ mg}}}{\underset{5}{250 \text{ mL}}} = 4 \text{ mg/5 mL}$$

2. Change mg to mcg.

   4 mg = 4000 mcg

   Solution is 4000 mcg/5 mL.

3. Reduce the number in the solution.

$$\frac{\overset{800}{4000 \text{ mcg}}}{\underset{1}{5 \text{ mL}}} = 800 \text{ mcg/mL}$$

> **Learning Aid**
>
> D = 160 mcg/min
>
> H = 800 mcg
>
> S = 60 gtt

4. Substitute 60 gtt for the mL.

   800 mcg/60 gtt

5. $\frac{D}{H} \times S = A$

Formula Method

$$\frac{\overset{2}{\cancel{160}} \text{ mcg/min}}{\underset{1}{\cancel{800}} \text{ mcg}} \times \cancel{60} \text{ gtt} = 12$$

$$12 \text{ gtt/min} = 12 \text{ mL/hr}$$

Ratio Method

$$60 : 800 : : x \text{ mL} : 160$$

$$800x = 9600$$

$$x = \frac{9600}{800}$$

$$x = 12 \text{ mL}$$

Proportion Method

$$\frac{x \text{ mL}}{160 \text{ mg/min}} \times \frac{60 \text{ gtt}}{800 \text{ mcg}}$$

Set the pump: total # mL = 250 (standard solution); mL/hr = 12 mL/hr

Milliunits/min—Rule and Calculation

In obstetrics, labor can be initiated using a pitocin drip. The standard solution is 15 units in 250 mL. Because 1 unit = 1000 milliunits, these problems are solved in the same way as mcg/min.

Example Order: pitocin drip 2 milliunits/min IV

Supply: infusion pump, standard solution 15 units in NS 250 mL

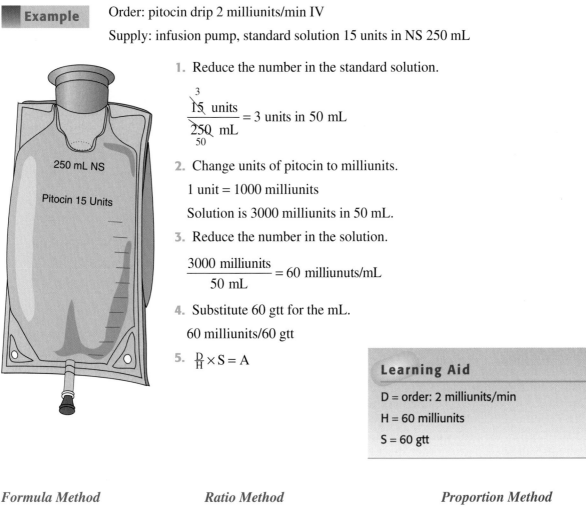

250 mL NS

Pitocin 15 Units

1. Reduce the number in the standard solution.

$$\frac{\overset{3}{\cancel{15}} \text{ units}}{\underset{50}{\cancel{250}} \text{ mL}} = 3 \text{ units in 50 mL}$$

2. Change units of pitocin to milliunits.

   1 unit = 1000 milliunits

   Solution is 3000 milliunits in 50 mL.

3. Reduce the number in the solution.

$$\frac{3000 \text{ milliunits}}{50 \text{ mL}} = 60 \text{ milliunuts/mL}$$

4. Substitute 60 gtt for the mL.

   60 milliunits/60 gtt

5. $\frac{D}{H} \times S = A$

Learning Aid

D = order: 2 milliunits/min

H = 60 milliunits

S = 60 gtt

Formula Method

$$\frac{2 \text{ milliunits/min}}{\underset{}{\cancel{60} \text{ milliunits}}} \times \cancel{60} \text{ gtt} =$$

$$2 \text{ gtt/min} = 2 \text{ mL/hr}$$

Ratio Method

$$60 : 60 : : x \text{ mL} : 2 \text{ milliunits}$$

Proportion Method

$$\frac{x \text{ mL}}{2 \text{ milliunits}} \times \frac{60 \text{ gtt}}{60 \text{ milliunits}}$$

$$60x = 120$$

$$x = 2 \text{ mL/hr}$$

Set the pump: total # mL = 250 mL; mL/hr = 2 mL/hr

SELF-TEST 3	Infusion Rates for Drugs Ordered in mcg/min, mcg/kg/min, milliunits/min

Calculate the number of mL to infuse and the rate of infusion. Answers are given at the end of the chapter.

1. Order: dopamine double strength, 800 mcg/min IV
   Supply: standard solution 800 mg in 250 mL D5W, infusion pump

2. Order: norepinephrine bitartrate, 12 mcg/min IV
   Supply: standard solution of 4 mg in 250 mL D5W, infusion pump

3. Order: dobutamine 5 mcg/kg/min IV
   Supply: patient weight, 220 lb; standard solution of 1 g in 250 mL D5W, infusion pump

4. Order: dobutamine 7 mcg/kg/min IV
   Supply: patient weight, 70 kg; standard solution of 500 mg in 250 mL D5W, infusion pump

5. Order: nitroglycerin 10 mcg/min IV
   Supply: standard solution of 50 mg in 250 mL D5W, infusion pump

6. Order: pitocin drip 1 milliunit/min IV
   Supply: infusion pump, standard solution 15 units in 250 mL NS

7. Order: isoproterenol titrated at 4 mcg/min IV
   Supply: infusion pump, solution 2 mg/in 250 mL D5W

8. Order: esmolol 50 mcg/kg/min IV
   Supply: infusion pump, 2.5 g in 250 mL D5W; weight, 58 kg

9. Order: nipride 2 mcg/kg/min IV
   Supply: patient weight, 80 kg; nipride 50 mg in 250 mL D5W, infusion pump

10. Order: amrinone 200 mcg/min
    Supply: amrinone 0.1 g in 100 mL NS, infusion pump

Body Surface Nomogram

Antineoplastic drugs used in cancer chemotherapy have a narrow therapeutic range. Dosage errors can lead to devastating effects. Calculation of these drugs is based on BSA in square meters. This method is considered more precise than mg/kg/body weight.

BSA can be estimated by using a three-column chart called a *nomogram* (Fig. 9-2). Height is marked in the first column; weight in the third column. A line is drawn between these two marks. The point at which the line intersects the middle column indicates estimated body surface in meters squared. A different BSA chart is used for children because of differences in growth (see Chapter 10).

The oncologist, a physician who specializes in treating cancer, lists the patient's height, weight, and BSA; gives the protocol (drug requirement based on BSA in m^2); and then gives the order. Figure 9-3 shows a partial order sheet for chemotherapy. The pharmacist and the nurse validate the order before preparation.

Determination of BSA in m^2 is easier, faster, and more accurate using either a manual sliding calculator or a battery-operated calculator. These can be purchased commercially or obtained from companies manufacturing antineoplastics. A good website that calculates BSA is www.halls.md/body-surface-area/bsa.htm.

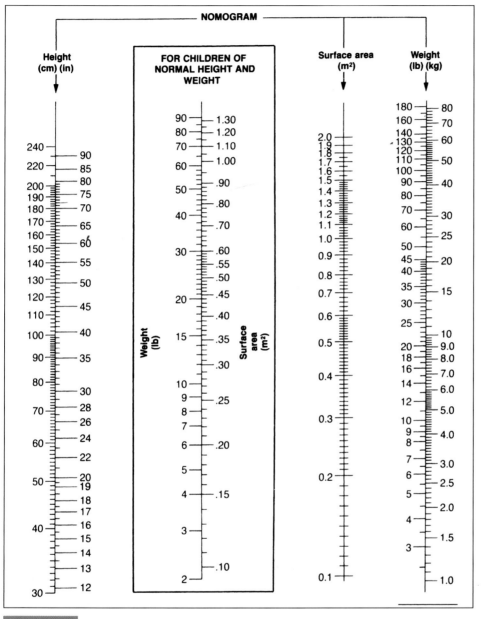

NOMOGRAM

| Height (cm) (in) | FOR CHILDREN OF NORMAL HEIGHT AND WEIGHT | Surface area (m²) | Weight (lb) (kg) |

FIGURE 9-2

Body surface area (BSA) is critical when calculating dosages for pediatric patients or for drugs that are extremely potent and need to be given in precise amounts. The nomogram shown here lets you plot the patient's height and weight to determine the BSA. Here's how it works:

1. Locate the patient's height in the left column of the nomogram and the weight in the right column.

2. Use a ruler to draw a straight line connecting the two points. The point where the line intersects the surface area column indicates the patient's BSA in square meters.

3. For an average-sized child, use the simplified nomogram in the box. Just find the child's weight in pounds on the left side of the scale, and then read the corresponding BSA on the right side.

during which the patient cannot initiate another dose after giving a self-dose. Lockout prevents overdosage. Total hourly dose is the maximum amount of medication the patient can receive in an hour. All this information is written by the physician on an order form.

Figure 9-5 shows a narcotic PCA medication record. Morphine concentration is 1 mg/mL. The pharmacy dispenses a 100-mL NS bag with 100 mL morphine. The patient continuously receives 0.5 mg by infusion pump and can give herself 1.5 mg by pressing the PCA button. Eight minutes must elapse before another PCA dose can be delivered. Note that at 12 NOON, the nurse charted that the patient made three attempts but received only two injections. This indicates that 8 minutes had not elapsed before one of the attempts.

The nurse's responsibility is to assess the patient every hour, noting how the patient scores her pain, the number of PCA attempts, and the total hourly dose received, as well as the cumulative dose, the patient's level of consciousness, and side effects and respirations.

Saint Vincent's Hospital and Medical Center
NARCOTIC / PCA
MEDICATION ADMINISTRATION RECORD

PCA Charting Legend

Pain	Sedation Scale	Side Effects
0 ——— 10	0 - alert	N - nausea
0 - no pain	1 - sleepy but arousable	V - vomiting
10 - excruciating	2 - somnolent, difficult to arouse	I - itching
	3 - minimal or no response	R - respiratory depression
		U - urinary retention

Date: From 8 a.m....   To 8 a.m....   **PHYSICIAN'S ORDER**

INIT.	TIME	Drug	Concentration	Basal Rate	PCA Dose	Delay	I Hour Limit
ṁ	114	Morphine	1 mg/cc	0.5 mg	1.5 mg	8 min	11.5 mg

4 Patient Identified Pain Score Goal

NURSING ASSESSMENT

Time	Pain Score	PCA Injections/Attempts	Total Dose This Hour	Cumulative Dose	Level of Consciousness	Side Effects	Respirations	Comments	Initials
12 N	7	2 - 3	3.5 mg	3.5 mg	0	0	18		m
1 P	7	1 - 3	2 mg	5.5 mg	0	0	18		m
2 P	7	3 - 4	5 mg	10.5 mg	0	0	18		m
3 P	8	2 - 2	3.5 mg	14 mg	0	0	18		m
4 P	8	3 - 6	5 mg	19 mg	0	N	18		m
5 P	6	4 - 7	6.5 mg	25.5 mg	0	N	18		m
6 P	6	3 - 5	5 mg	30.5 mg	0	N	18		m
7 P	8	3 - 3	5 mg	35.5 mg	0	V	18		m
8 P	8	4 - 5	6.5 mg	42 mg	I	0	18		m
9 P	8	2 - 3	3.5 mg	45.5 mg	I	0	18		m
10 P	7	3 - 5	5 mg	50.5 mg	I	0	18		m
11 P	7	5 - 6	8 mg	58.5 mg	I	0	18		m
12 m	7	4 - 4	6.5 mg	65 mg	I	0	18		m
1 A	6	3 - 3	5 mg	70 mg	I	0	18		m
2 A	6	2 - 3	3.5 mg	73.5 mg	I	0	16		m
3 A	5	1 - 1	2 mg	75.5 mg	I	U	16		m
4 A	4	0 - 0	0	75.5 mg	I	U	16		m
5 A	4	0 - 0	0	75.5 mg	I	0	16		m
6 A	4	0 - 0	0	75.5 mg	0	0	16		m
7 A	4	3 - 4	5 mg	80.5 mg	0	0	18		m
8 A	5	3 - 3	5 mg	85.5 mg	0	0	20		m
9 A	4	2 - 3	3.5 mg	89 mg	0	0	20		m
10 A	4	2 - 2	3.5 mg	92.5 mg	0	0	20		m
11 A	4	2 - 2	3.5 mg	96 mg	0	0	20		m

Initials	Signature				Initials	Signature	
m	Josephine Musto						

FIGURE 9-5

Sample PCA medication record. (Courtesy of Saint Vincent's Hospital and Medical Center.)

SELF-TEST 5   Infusion Problems

Solve these problems. Answers are given at the end of the chapter.

1. Order: start labetalol 0.5 mg/min on pump
   Supply: infusion pump, standard solution of 200 mg in 200 mL D5W
   What is the pump setting?

2. Order: aminophylline 250 mg in 250 mL D5W at 75 mg/hr IV
   Supply: infusion pump, vial of aminophylline labeled 250 mg/10 mL

   a. How much drug is needed?
   b. What is the pump setting?

3. Order: Bretylol 2 g in 500 mL D5W at 4 mg/min IV
   Supply: infusion pump, standard solution of 2 g in 500 mL D5W
   What is the pump setting?

4. Order: acyclovir 400 mg in 100 mL D5W over 2 hr
   Supply: infusion pump, 500-mg vials of acyclovir with 10 mL diluent; makes 50 mg/mL

   a. How much drug is needed?
   b. What is the pump setting?

5. Order: urokinase 5000 units/hr for 5 hr IV
   Supply: infusion pump, vials of 5000 units
   Directions: Dissolve urokinase in 1 mL sterile water. Add to 250 mL D5W.

   a. How much drug is needed?
   b. What is the pump setting?

6. Order: Magnesium Sulfate 4 g in 100 mL D5W to infuse over 30 min IV
   Supply: infusion pump, 50% solution of Magnesium Sulfate

   a. How much drug is needed?
   b. What is the pump setting?

7. Order: nitroglycerin 80 mcg/min IV
   Supply: infusion pump, standard solution of 50 mg in 250 mL D5W
   What is the pump setting?

8. Order: dobutamine 6 mcg/kg/min IV
   Supply: infusion pump, solution 500 mg/250 mL D5W; weight, 180 lb
   Change pounds to kilograms. What is the pump setting?

9. Order: pitocin 2 milliunits/min IV
   Supply: infusion pump, solution of 9 units in 150 mL NS
   What is the pump setting?

10. Hgt, 60″; wgt, 110 lb; BSA, 1.55 m^2
    Order: cisplatin 124 mg (80 mg/m^2) in 1 L NS to infuse over 4 hr

    a. Is dose correct?
    b. How should the pump be set?

CRITICAL THINKING: TEST YOUR CLINICAL SAVVY

A 65-year-old NIDDM patient with a 10-year history of congestive heart failure is admitted to the intensive care unit with chest pain of more than 24 hours. The patient is receiving heparin, insulin, calcium gluconate, and potassium chloride, all intravenously.

a. Why would an infusion pump be needed with these medications?

b. Why would medications that are based on body weight require the use of a pump? Why would medications based on BSA require an infusion pump?

c. Can any of these medications be regulated with standard roller clamp tubing? What would be the advantage? What would be the contraindication?

d. What other information would you need to calculate the drip rates of these medications?

e. Why would it be necessary to calculate how long each infusion will last?

Name: _____

Solve these problems. Aim at a high degree of accuracy. Answers are given on page 433.

1. Order: regular insulin 15 units/hr IV
   Supply: infusion pump, standard solution 125 units in 250 mL NS
   What is the pump setting?

2. Order: heparin sodium 1500 units/hr IV
   Supply: infusion pump, standard solution 25,000 units in 500 mL D5W IV
   What is the pump setting?

3. Order: bretylium tosylate 2 g in 500 mL D5W at 2 mg/min IV
   Supply: infusion pump, standard solution of 2 g in 500 mL D5W
   What is the pump setting?

4. Order: diltiazem 125 mg in 100 mL D5W at 5 mg/hr IV
   Supply: infusion pump, vial of diltiazem labeled 5 mg/mL

   a. What is the pump setting?
   b. How much drug is needed?

5. Order: lidocaine 4 mg/min IV
   Supply: infusion pump, standard solution of 2 g in 500 mL D5W
   What is the pump setting?

6. Order: KCl 40 mEq/L at 10 mEq/hr IV
   Supply: infusion pump, vial of KCl labeled 20 mEq/10 mL in D5W 1000 mL
   a. How much KCl should be added?
   b. What is the pump setting?

7. Order: procainamide 1 mg/min IV
   Supply: infusion pump, standard solution of 2 g in 500 mL D5W
   What is the pump setting?

8. Order: amphotericin B 50 mg in 500 mL D5W over 6 hr IV
   Supply: infusion pump, vial of 50 mg

   a. How should the drug be added to the IV?
   b. What is the pump setting?

9. Order: vasopressin 18 units/hr IV, solution 200 units in 500 mL D5W
   Supply: infusion pump, vial of vasopressin labeled 20 units/mL

   a. How much drug is needed?
   b. What is the pump setting?

10. Order: dobutamine 250 mcg/min IV
    Supply: infusion pump, solution of 500 mg in 500 mL D5W
    What is the pump setting?

11. Order: renal dose dopamine 2.5 mcg/kg/min
    Supply: infusion pump, solution 400 mg in 250 mL D5W; wgt, 60 kg
    What is the pump setting?

12. Order: pitocin 2 milliunits/min IV
    Supply: infusion pump, solution of 9 units in 150 mL NS
    What is the pump setting?

(continued)

13. Hgt, 5′3″; wgt, 143 lb; BSA, 1.7 m²
    Order: Ara-C 170 mg (100 mg/m²) in 1 L D5W over 24 hr

    a. Is dose correct?
    b. How should the pump be set?

14. Order: nipride 5 mcg/kg/mm IV
    Supply: patient weight = 90 kg; nipride 50 mg in 250 mL D5W, infusion pump
    What is the pump setting?

15. Order: epinephrine 2 mcg/min
    Supply: epinephrine 4 mg in 250 mL D5W, infusion pump
    What is the pump setting?

Answers

Self-Test 1 Infusion Rates

Formula Method

1. $\frac{D}{H} \times S = A$

$$\frac{\overset{8}{\cancel{800}} \text{ units/hr}}{\underset{\underset{1}{100}}{\cancel{25,000}} \text{ units}} \times \overset{1}{\cancel{250}} \text{ mL}$$

$= 8$ mL/hr on a pump

$\dfrac{\# \text{ mL}}{\# \text{ mL/hr}}$

$$\frac{250 \text{ mL}}{8 \text{ mL/hr}} \quad \begin{array}{r} 31.2 \\ \overline{)250.0} \\ \underline{24} \\ 10 \\ \underline{8} \\ 2.0 \end{array}$$

approximately 31 hours; hospital policy states that IV bags be changed after 24 hours

Ratio Method

250 mL : 25000 units : : x mL : 800 units

Proportion Method

$$\frac{x \text{ mL}}{800 \text{ units}} = \frac{250 \text{ mL}}{25000 \text{ units}}$$

$$25000x = 200000$$

$$x = \frac{200,000}{25000}$$

$$x = 8 \text{ mL/hr}$$

2. Add 500 mg acyclovir to 100 mL D5W using a reconstitution device (see Chapter 8).

$\dfrac{\# \text{ mL}}{\# \text{ hr}} = \text{mL/hr}$

$\dfrac{100 \text{ mL}}{1 \text{ hr}}$ No math is necessary. Set the pump at 100 mL/hr.

3. a. Add amicar to IV.

Formula Method

$\frac{D}{H} \times S = A$

$$\frac{24 \text{ g}}{5 \text{ g}} \times \overset{4}{\cancel{20}} \text{ mL} = 96 \text{ mL}$$

Ratio Method

20 mL : 5 g : : x mL : 24 g

Proportion Method

$$\frac{x \text{ mL}}{24 \text{ g}} = \frac{20 \text{ mL (cc)}}{5 \text{ g}}$$

$$5x = 24 \times 20$$

$$x = \frac{480}{5}$$

$$x = 96 \text{ mL}$$

(*Note:* Adding 96 mL to 1000 mL D5W = 1096 mL.)

Use five vials. Empty four completely.
Take 16 mL from the last vial.
20 mL × 4 vials = 80 mL + 16 mL = 96 mL
Remove 96 mL D5W from the IV bag before adding the amicar. This results in 1000 mL.

b. $\frac{\#\ mL}{\#\ hr} = mL/hr$

$$\frac{1000\ mL}{24\ hr}\quad \begin{array}{r} 41.6 \\ \overline{)1000.0} \\ \underline{96} \\ 40 \\ \underline{24} \\ 16.0 \\ \underline{14.4} \end{array}$$

Set pump at 42 mL/hr.

4. a. Add diltiazem to IV.

Formula Method	Ratio Method	Proportion Method

$\frac{D}{H} \times S = A$

$\dfrac{\overset{25}{\cancel{125\ mg}}}{\cancel{5\ mg}} \times 1\ mL = 25\ mL$

1 mL : 5 mg : : x mL : 125 mg

$\dfrac{x\ mL}{125\ mg} = \dfrac{1\ mL}{5\ mg}$

$x = \dfrac{125}{5}$

$x = 25\ mL$

(*Note:* Adding 25 mL to 100 mL D5W = 125 mL. Remove 25 mL D5W from the IV bag before adding the diltiazem. This results in 100 mL.)

Add 25 mL to IV bag.

Formula Method	Ratio Method	Proportion Method

b. $\frac{D}{H} \times S = A$

$\dfrac{\overset{2}{\cancel{10\ mg}}}{\underset{\underset{1}{5}}{\cancel{125\ mg}}} \times \overset{4}{\cancel{100}}\ mL = 8\ mL/hr$

100 mL : 125 mg : : x mL : 10 mg

$\dfrac{x\ mL}{10\ mg} = \dfrac{100\ mL}{125\ mg}$

$x = \dfrac{1000}{125}$

$x = 8\ mL/hr$

5. a. Add furosemide to IV.

Formula Method	Ratio Method	Proportion Method

$\frac{D}{H} \times S = A$

$\dfrac{\overset{10}{\cancel{100\ mg}}}{\underset{1}{\cancel{10\ mg}}} \times 1\ mL = 10\ mL$

1 mL : 10 mg : : x mL : 100 mg

$\dfrac{x\ mL}{100\ mg} = \dfrac{1\ mL}{10\ mg}$

$x = 10\ mL$

(*Note:* Adding 10 mL to 100 mL D5W = 100 mL. Remove 10 mL D5W from the IV bag before adding the furosemide. This results in 100 mL.)

Add 10 mL to the IV bag.

b. Logic: Because the solution is 100 mg/100 mL (1:1) and the order reads 4 mg/hr, the pump should be set at 4 mL/hr. Let's prove this!

Formula Method	*Ratio Method*	*Proportion Method*

$$\frac{D}{H} \times S = A$$

$$\frac{4 \text{ mg/hr}}{\overset{}{\underset{1}{100 \text{ mg}}}} \times \overset{1}{100} \text{ mL} = 4 \text{ mL/hr}$$

$$100 \text{ mL} : 100 \text{ mg} :: x \text{ mL} : 4 \text{ mg}$$

$$\frac{x \text{ mL}}{4 \text{ mg}} = \frac{100 \text{ mL}}{100 \text{ mg}}$$

$$x = 4 \text{ mL/hr}$$

6. a.

Formula Method	*Ratio Method*	*Proportion Method*

$$\frac{D}{H} \times S = A$$

$$\frac{15 \text{ units}}{125 \text{ units}} \times 250 \text{ mL}$$

$$250 \text{ mL} : 125 :: x \text{ mL} : 15 \text{ units}$$

$$\frac{x \text{ mL}}{15 \text{ units}} = \frac{250 \text{ mL}}{125}$$

$$0.12 \times 250 \text{ mL} = 30 \text{ mL/hr}$$

$$x \text{ mL} = 30 \text{mL/hr}$$

b. Logic: The total volume of medication is 125 units and the client receives 15 units/hr.

$$\frac{125}{15} \quad \overset{8.33}{\underset{}{\big)125.00}} = \text{ approximately 8 hours}$$
$$\underline{120}$$
$$5.0$$
$$\underline{4.5}$$
$$50$$

7. Logic: Nitroglycerin is prepared by the pharmacy as a standard solution of 50 mg in 250 mL/hr. We only need to calculate mL/hr.

Rule: $\frac{\# \text{ mL}}{\# \text{ hr}} = \text{mL/hr}$

$$\frac{250 \text{ mL}}{24 \text{ hr}} \quad \overset{10.4}{\underset{}{\big)250.0}}$$
$$\underline{24}$$
$$10\ 0$$
$$\underline{9\ 6} \qquad \text{Set pump at 10 mL/hr.}$$

8. a.

Formula Method	*Ratio Method*	*Proportion Method*

$$\frac{D}{H} \times S = A$$

$$\frac{\overset{}{\underset{5}{1200 \text{ units}}}}{\overset{}{25000 \text{ units}}} \times \overset{1}{500} \text{ mL} = 24 \text{ mL/hr}$$

$$500 \text{ mL} : 25,000 \text{ units} :: x \text{ mL} : 1200 \text{ units}$$

$$\frac{x \text{ mL}}{1200 \text{ units}} = \frac{500 \text{ mL}}{25,000 \text{ units}}$$

$$25,000x = 600,000$$

$$x = \frac{600,000}{25,000}$$

$$x = 24 \text{ mL/hr}$$

b. Rule: $\frac{\#\ mL}{\#\ mL/hr}$

$\frac{500\ mL}{24\ mL/hr} = 20.8$ or approximately 21 hours

9. a.

Formula Method   *Ratio Method*   *Proportion Method*

Rule: $\frac{D}{H} \times S = A$

$\frac{23\ units/hr}{250\ units} \times 250\ mL = 23\ mL/hr$ 250 mL : 250 units : : x mL : 23 units $\frac{x\ mL}{23\ units} = \frac{250\ mL}{250\ units}$

$x = 23\ mL/hr$

b. Rule: $\frac{\#\ mL}{\#\ mL/hr}$

$\frac{250mL}{23mL/hr} = 10.8$ or approximately 11 hours

10.

Formula Method   *Ratio Method*   *Proportion Method*

$\frac{D}{H} \times S = A$

$\frac{100,000\ units}{750,000\ units} \times 250\ mL = 33\ mL/hr$ 250 mL : 750000 : : x mL : 100000 $\frac{x\ mL}{100000\ units} = \frac{250\ mL}{750000\ units}$

$x = \frac{2500}{75}$

$x = 33\ mL/hr$

Self-Test 2 Infusion Rates for Drugs Ordered in mg/min

1. a. Order: 1 mg/min, D = 60 mg/hr (1 mg/min × 60 minutes)
Solution: 2 g in 250 mL
2 g = 2000 mg

Formula Method   *Ratio Method*   *Proportion Method*

Rule: $\frac{D}{H} \times S = A$

$\frac{60\ mg/hr}{2000\ mg} \times \overset{1}{250}\ mL$ 250 mL : 2000 mg : : x mL : 60 mg $\frac{x\ mL}{60\ mg} = \frac{250\ mL}{2000\ mg}$

$= 7.5\ mL/hr$ or 8 mL/hr

2000 x = 75000
x = 7.5 mL

Set pump at 8 mL/hr.

b. Rule: $\frac{\#\ mL}{\#\ mL/hr}$

$\frac{250\ mL}{8\ mL/hr} = 31.25$ or approximately 31 hours; hospital policy requires that IV bags be changed every 24 hours

2. a. Order: 3 mg/min, D = 180 mg/hr (3 mg/min × 60 minutes)
   Solution: 1 g in 250 mL
   1 g = 1000 mg

Formula Method	*Ratio Method*	*Proportion Method*

Rule: $\dfrac{D}{H} \times S = A$

$\dfrac{180 \text{ mg/hr}}{\underset{4}{\cancel{1000} \text{ mg}}} \times \cancel{250} \text{ mL} = 45 \text{ mL/hr}$

250 mL : 1000 mg :: x mL : 180 mg

$\dfrac{x \text{ mL}}{180 \text{ mg}} = \dfrac{250 \text{ mL}}{1000 \text{ mg}}$

$1000 \, x = 45000$

$x = 45$

Set pump at 45 mL/hr.

b. Rule: $\dfrac{\# \text{ mL}}{\# \text{ mL/hr}}$

$\dfrac{250 \text{ mL}}{45 \text{mL/hr}} = 5.5$ or approximately 6 hours

3. a. Order: 2 mg/min, D = 120 mg/hr (2 mg/min × 60 minutes)
   Solution: 1 g in 500 mL
   1 g = 1000 mg

Formula Method	*Ratio Method*	*Proportion Method*

Rule: $\dfrac{D}{H} \times S = A$

$\dfrac{120 \text{ mg/hr}}{\underset{2}{\cancel{1000} \text{ mg}}} \times \overset{1}{\cancel{500}} \text{ mL} = 60 \text{ mL/hr}$

500 mL : 1000 mg :: x mL : 120 mg

$\dfrac{x \text{ mL}}{120 \text{ mg}} = \dfrac{500 \text{ mL}}{1000 \text{ mg}}$

$1000x = 60000$

$x = 60 \text{ mL/hr}$

Set pump at 60 mL/hr.

b. Rule: $\dfrac{\# \text{ mL}}{\# \text{ mL/hr}}$

$\dfrac{500 \text{ mL}}{60 \text{mL/hr}} = 8.3$ or approximately 8 hours

4. Order: 1 mg/min, D = 60 mg/hr (1 mg/min × 60 minutes)
   Solution: 450 mg in 250 mL

Formula Method	*Ratio Method*	*Proportion Method*

Rule: $\dfrac{D}{H} \times S = A$

$\dfrac{60 \text{ mg/hr}}{\underset{9}{\cancel{450} \text{ mg}}} \times \overset{5}{\cancel{250}} \text{ mL} = 33.33 \text{ or } 33 \text{ mL/hr}$

250 mL : 450 mg :: x mL : 60 mg

$\dfrac{x \text{ mL}}{60 \text{ mg}} = \dfrac{250 \text{ mL}}{450 \text{ mg}}$

$45x = 1500$

$x = \dfrac{1500}{45}$

$x = 33.33$

Set the pump at 33 mL/hr. Run for 6 hours.

5. a. Order: 1 mg/min, D = 60 mg/hr (1 mg/min × 60 minutes)

Solution: 2 g in 500 mL

2 g = 2000 mg

Formula Method   *Ratio Method*   *Proportion Method*

Rule: $\frac{D}{H} \times S = A$

$$\frac{60 \overset{}{\text{mg/hr}}}{\underset{4}{2000 \text{ mg}}} \times 5\overset{1}{0}0 \text{ mL} =$$

500 mL : 2000 mg :: x mL : 60 mg

$$\frac{x \text{ mL}}{60 \text{ mg}} = \frac{500 \text{ mL}}{2000 \text{ mg}}$$

15 mL/hr

$$2000x = 30000$$

$$x = 15 \text{ mL/hr}$$

Set the pump at 15 mL/hr.

b. Rule: $\frac{\# \text{ mL}}{\# \text{ mL/hr}}$

$\frac{500 \text{ mL}}{15 \text{ mL/hr}}$ = 33.3 or approximately 33 hours; hospital policy requires that IV bags be changed

every 24 hours

Self-Test 3 Infusion Rates for Drugs Ordered in mcg/min, mcg/kg/min, milliunits/min

1. Order: 800 mcg/min

Standard solution: 800 in 250 mL D5W

Step 1. $\dfrac{\overset{16}{800} \text{ mg}}{\underset{5}{250} \text{ mL}} = 16 \text{ mg/5 mL}$

Step 2. 16 mg = 16,000 mcg

16,000 mcg/5 mL

Step 3. $\dfrac{\overset{3200}{16{,}000 \text{ mcg}}}{\underset{1}{5 \text{ mL}}} = 3200 \text{ mcg/mL}$

Step 4. 3200 mcg/60 gtt

Formula Method   *Ratio Method*   *Proportion Method*

Step 5. $\dfrac{\overset{1}{800} \text{ mcg/min}}{\underset{\underset{1}{4}}{3200 \text{ mcg}}} \times 6\overset{15}{0} \text{ gtt} = 15 \text{ gtt/min}$

60 gtt : 3200 mcg :: x mL : 800 mcg

$$\frac{x \text{ mL}}{800 \text{ mcg}} = \frac{60 \text{ gtt}}{3200 \text{ mcg}}$$

= 15 mL/hr

$$3200x = 48000$$

$$x = 15 \text{ mL/hr}$$

Set the pump: total # mL = 250 (standard solution); mL/hr = 15

2. Order: 12 mcg/min

Standard solution: 4 mg in 250 mL D5W

Step 1. Skip this step for easier calculation.

Step 2. 4 mg = 4000 mcg

Solution is 4000 mcg/250 mL.

Step 3. $\dfrac{\overset{\overset{16}{\overset{80}{4000}}}{\text{mcg}}}{\underset{\underset{1}{5}}{250\ \text{mL}}} = 16$ mcg/mL

Step 4. 16 mcg/60 gtt

Formula Method	*Ratio Method*	*Proportion Method*

Step 5. $\dfrac{\overset{3}{12\ \text{mcg/min}}}{\underset{\underset{1}{4}}{16\ \text{mcg}}} \times \overset{15}{60}\ \text{gtt} = 45$

60 gtt : 16 mcg : : x mL : 12 mcg

$\dfrac{\text{x mL}}{12\ \text{mcg}} = \dfrac{60\ \text{gtt}}{16\ \text{mcg}}$

45 gtt/min = 45 mL/hr
Set the pump: total # mL = 250; mL/hr = 45

16x = 720

x = 45 mL/hr

3. Order: 5 mcg/kg/min

Weight, 220 lb

Standard solution: 1 g in 250 mL

Convert lb to kg.

$\dfrac{220\ \text{lb}}{2.2\ \text{kg}}$ $\dfrac{100.0}{\overline{)220.0}} = 100$ kg

To obtain the order in mcg:

multiply 100 kg

$\begin{array}{r} 100\ \text{kg} \\ \times\ 5\ \text{mcg/kg/min} \\ \hline 500\ \text{mcg/min (order)} \end{array}$

Step 1. 1 g = 1000 mg

Solution is 1000 mg/250 mL.

$\dfrac{\overset{4}{1000}\ \text{mg}}{\underset{1}{250\ \text{mL}}} = 4$ mg/mL

Step 2. 4 mg = 4000 mcg

Solution is 4000 mcg/mL.

Step 3. Not needed

Step 4. 4000 mcg/60 gtt

Formula Method   *Ratio Method*   *Proportion Method*

Step 5. $\dfrac{\overset{5}{\cancel{500\ \text{mcg/min}}}}{\underset{2}{\cancel{4000\ \text{mcg}}}} \times \overset{3}{\cancel{60}}\ \text{gtt}$ $60\ \text{gtt} : 4000\ \text{mcg} :: x\ \text{mL} : 500\ \text{mcg}$ $\dfrac{x\ \text{mL}}{500\ \text{mcg}} = \dfrac{60\ \text{gtt}}{4000\ \text{mcg}}$

$= \frac{15}{2} = 7.5 = 8\ \text{gtt/min}$

$8\ \text{gtt/min} = 8\ \text{mL/hr}$ $4000x = 30000$

$x = 7.5$

Set the pump: total # mL = 250 (standard solution); mL/hr = 8

4. Order: 7 mcg/kg/min

Standard solution: 500 mg in 250 mL D5W

Patient's weight, 70 kg

$$\text{The patient weights}\ \begin{array}{r} 70\ \text{kg} \\ \times 7\ \text{mcg/kg/min} \\ \hline 490\ \text{mcg/min} \end{array}$$

Step 1. $\dfrac{\overset{2}{\cancel{500\ \text{mg}}}}{\underset{1}{\cancel{250\ \text{mL}}}} = 2\ \text{mg/mL}$

Step 2. 2 mg = 2000 mcg

Solution is 2000 mcg/mL.

Step 3. Not needed

Step 4. 2000 mcg/60 gtt

Formula Method   *Ratio Method*   *Proportion Method*

Step 5. $\dfrac{\overset{}{\cancel{490\ \text{mcg/min}}}}{\underset{\underset{10}{\cancel{100}}}{\cancel{2000\ \text{mcg}}}} \times \overset{3}{\cancel{60}}\ \text{gtt} = 49 \times 3$ $60\ \text{gtt} : 2000\ \text{mcg} :: x\ \text{mL} : 490\ \text{mcg}$ $\dfrac{x\ \text{mL}}{490\ \text{mcg}} = \dfrac{60\ \text{gtt}}{2000\ \text{mcg}}$

$= \frac{147}{10} = 14.7 = 15$ $2000x = 29400$

$15\ \text{gtt/min} = 15\ \text{mL/hr}$ $14.7\ \text{or}\ 15\ \text{mL/hr}$

Set the pump: total # mL = 250 (standard solution); mL/hr = 15

5. Order: 10 mcg/min

Standard solution: 50 mg in 250 mL

Step 1. $\dfrac{\overset{1}{\cancel{50\ \text{mg}}}}{\underset{5}{\cancel{250\ \text{mL}}}} = 1\ \text{mg/5 mL}$

Step 2. 1 mg = 1000 mcg

Solution is 1000 mcg/5 mL

Step 3. $\dfrac{\overset{200}{\cancel{1000\ \text{mcg}}}}{\underset{1}{\cancel{5\ \text{mL}}}} = 200\ \text{mcg/mL}$

Step 4. 200 mcg/60 gtt

Formula Method	*Ratio Method*	*Proportion Method*

Step 5. $\dfrac{\cancel{10}\ \text{mcg/min}}{\cancel{200}\ \text{mcg}} \times \cancel{60}\ \overset{3}{\text{gtt}} = 3$ 60 gtt : 200 mcg : : x mL : 10 mcg $\dfrac{x\ \text{mL}}{10\ \text{mcg}} = \dfrac{60\ \text{gtt}}{200\ \text{mcg}}$

3 gtt/min = 3 mL/hr

Set the pump: total # mL = 250; mL/hr = 3

$200x = 600$

$x = 3\ \text{mL/hr}$

6. Order: 1 milliunit/min

Standard solution: 15 units in 250 mL NS

Step 1. $\dfrac{\overset{3}{\cancel{15}\ \text{units}}}{\underset{50}{\cancel{250}\ \text{mL}}} = 3\ \text{units}/\ 50\ \text{mL}$

Step 2. 1 unit = 1000 milliunits

Solution is 3000 milliunits in 50 mL.

Step 3. $\dfrac{3000\ \text{milliunits}}{50\ \text{mL}} = 60\ \text{milliunits/mL}$

Step 4. 60 milliunits/60 gtt

Formula Method	*Ratio Method*	*Proportion Method*

Step 5. $\dfrac{1\ \cancel{\text{milliunit}}\ \text{/min}}{\cancel{60}\ \cancel{\text{milliunits}}} \times \cancel{60}\ \text{gtt}$ 60 gtt : 60 milliunits : : x mL : 1 milliunits $\dfrac{x\ \text{mL}}{1\ \cancel{\text{milliunits}}} = \dfrac{\cancel{60}\ \cancel{\text{gtt}}}{\cancel{60}\ \cancel{\text{milliunits}}}$

1 gtt/min = 1 mL/hr

Set the pump: total # mL = 250; mL/hr = 1

$x = 1\ \text{mL/hr}$

7. Order: 4 mcg/min

Solution: 2 mg in 250 mL

Step 1. Not necessary; math easier

Step 2. 2 mg = 2000 mcg

Solution is 2000 mcg/250 mL.

Step 3. $\dfrac{\overset{8}{\cancel{2000}\ \text{mcg}}}{\underset{1}{\cancel{250}\ \text{mL}}} = 8\ \text{mcg/mL}$

Step 4. 8 mcg/60 gtt

Formula Method	*Ratio Method*	*Proportion Method*

Step 5. $\dfrac{4\ \cancel{\text{mcg}}\ \text{/min}}{\underset{\underset{1}{2}}{\cancel{8}\ \cancel{\text{mcg}}}} \times \cancel{60}\ \overset{30}{\text{gtt}} = 30$ 60 gtt : 8 mcg : : x mL : 4 mcg $\dfrac{x\ \text{mL}}{4\ \text{mcg}} = \dfrac{60\ \text{gtt}}{8\ \text{mcg}}$

30 gtt/min = 30 mL/hr

Set the pump: total # mL = 250; mL/hr = 30

$8x = 240$

$x = 30\ \text{mL/hr}$

8. Order: 50 mcg/kg/min

Solution: 2.5 g in 250 mL

Weight: 58 kg

$$58 \text{ kg} \times 50 \text{ mcg} = 2900 \text{ mcg (order)}$$

Step 1. $2.5 \text{ g} = \dfrac{\overset{10}{\cancel{2500} \text{ mg}}}{\underset{1}{\cancel{250} \text{ mL}}} = 10 \text{ mg/mL}$

Step 2. 10 mg = 10,000 mcg

Solution is 10,000 mcg/mL.

Step 3. Not needed

Step 4. 10,000 mcg/60 gtt

Formula Method   *Ratio Method*   *Proportion Method*

Step 5. $\dfrac{2900 \text{ mcg/min}}{10,000 \text{ mcg}} \times 60 \text{ gtt} = \dfrac{174}{10} = 17.4$ 60 gtt : 10,000 :: x mL : 2900 mg $\dfrac{\text{x mL}}{2900 \text{ mcg}} = \dfrac{60 \text{ gtt}}{10,000 \text{ mcg}}$

$17 \text{ gtt/min} = 17 \text{ mL/hr}$

$$10,000\text{x} = 174000$$

Set the pump: total # mL = 250; mL/hr = 17

$$\text{x} = 17.4 \text{ or } 17 \text{ mL/hr}$$

9. Order: 2 mcg/kg/min

Solution: 50 mg in 250 mL

Weight: 80 kg

$$80 \text{ kg} \times 2 \text{ mcg} = 160 \text{ mcg (order)}$$

Step 1. $\dfrac{50 \text{ mg}}{250 \text{ mL}} = 0.2 \text{ mg/mL}$

Step 2. 0.2 mg = 200 mcg

Solution is 200 mcg/mL.

Step 3. Not needed

Step 4. 200 mcg/60 gtt

Formula Method   *Ratio Method*   *Proportion Method*

Step 5. $\dfrac{160 \text{ mcg}}{200 \text{ mcg}} \times 60 \text{ gtt} = 48 \text{ gtt/min or } 48 \text{ mL/hr}$ 60 gtt : 200 mcg :: x mL : 160 mcg $\dfrac{\text{x mL}}{160 \text{ mcg}} = \dfrac{60 \text{ gtt}}{200 \text{ mcg}}$

$$200\text{x} = 9600$$

Set the pump: total # mL = 250; mL/hr = 48

$$\text{x} = 48$$

10. Order: 200 mcg/min

Solution: 0.1 g in 100 mL

100 mg in 100 mL

Step 1. $\dfrac{100 \text{ mg}}{100 \text{ mL}} = 1 \text{ mg/mL}$

Step 2. 1 mg = 1000 mcg

1000 mcg/1 mL

Step 3. Not needed; math easier

Step 4. 1 mg/60 gtt = 1000 mg/60 gtt

Formula Method	*Ratio Method*	*Proportion Method*
Step 5. $\dfrac{200 \text{ mcg/min}}{1000 \text{ mcg}} \times 60 \text{ gtt}$	60 gtt : 1000 mcg : : x mL : 200 mcg	$\dfrac{\text{x mL}}{200 \text{ mcg}} = \dfrac{60 \text{ gtt}}{1000 \text{ mg}}$
12 gtt/min or 12 mL/hr		$1000x = 12000$ $x = 12$

Set the pump: total # mL = 100; mL/hr = 12

Self-Test 4 Use of Nomogram

1. **a.** Dose is correct; $20 \text{ mg/m}^2 \times 1.96 = 39 \text{ mg}$
   b. Order calls for 250 mL over ½ hour, but pump is set in mL/hr. Double 250 mL.
   Setting: total # mL = 250; mL/hr = 500.
   The pump will deliver 250 mL in ½ hour.

2. **a.** Correct; $130 \text{ mg/m}^2 \times 1.77 = 230 \text{ mg}$
   b. Pour two 100-mg tabs and three 10-mg tabs.

3. **a.** Correct; $40 \text{ mg/m}^2 \times 2 = 80 \text{ mg}$
   b. Rapidly flowing IV is the primary line. Set the secondary pump: total # mL, 80; mL/hr, 80 (see Chapter 8 for IVPB).

4. **a.** Correct; $200 \text{ mg/m}^2 \times 2 = 400 \text{ mg}$

Formula Method	*Ratio Method*	*Proportion Method*
b. Rule: $\dfrac{D}{H} \times S = A$	1 capsule : 50 mg : : x mL : 400 mg	$\dfrac{\text{x capsule}}{400 \text{ mg}} = \dfrac{1 \text{ capsule}}{50 \text{ mg}}$
$\dfrac{\overset{8}{400 \text{ mg}}}{50 \text{ mg}} \times 1 \text{ capsule} = 8 \text{ capsules}$	$50x = 400$ $x = 8 \text{ capsules}$	

5. **a.** Correct; $135 \text{ mg/m}^2 \times 1.6 = 216 \text{ mg}$

   b. ½ L = 500 mL over 3 hr; $\dfrac{500}{3}$ $\quad 500 \overline{\smash{)}\,166.6} = 167$

   Set the pump: total # mL = 500; mL/hr = 167

Self-Test 5 Infusion Problems

1. Logic: A pump is needed. This is set in mL/hr. The order calls for 0.5 mg/min. Because there are 60 minutes in an hour, multiply 0.5 mg × 60 = 30 mg/hr. The standard solution is 200 mg in 200 mL. This is a 1:1 solution, so 30 mg/hr = 30 mL/hr.

8. Order: 6 mcg/kg/min

   Solution: 500 mg/250 mL

   Weight: 180 lb

   a. Change lbs to kg $\dfrac{180\ lbs}{2.2}$ $\dfrac{81.8}{2.2\,\overline{)180.00}} = 82\ kg$

   $$\begin{array}{r}176\\ \hline 4\ 0\\ 2\ 2\\ \hline 1\ 80\end{array}$$

   b. 6 mcg/kg × 82 kg = 492 mcg (order now)

   Step 1. $\dfrac{\overset{2}{\cancel{500\ mg}}}{\underset{1}{\cancel{250\ mL}}} = 2\ mg/mL$

   Step 2. 2 mg = 2000 mcg

   Solution is 2000 mcg/mL.

   Step 3. Not necessary

   Step 4. 2000 mcg/60 gtt

   Formula Method   *Ratio Method*   *Proportion Method*

   Step 5. $\dfrac{492\ \cancel{mcg}/min}{\underset{100}{\cancel{2000}}\ \cancel{mcg}} \times \overset{3}{\cancel{60}}\ gtt = \dfrac{1476}{100}$ $\dfrac{14.76}{100\,\overline{)1476.00}}$ 60 gtt : 2000 mcg : : x mL : 492 mg $\dfrac{x\ mL}{492\ mcg} = \dfrac{60\ gtt}{2000\ mg}$

   $= 15$ $2000x = 2952$

   15 gtt/min = 15 mL/hr $x = 15\ mL/hr$

   Set pump: total # mL = 250; mL/hr = 15

9. Order: 2 milliunits/min

   Supply: 9 units in 150 mL NS

   Step 1. $\dfrac{\overset{3}{\cancel{9\ units}}}{\underset{50}{\cancel{150\ mL}}} = 3\ units/\ 50\ mL$

   Step 2. 1 unit = 1000 milliunits

   Solution is 3000 milliunits/50 mL.

   Step 3. $\dfrac{3000\ milliunits}{50\ mL} = 60\ milliunits/mL$

   Step 4. 60 milliunits/60 gtt

Formula Method   *Ratio Method*   *Proportion Method*

Step 5. $\frac{D}{H} \times S = A$

$$\frac{2 \text{ milliunits}}{60 \text{ milliunits}} \times 60 \text{ gtt} =$$ 60 gtt : 60 milliunits : : x mL : 2 milliunits $$\frac{x \text{ mL}}{2 \text{ milliunits}} = \frac{60 \text{ gtt}}{60 \text{ milliunits}}$$

2 gtt/min = 2 mL/hr

$$60x = 120$$
$$x = 2 \text{ mL/hr}$$

Set pump: total # mL = 150 mL; mL/hr = 2

10. a. Correct; 1.55 BSA × 80 mg

   b. 1 L = 1000 mL

$$\frac{\# \text{ mL}}{\# \text{ hr}} = \frac{\overset{250}{\cancel{1000} \text{ mL}}}{\underset{1}{\cancel{4} \text{ hr}}} = 250 \text{ mL/hr}$$

Set the pump: total # mL = 1000; mL/hr = 250

CHAPTER 10

Dosage Problems for Infants and Children

In previous chapters we discussed calculations for adult medications administered orally and parenterally. This chapter considers dosage for infants and children. Wide variations in age, weight, growth, and development within this group require special care in computation. Pediatric doses are lower than adult doses and are more narrow in dosage range. A slight error can result in serious harm.

Before preparing and administering a pediatric medication, the nurse determines that the dose is safe for the child. Safe means that the amount ordered is not an overdose or an underdose. An overdose can product toxic effects; an underdose may lead to therapeutic failure. When a discrepancy is noted, the nurse consults the physician or health care provider who ordered the drug.

Children's medications are usually given by mouth in a liquid form or intravenously. Subcutaneous and IM injections are given less often but are included in this chapter. Immunizations are given subcutaneously and IM. Pediatric injections are calculated to the nearest hundredth and are often administered using a 1-mL precision (formerly called *tuberculin*) syringe. For IV therapy, microdrip, Buretrols, or other volume control sets and infusion pumps are used. Most institutions will have guidelines for pediatric infusions. When guidelines are not available, the nurse must consult a reliable *pediatric* reference. Adult guidelines are not safe for children.

A brief overview of pediatric medication administration is discussed in Chapter 13. More information about pediatric medication administration, such as needle size and injection sites, can be found in pediatric nursing textbooks. Also, institutional policy must be followed.

A word about calculators. Because pediatric doses must be accurate, the use of a calculator is advisable. However, it is still the responsibility of the nurse to know what numbers to enter into the calculator to calculate the correct amount. Double- or triple-checking the answer is suggested.

Recall these equivalents as you begin this chapter:

1 g = 1000 mg	16 oz = 1 lb
1 kg = 2.2 lb	microdrip = 60 gtt/mL
1 mg = 1000 mcg	> = greater than
1 tsp = 5 mL	< = less than
1 oz = 30 mL	q4° = every four hours

Dosage Based on mg/kg and Body Surface Area

The dose of most pediatric drugs is based on mg/kg body weight or BSA in meters squared. We will learn how to convert pounds to kilograms, to use a nomogram to calculate BSA, to estimate the safety of a dose, and, finally, to determine the dose. *The use of a calculator is advisable.*

Converting Ounces to Pounds

Example An infant weighs 20 lb 12 oz. Convert the ounces to pounds.

Step 1: Because there are 16 oz in 1 lb, divide the 12 oz by 16. You should get a decimal.

$$\frac{12}{16} \quad 16\overline{)12.00}$$

$$\begin{array}{r} 0.75 \\ 16\overline{)12.00} \\ \underline{11\ 2} \\ 80 \\ \underline{80} \\ 0 \end{array}$$

Step 2: Add the answer to the pounds to get the total number of pounds.

$$20 + 0.75 = 20.75 \text{ lb}$$

Example An infant weighs 25 lb 6 oz. Convert the ounces to pounds.

Step 1: Divide 6 by 16.

$$\frac{6}{16} \quad \begin{array}{r} 0.375 \\ 16\overline{)6.0} \\ \underline{4\ 8} \\ 120 \\ \underline{112} \\ 80 \\ \underline{80} \\ 0 \end{array}$$

Step 2: Add the answer to the pounds.

$$25 + 0.375 = 25.375 \text{ lb}$$

Converting Pounds to Kilograms

Example A child weighs 33 lb. How many kilograms?

Step 1: Because there are 2.2 lb per 1 kg, divide the 33 lb by 2.2. Round off to the nearest hundredth.

$$\frac{33}{2.2} \quad \begin{array}{r} 15 \\ 2.2\overline{)33.0} \\ \underline{22} \\ 11\ 0 \\ \underline{11\ 0} \\ 0 \end{array}$$

The child weighs 15 kg.

Example	An infant weighs 18 lb 12 oz. How many kilograms?

Step 1: Convert ounces to pounds first.

$$\frac{12}{16} \quad \begin{array}{r} 0.75 \\ 16\overline{)12.0} \\ \underline{11\ 2} \\ 80 \\ \underline{80} \\ 0 \end{array}$$

Step 2: Add the answer to the pounds.

$$18 + 0.75 = 18.75 \text{ lb}$$

Step 3: Convert to kilograms. Round off to the nearest hundredth.

$$\frac{18.75}{2.2} \quad \begin{array}{r} 8.522 \\ 2.2\overline{)18.75} \\ \underline{17\ 6} \\ 1\ 15 \\ \underline{1\ 10} \\ 50 \\ \underline{44} \\ 60 \\ 44 \end{array}$$

The infant weighs 8.52 kg.

SELF-TEST 1	Converting Pounds to Kilograms

Convert pounds to kilograms. Use a calculator. Round the final answer to the nearest hundredths place. Answers are given at the end of the chapter.

1. 30 lb = _____ kg	**6.** 4 lb 5 oz = _____ kg
2. 15 lb 5 oz = _____ kg	**7.** 75 lb = _____ kg
3. 7¼ lb = _____ kg	**8.** 12 lb 3 oz = _____ kg
4. 22 lb = _____ kg	**9.** 66 lb = _____ kg
5. 54 lb 8 oz = _____ kg	**10.** 10½ lb = _____ kg

Steps and Rule—mg/kg Body Weight

Example	A child weighing 33 lb is ordered Augmentin 150 mg po q8h. Figure 10-1 shows the label for Augmentin, which comes as a dry powder. The accompanying prescribing information states that children ≤ 40 kg receive 6.7 to 13.3 mg/kg q8h. We need to convert 33 lb to kg, calculate the low and high safe dose, determine whether the dose ordered is within the safe range, and prepare the dose. These are the steps:

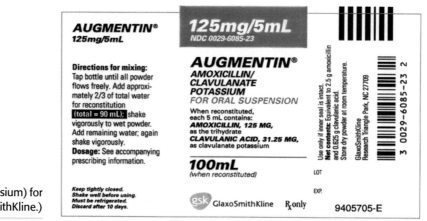

Label for amoxicillin (clavulanate potassium) for oral suspension. (Courtesy of GlaxoSmithKline.)

STEP 1.	Convert lb to kg by dividing by 2.2.
STEP 2.	Determine the safe dose range in milligrams per kilograms using a reference.
STEP 3.	Decide whether the ordered dose is safe by comparing the order with the safe dose range listed in the reference.
STEP 4.	Calculate the dose needed.

Step 1. Convert lb to kg. Divide the number of pounds by 2.2.

$$\begin{array}{r} 1\,5. \\ 2.2\overline{\smash{)}33.0} \\ \underline{22} \\ 11\ 0 \\ \underline{11\ 0} \end{array}$$

The child weighs 15 kg.

> **Learning Aid**
>
> 2.2 lb = 1 kg
>
> $$\frac{2.2\ lb}{1\ kg} = \frac{33\ lb}{x\ kg}$$
>
> 2.2x = 33
>
> $$x = \frac{33}{2.2}$$
>
> Therefore, to obtain kg divide lb by 2.2.

Step 2. Determine the safe dose range. The literature states that the dose should range from 6.7 to 12.3 mg/kg q8h.

Low Dose

$$\begin{array}{r} 6.7\ mg \\ \times\ 15\ kg \\ \hline 100.5\,(\text{calculator}) \end{array}$$

High Dose

$$\begin{array}{r} 13.3\ mg \\ \times\ 15\ kg \\ \hline 199.5 = 200\ mg\,(\text{calculator}) \end{array}$$

Step 3. Is the dose safe? The safe range is 100 to 200 mg q8h. The dose ordered (150 mg q8h) is safe because it falls within the 100- to 200-mg range.

Step 4.   Calculate the dose.

The label states that 90 mL water should be added gradually (see Fig. 10-1) to make a concentration of 125 mg/5 mL.

Formula Method   *Ratio Method*   *Proportion Method*

Rule: $\frac{D}{H} \times S = A$

$$\frac{\overset{6}{\cancel{150\ mg}}}{\underset{\underset{1}{5}}{\cancel{125\ mg}}} \times \overset{1}{\cancel{5}}\ mL = 6\ mL$$

$$5\ mL : 125\ mg :: x : 150\ mg$$

$$\frac{5\ mL}{125\ mg} \times \frac{x\ mL}{150\ mg}$$

$$150 \times 5 = 125x$$

$$750 = 125x$$

$$\frac{750}{125} = x$$

$$6\ mL = x$$

Give 6 mL.

This dose can be measured with a calibrated safety dropper or oral syringe. See Figure 10-2 for examples of this equipment.

Example   A child weighing 16 lb 10 oz is ordered Lasix 15 mg po bid (Fig. 10-3). Is the dose safe? What amount should be poured?

Step 1.   Convert lb to kg.

a. Change the ounces to part of a pound.

$$\begin{array}{r} 0.625 \\ 6\ )\overline{10.0} \\ \underline{9\,6} \\ 40 \\ \underline{32} \\ 80 \\ \underline{80} \\ 0 \end{array}$$

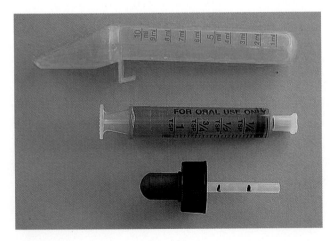

FIGURE 10-2

Examples of equipment used to obtain pediatric doses: (*top*) a medication spoon calculated in mL and teaspoons; (*center*) an oral syringe calculated in teaspoons; (*bottom*) a safety dropper calibrated in mL.

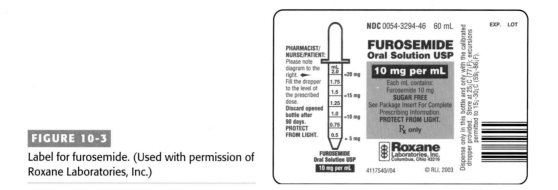

FIGURE 10-3

Label for furosemide. (Used with permission of Roxane Laboratories, Inc.)

The child's weight is $16 + 0.625 = 16.625$ lb.

b. Change pounds to kilograms. Round off to the nearest hundredth.

$$
\begin{array}{r}
7.556 \\
2.2\overline{)16.625} \\
\underline{15\ 4} \\
1\ 22 \\
\underline{1\ 10} \\
125 \\
\underline{110} \\
150 \\
\underline{110}
\end{array}
$$

The child weighs 7.56 kg.

Step 2. Determine the safe dose range in mg/kg. The package insert states: The initial dose of oral Lasix (furosemide) in infants and children is 2 mg/kg body weight, given as a single dose. If the diuretic response is not satisfactory after the initial dose, dosage may be increased by 1 or 2 mg/kg no sooner than 6 to 8 hours after the previous dose. Doses greater than 6 mg/kg body weight are not recommended.

Single Dose	*High Range*
7.56 kg	7.56 kg
$\times$ 2 mg	$\times$ 6
15.12 mg/day	45.36 mg/day

Step 3. Decide whether the ordered dose is safe. The order is 15 mg po bid. The 15 mg meets the requirement for a single dose. The order is bid, which means twice in a day, so $15\ \text{mg} \times 2 = 30\ \text{mg}$. The child will receive 30 mg in a day. The high range is 45 mg, so the dose is safe.

Step 4. Calculate the dose needed. The supply is 10 mg/mL (Fig. 10-3).

Formula Method   *Ratio Method*   *Proportion Method*

$$\frac{D}{H} \times S = A$$

$$\frac{\overset{3}{\cancel{15\,mg}}}{\underset{2}{\cancel{10\,mg}}} \times 1\,mL = \frac{3}{2} = 1.5\,mL$$ $$1\,mL : 10\,mg :: x : 15\,mg$$ $$\frac{1\,mL}{10\,mg} \times \frac{x}{15\,mg}$$

$$15 = 10x$$

$$\frac{15}{10} = x$$

$$1.5\,mL = x$$

The label states that Lasix comes with a calibrated safety dropper. The dropper can be used to obtain the dose of 1.5 mL.

| **Example** | A premature infant weighing 1500 g is ordered digoxin 37.5 mcg po × 1. Is the dose safe? What amount should be given? |

Step 1. Convert grams to kilograms.

$$\frac{1500}{1000} = 1.5\,kg$$

> **Learning Aid**
>
> 1000 grams = 1 kg

Step 2. Determine the safe dose range in mg/kg.

The *Nursing Drug Guide* states: Loading dose (oral) for the premature infant is 20 to 30 mcg/kg.

a. Convert mcg to mg.

$$\frac{20\,mcg}{1000} = 0.02\,mg$$

$$\frac{30\,mcg}{1000} = 0.03\,mg$$

> **Learning Aid**
>
> 1000 mcg = 1 mg

b.

Low Range	*High Range*
1.5 kg	1.5 kg
×0.02 mg	× 0.03 mg
0.03 mg	0.045 mg

Step 3. The ordered dose is 37.5 mcg. Convert to mg.

$$\frac{37.5\,mcg}{1000} = 0.0375\,mg$$

The dosage ordered is safe.

Step 4.   Calculate the dose. Digoxin elixir (Fig. 10-4) comes 0.125 mg/2.5 mL

| *Formula Method* | *Ratio Method* | *Proportion Method* |

$$\frac{\overset{0.3}{\cancel{0.0375}\text{ mg}}}{\underset{1}{\cancel{0.125}\text{ mg}}} \times 2.5\text{ mL} = 0.75\text{ mL}$$

$$2.5\text{ mL} : 0.125\text{ mg} :: x : 0.0375\text{ mg}$$

$$\frac{25\text{ mL}}{0.125} \times \frac{x}{0.0375\text{ mg}}$$

$$2.5 \times 0.0375 = 0.125x$$

$$\frac{0.09375}{0.125} = x$$

$$0.75\text{ mL} = x$$

Use a calibrated safety dropper or oral syringe (1 mL) to draw up 0.75 mL.

Example   A child weighing 66 lb is prescribed epinephrine subcutaneous injection for an allergic reaction. The dosage prescribed is 0.3 mg. Is the dose safe? What amount should be given?

Step 1.   Convert pounds to kilograms.

$$\frac{66}{2.2}\overset{30.}{\overline{)66.0}}$$
$$\underline{66}$$
$$0$$

The child weighs 30 kg.

Step 2.   Determine the safe dose range in mg/kg.

The *Nursing Drug Guide* states 0.01 mg/kg subcutaneous every 20 minutes. Do not exceed 0.5 mg in a single dose.

Step 3.   The ordered dose is 0.3 mg.

$$30\text{ kg}$$
$$\underline{\times\ 0.01\text{ mg/kg}}$$
$$0.3\text{ mg}$$

The dosage is safe.

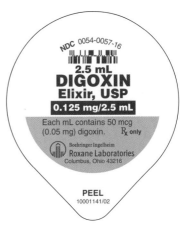

FIGURE 10-4
Label for Digoxin Elixir. (Courtesy of Roxane Laboratories, Inc.)

Step 4. Calculate the dose. Figure 10-5 shows a concentration of 1 mg/mL. Therefore, 0.3 mg = 0.3 mL. Use a 1-mL precision syringe for the dose.

Example A child weighing 50 lb is ordered promethazine IM 20 mg for nausea and vomiting. Is the dose safe? What amount should be given?

Step 1. Convert pounds to kilograms.

$$
\begin{array}{r}
\frac{50}{2.2\,}\begin{array}{l}22.727\\\overline{)50.00}\end{array}\\
\end{array}
$$

$$
\begin{array}{r}
22.727\\
2.2\,\overline{)50.00}\\
\underline{44}\\
60\\
\underline{44}\\
16\,0\\
\underline{15\,4}\\
60\\
\underline{44}\\
160
\end{array}
$$

The child weighs 22.73 kg.

Step 2. Determine the safe dosage range. The *Nursing Drug Guide* states 1 mg/kg IM q4–6h as needed. The safe dosage range is 10 to 25 mg.

Step 3. The ordered dose is 20 mg.

$$
\begin{array}{r}
22.73\text{ kg}\\
\times\quad 1\text{ mg/kg}\\
\hline
22.73\text{ mg}
\end{array}
$$

A total of 22.73 mg is the calculated dose; however, the ordered dose is used and is within the safe range.

Step 4. Calculate the dose.

Promethazine is available 25 mg/mL (Fig. 10-6).

Formula Method	*Ratio Method*	*Proportion Method*
$\frac{20\text{ mg}}{25\text{ mg}}\times 1\text{ mL}=0.8\text{ mL}$	1 mL : 25 mg : : x : 20 mg	$\dfrac{1\text{ mL}}{25\text{ mg}}\times\dfrac{\text{x}}{20\text{ mg}}$

$$20=25\text{x}$$
$$\frac{20}{25}=0.8\text{ mL}$$

Use a 1-mL precision syringe to draw up and administer the dose.

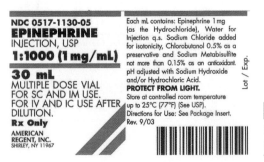

NDC 0517-1130-05
EPINEPHRINE
INJECTION, USP
1:1000 (1 mg/mL)

30 mL
MULTIPLE DOSE VIAL
FOR SC AND IM USE.
FOR IV AND IC USE AFTER
DILUTION.
Rx Only
AMERICAN
REGENT, INC.
SHIRLEY, NY 11967

Each mL contains: Epinephrine 1 mg (as the Hydrochloride), Water for Injection q.s. Sodium Chloride added for isotonicity, Chlorobutanol 0.5% as a preservative and Sodium Metabisulfite not more than 0.15% as an antioxidant. pH adjusted with Sodium Hydroxide and/or Hydrochloric Acid.
PROTECT FROM LIGHT.
Store at controlled room temperature up to 25°C (77°F) (See USP).
Directions for Use: See Package Insert.
Rev. 9/03

FIGURE 10-5

Label for subcutaneous and intramuscular epinephrine. (Courtesy of American Regent, Inc.)

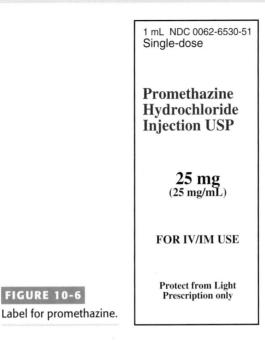

1 mL NDC 0062-6530-51
Single-dose

**Promethazine
Hydrochloride
Injection USP**

25 mg
(25 mg/mL)

FOR IV/IM USE

Protect from Light
Prescription only

FIGURE 10-6

Label for promethazine.

SELF-TEST 2   Dosage Calculations

*In these practice problems, determine whether the doses are safe and calculate the amount needed.
Answers are given at the end of the chapter. Use a calculator.*

1. Order: Amoxil 60 mg po q8h
   Patient: child weighing 20 lb
   Supply: amoxil 125 mg/5 mL; label states 20 to 40 mg/kg/day in divided doses q8h

2. Order: Augmentin 175 mg po q8h
   Patient: child weighing 29 lb
   Supply: Literature states 40 mg/kg/day in divided doses; bottle of 125 mg/5 mL

3. Order: Ferrous sulfate 200 mg po tid
   Patient: child is 9 years old and weighs 30 kg
   Supply: bottle of 125 mg/5 mL
   Literature states: children 6 to 12 years old, 600 mg divided doses tid

4. Order: Tylenol 80 mg po q4° prn for temp 100.9°F and above
   Patient: child is 6 years old and weighs 20.5 kg
   Supply: chewable tablets 80 mg
   Literature states: for child 6 to 8 years give four chewable tablets. May repeat four or five
   times daily. Not to exceed five doses in 24 hours. Is the dose safe?

5. Order: diazepam 1 mg IM q3–4h prn
   Patient: infant 30 days old
   Supply: vial 5 mg/1 mL
   Literature states: child < 6 mo IM 1 to 2.5 mg tid or qid

(continued)

SELF-TEST 2   Dosage Calculations (Continued)

6. Order: Demerol 15 mg subcutaneous q3–4h for relief of pain
   Patient: child is 3 years old and weighs 14 kg
   Supply: injection 10 mg/mL or 25 mg/mL
   Literature states Demerol 1.1 mg/kg/dose q3–4h not to exceed 100 mg/dose

7. Order: dimenhydrinate 25 mg IM q6h as needed
   Patient: child is 10 years old and weighs 30 kg
   Supply: injection labeled 50 mg/mL
   Literature states 1.25 mg/kg qid not to exceed 300 mg/day

8. Order: cloxacillin 250 mg po q6h
   Patient: child weighs 48 lbs
   Supply: liquid labeled 125 mg in 5 mL
   Literature states for children more than 20 kg, the dose should be 250 to 500 mg q6h.

9. Order: Zithromax po 300 mg × 1 dose
   Patient: child is 10 years old and weighs 30 kg
   Supply: oral suspension 100 mg/5 mL in 15-mL bottle
   Literature states for children 2 to 15 years, 10 mg/kg (not more than 500 mg/dose) on day 1.

10. Order: Dilantin po 60 mg bid
    Patient: infant weighs 12 lb 8 oz
    Supply: Dilantin suspension 30 mg/5 mL
    Literature states 4 to 8 mg/kg/day divided into two doses. Maximum dose is 300 mg/day.

Determining BSA in m²

A second method to determine pediatric dosage is to calculate BSA in meters squared (m^2) using a chart called a nomogram (Fig. 10-7). Height is marked in the left column, weight in the right column. A line is drawn between these two marks. The point at which the line intersects the middle column indicates BSA in m^2.

Because of differences in growth, different charts are used for infants and young children than for older children and adults. If a child weighs more than 65 lb or is more than 3 ft tall, the adult nomogram should be used (Fig. 10-8).

Example
1. An infant with a height of 12 in weighing 15 lb has a BSA of 0.19 m^2.
2. A child 4′2″ weighing 130 lb has a BSA of 1.55 m^2.

Determining BSA is easier and faster with a battery-operated calculator or with a manual slide calculator. Figure 10-9 shows how a slide calculator is used.

BSA is used mainly in calculating chemotherapy dosages. A useful website for calculating BSA is www.halls.md/body-surface-area/bsa.htm.

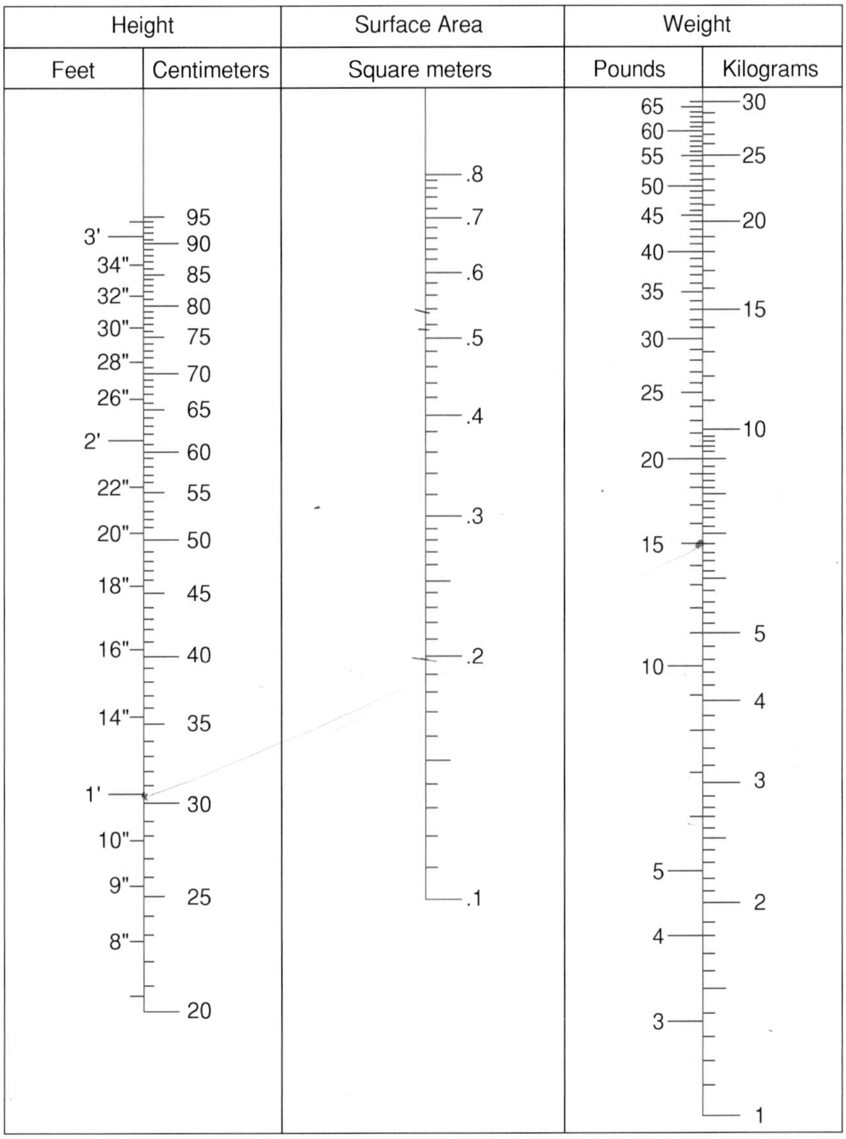

Height		Surface Area	Weight	
Feet	Centimeters	Square meters	Pounds	Kilograms

FIGURE 10-7

Nomogram for infants and toddlers.

SELF-TEST 3   **Determining BSA**

Convert height and weight to BSA in m² using Figure 10-7 or 10-8. Answers are given at the end of this chapter.

Height	Weight	BSA in m²
1. 36 in	26 lb	_____
2. 80 cm	13 kg	_____
3. 50 in	75 lb	_____
4. 17 in	9 lb	_____

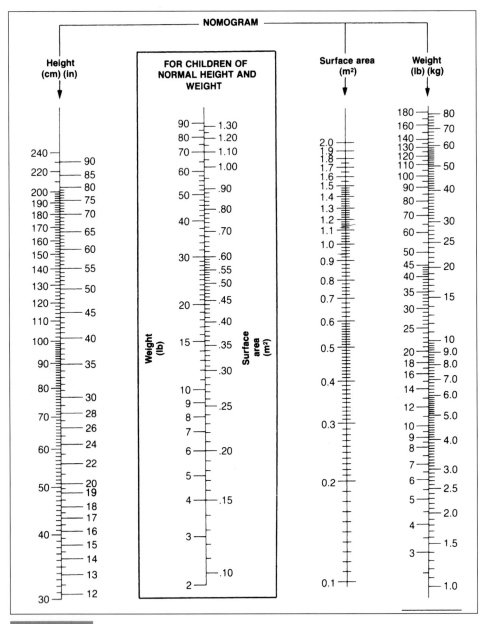

FIGURE 10-8

Nomogram for adults and children. To determine the surface area, draw a straight line between the point representing the patient's height on the left vertical scale to the point representing the patient's weight on the right vertical scale. The point at which this line intersects the middle vertical scale represents the surface area in square meters.

Steps and Rule—m² Medication Orders

STEP 1. Find the BSA in m².

STEP 2. Determine the safe dose using a reference.

STEP 3. Decide whether the ordered dose is safe.

STEP 4. Calculate the dose needed.

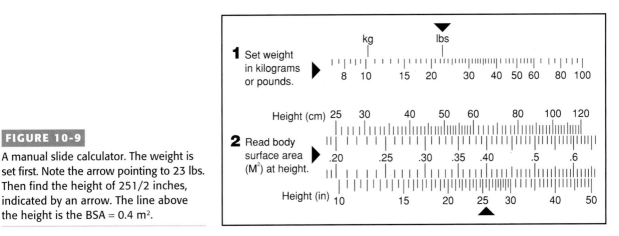

FIGURE 10-9

A manual slide calculator. The weight is set first. Note the arrow pointing to 23 lbs. Then find the height of 251/2 inches, indicated by an arrow. The line above the height is the BSA = 0.4 m².

Example
A 2-year-old child weighing 27 lb 12 oz; height, 35 in; is prescribed leucovorin calcium 5.5 mg po q6h × 72 hr.

Literature states dose for rescue after methotrexate therapy is 10 mg/m²/dose q6h × 72 hours.

Supply: 1 mg/mL reconstituted by the pharmacy

Step 1. Use Figure 10-7.
Height, 35 in; weight, 27 lb 12 oz
Make weight 27¾ lbs.
BSA = 0.55

Learning Aid

To use the nomogram convert oz to lb.
16 oz = 1 lb

$$\frac{\overset{3}{\cancel{12}}}{\underset{4}{\cancel{16}}} = 3/4 \text{ lb}$$

Step 2. Safe dose is 10 mg/m²/dose q6h.

$$\begin{array}{r} 10 \text{ mg} \\ \times\, 0.55 \text{ m}^2 \\ \hline 5.5 \text{ mg} = \text{safe dose q6h} \end{array}$$

Step 3. Order is 5.5 mg q6h. Dose is safe.

Step 4.

Formula Method

$\frac{D}{H} \times S = A$

$\frac{5.5\, mg}{1\, mg} \times 1 \text{ mL} = 5.5 \text{ mL}$

Give 5.5 mL po q6h.

Ratio Method

1 mL : 1 mg : : x : 5.5 mg

5.5 = x

Proportion Method

$\frac{1 \text{ mL}}{1 \text{ mg}} \times \frac{x}{5.5 \text{ mg}}$

Example
A 6-year-old child weighing 40 lb; height, 45 in; is prescribed methotrexate 7.5 mg po twice weekly.

Literature states methotrexate 7.5 to 30 mg/m²/dose twice weekly

Supply: 2.5-mg tablets

Step 1: Use Figure 10-8.

Height, 45 in; weight, 40 lb

BSA = 0.75

Step 2. Safe dose is 7.5 to 30 mg/m²/dose twice weekly

$$\begin{array}{cc} 7.5 \text{ kg} & 30 \text{ mg} \\ \underline{\times 0.75 \text{ m}^2} & \underline{\times 0.55 \text{ m}^2} \\ 5.625 \text{ mg} & 16.5 \text{ mg} \end{array}$$

Step 3: Order is 7.5 mg po twice weekly. Dose is safe.

Step 4:

Formula Method

$$\frac{\overset{3}{\cancel{7.5 \text{ mg}}}}{\underset{1}{\cancel{2.5 \text{ mg}}}} \times 1 \text{ tablet} = 3 \text{ tablets}$$

Ratio Method

$$1 \text{ tablet} : 2.5 \text{ mg} :: x : 7.5 \text{ mg}$$

Proportion Method

$$\frac{1 \text{ tablet}}{2.5 \text{ mg}} \times \frac{x}{7.5 \text{ mg}}$$

$$7.5 = 2.5x$$

$$\frac{7.5}{2.5} = x$$

Give 3 tablets po twice weekly.   3 tablets

SELF-TEST 4   Use of the Nomogram

In these problems, determine whether the dose is safe using the nomogram in Figure 10-7 or 10-8 and calculate the amount needed. Answers are given at the end of the chapter. You will find it helpful to use a calculator.

1. Child: 8 years; height, 50 in; weight, 55 lb
   Order: flecainide 50 mg po q8h
   Literature: dose 100 to 200 mg/m²/24 hours divided q8–12h
   Supply: 50-mg tablets

2. Child: 12 years; height, 59 in; weight, 88 lb
   Order: methotrexate 12.5 mg po q week
   Literature: 10 mg/m²/dose as needed weekly to control fever and joint inflammation in rheumatoid arthritis
   Supply: 2.5-mg tablets

3. Infant: 12 months; height, 30 in; weight, 22 lb 8 oz
   Order: prednisone 5 mg po q12h
   Literature: immunosuppressive dose 6–30 mg/m²/24 hours
   Supply: 5 mg/5 mL syrup

4. Child: 10 years; height, 50 in; weight, 35 kg
   Order: Dronabinol po 5 mg × 1
   Literature: dose 5 mg/m² 1 to 3 hours before chemotherapy
   Supply: 2.5 mg capsules

5. Child: 12 years; height, 60 in; weight, 100 lb
   Order: quinidine po 250 mg/dose
   Literature: dose 900 mg/m²/day in 5 divided doses
   Supply: 200-mg, 300-mg tablets

Administering Intravenous Medications

IV medications are administered when a child cannot maintain an oral fluid intake, has fluid electrolyte imbalances, or requires IV medication. Dosages for IV medications are calculated in mg/kg.

IVP (IV push) medications are calculated according to weight and are then given per protocol from a drug handbook or hospital policy. Continuous IV medications are also calculated according to weight and are then infused through an infusion pump.

IVPB medications are administered in small amounts of diluent. A pediatric reference or institutional manual must be consulted to determine the minimum safe amount. *Drugs for IVPB must be initially diluted following the manufacturer's directions.* Once the initial dilution is made, the amount of drug required to obtain the dose is withdrawn from the vial and is then further diluted. IV solutions in pediatrics usually range from 10 to 20 mL for smaller children and infants requiring IVPB medications. This amount of fluid will fill the tubing from the Buretrol to the patient. When the Buretrol is empty of the IV medication, most of the drug will be in the tubing. For this reason an IV flush of 20 mL must be added to the Buretrol *after* the medication is infused to ensure that the patient receives the drug.

Buretrols or other volume control units are used to administer IV fluids. They are calibrated and hold no more than 100 to 150 mL at a time. This reduces the possibility of fluid overload. Infusion pumps are also used to provide a second safeguard (Fig. 10-10). In neonatal areas, syringe pumps can deliver IV fluid ranging from 1 to 60 mL.

In this section we consider the calculation of pediatric doses for IV and IVPB administration. These problems may seem complex; however, their solution requires a step-by-step analysis that is easily learned and applied.

STEPS TO SOLVING PARENTERAL PEDIATRIC MEDICATIONS IVP

STEP 1.   Convert lb to kg.

STEP 2.   Determine the safe dose range in mg/kg using a reference.

STEP 3.   Decide whether the ordered dose is safe by comparing the order with the safe dose range listed in the reference.

STEP 4.   Calculate the dose needed.

STEP 5.   Check the reference for diluent and duration for administration.

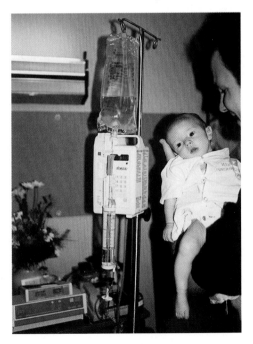

FIGURE 10-10

An infusion pump with a volume control unit. (With permission from Pillitteri, A. [2002]. *Maternal and child health nursing* [4th ed.]. Philadelphia: Lippincott Williams & Wilkins, p. 1106.)

| Example | Child: | 5 years; weight, 44 lb |

Child: 5 years; weight, 44 lb

Order: famotidine 5 mg IV bid

Literature: 0.25 mg/kg q12h IV up to 40 mg/day

Dilute to 5 or 10 mL with 5% dextrose or 0.9% sodium chloride and injected over at least 2 minutes.

Supply: See label (Fig. 10-11).

Step 1. Convert pounds to kg.

$$\frac{44}{2.2} \quad \frac{2\,0.}{\big)44.0}$$
$$\underline{44}$$
$$0$$

The child weighs 20 kg.

Step 2. Determine the safe dose.

$$\begin{array}{r}20 \text{ kg} \\ \times 0.25 \text{ mg/kg} \\ \hline 5 \text{ mg}\end{array}$$

Step 3. The dose is safe. It meets the mg/kg rule and does not exceed 40 mg/day.

5 mg bid = total 10 mg/day

Step 4. Calculate the dose.

Formula Method

$$\frac{\overset{1}{5 \text{ mg}}}{\underset{2}{10 \text{ mg}}} \times 1 \text{ mL} = 0.5 \text{ mL}$$

Ratio Method

$$1 \text{ mL} : 10 \text{ mg} :: x : 5 \text{ mg}$$

Proportion Method

$$\frac{1 \text{ mL}}{10 \text{ mg}} \times \frac{x}{5 \text{ mg}}$$

$$5 = 10x$$

$$\frac{5}{10} = x$$

$$0.5 \text{ mL}$$

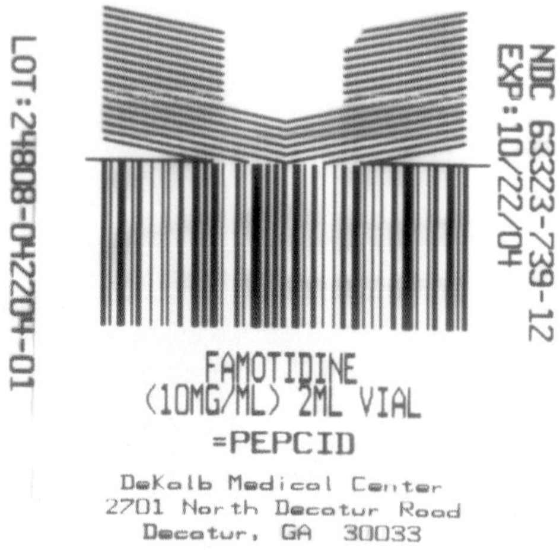

LOT: 24808-042204-01

NDC 63323-739-12
EXP: 10/22/04

FAMOTIDINE
(10MG/ML) 2ML VIAL
=PEPCID

DeKalb Medical Center
2701 North Decatur Road
Decatur, GA 30033

FIGURE 10-11

Famotidine. (Courtesy of DeKalb Medical Center, Decatur, GA.)

Step 5. Dilute with 5 or 10 mL suggested diluent. Inject over 2 minutes.

Example   Child: 10 years; weight, 40 kg.

Order: furosemide 40 mg IV bid

Literature: 1 mg/kg q12h IV, no more than 6 mg/kg/day

Inject directly or into tubing of actively running IV; inject slowly over 1 to 2 minutes.

Supply: See label (Fig. 10-12).

Step 1. Weight is in kg: 40 kg

Step 2. 1 mg/kg

40 kg = 40 mg

Step 3. 40 mg bid would be a total of 80 mg

Maximum dose: 6 mg/kg/day

40 kg × 6 = 240 mg

The dosage is safe.

FIGURE 10-12

Furosemide. (Courtesy of DeKalb Medical Center, Decatur, GA.)

Step 4. Calculate the dose needed.

Formula Method

$$\frac{\overset{4}{40}\ \text{mg}}{\underset{1}{10}\ \text{mg}} \times 1\ \text{mL} = 4\ \text{mL}$$

Ratio Method

1 mL : 10 mg : : x : 40 mg

$$40 = 10x$$

$$\frac{40}{10} = x$$

4 mL

Proportion Method

$$\frac{1\ \text{mL}}{10\ \text{mg}} \times \frac{\text{x}}{40\ \text{mg}}$$

Step 5. Check the reference for diluent and duration for administration.

STEPS TO SOLVE PARENTERAL PEDIATRIC MEDICATIONS IVPB

1. Decide whether the dose is safe; check a pediatric reference.
2. Decide whether the dilution ordered meets the minimum pediatric safety standard.
3. Prepare the medication according to directions.
4. Draw up the dose and dilute further as needed.
5. Set the pump in mL/hr. If the infusion time is 30 minutes, set the pump for double the amount because the pump delivers mL/hr.

   Example   The order is 10 mL over 30 minutes. Set the pump for 20 mL/hr. It will deliver 10 mL in 30 minutes.

6. When the IV is completed, add a flush of 20 mL to the Buretrol to clear the tubing of the medication. Be sure to chart the flush as fluid intake. Follow institutional requirements regarding IV flush.

| **Example** | Child: 4 years; weight, 17 kg |

Order: fortaz 280 mg IV q8h in 10 mL D5⅓NS

Literature: Safe dose 30 to 50 mg/kg/day
Concentration for IV use: 50 mg/mL over 30 minutes

Supply: 1 g powder. Directions: Dilute with 10 mL sterile water for injection to make 95 mg/mL; stable for 7 days if refrigerated (Fig. 10-13).

1. Safe dose is 30 to 50 mg/kg/day.

Low Range	*High Range*
30 mg	50 mg
× 17 mg	× 17 mg
510 mg/day	850 mg/day

Order is 280 mg q8h (three doses).

280 mg × 3 = 840 mg

Dose falls within the range and is safe.

2. Minimum safe dilution is 50 mg/mL. Dose is 280 mg.

$$50\overline{)280.}$$

5.6 = 6 mL, the minimum dilution. The order of 10 mL is safe because it is more than the minimum.

$$
\begin{array}{r}
5.6 \\
50\overline{)280.} \\
\underline{250} \\
300 \\
\underline{300}
\end{array}
$$

3. Dilute 1 g with 10 mL sterile water to make 95 mg/mL.

Formula Method

$\frac{D}{H} \times S = A$

$\frac{280 \text{ mg}}{95 \text{ mg}} \times 1 \text{ mL} = 2.9 \text{ mL}$

Withdraw 2.9 mL; label the vial and store in the refrigerator.

Ratio Method

1 mL : 95 mg :: x : 280 mg

Proportion Method

$\frac{1 \text{ mL}}{95 \text{ mg}} \times \frac{x}{280 \text{ mg}}$

280 = 95x

$\frac{280}{95} = x$

2.9 mL

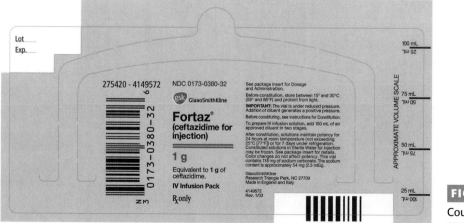

FIGURE 10-13

Courtesy of GlaxoSmithKline.

4. Run about 5 mL D5⅓NS into the Buretrol. Add the 2.9 mL drug. Add more D5⅓NS to make 10 mL.

5. Set the pump at 20. This is 20 mL/hr. The pump will deliver 10 mL in 30 minutes.

6. When the IV is completed, add a 20-mL flush of D5⅓NS to clear the IV tubing of medication.

Example

Infant: 4.3 kg

Order: ampicillin 100 mg IV q6h in 10 mL D5⅓NS

Literature: The safe dose is 75 to 200 mg/kg/24 hours given q6 to 8h IV.

Concentration for IV use: 50 mg/mL over 10 to 30 minutes

Supply: Vial of powder labeled 500 mg. Directions: Add 1.8 mL sterile water for injection to make 250 mg/mL; use within 1 hour.

1. Safe dose is 75 to 200 mg/kg/24 hours given q6–8h.

Low Range	*High Range*
75 mg	200 mg
× 4.3 kg	× 4.3 kg
322.5 mg/24 hr	860 mg/24 hr

Order is 100 mg q6h (four doses).

100 mg × 4 doses = 400 mg.

This is within the range. The dose is safe.

2. Minimum safe dilution is 50 mg/mL (Table 10-1). Dose is 100 mg.

$$50\overline{)100}^{2}$$ 2 mL is the minimum dilution; 10 mL is safe.

3. Add 1.8 mL sterile water for injection to 500 mg powder to make 250 mg/mL.

TABLE 10-1   Sample of a Dilution Table for Pediatric Antibiotics

Antibiotic	Recommended Final Concentration IV	Recommendation Duration of IV
Ampicillin	50 mg/mL	10–30 min
Cefotaxime	50 mg/mL	10–30 min
Clindamycin	6–12 mg/mL	15–30 min
Gentamicin	2 mg/mL	15–30 min
Penicillin G	Infants: 50,000 units/mL	10–30 min
	Large child: 100,000 units/mL	
Pentamidine	2.5 mg/mL	1 hr

Formula Method	*Ratio Method*	*Proportion Method*

$$\frac{D}{H} \times S = A$$

$$\frac{100 \ \cancel{mg}}{250 \ \cancel{mg}} \times 1 \ mL = \frac{2}{5} = 0.4 \ mL \qquad\qquad 1 \ mL : 250 \ mg :: x : 100 \ mg \qquad\qquad \frac{1 \ mL}{250 \ mg} \times \frac{x}{100 \ mg}$$

$$100 = 250x$$

$$\frac{100}{250} = x$$

$$0.4 \ mL = x$$

Withdraw 0.4 mL from the vial. Discard the remainder (directions say to use within 1 hour).

4. Add about 5 mL D5⅓NS to the Buretrol. Add 0.4 mL drug. Add more D5⅓NS to make 10 mL.

5. Set the pump at 20. This means 20 mL/hr. The pump will deliver 10 mL in 30 minutes.

6. When the IV is finished, add a 20-mL flush of D5⅓NS to the Buretrol to clear the tubing of medication.

General Guidelines for Continuous IV Medications

1. Continuous IV medications for children and infants are calculated with the methods and formulas used in Chapter 9.

2. Continuous IV dosages are based on weight in kilograms.

3. An infusion pump and/or volume control sets are always used.

4. Small bags of fluid are used to prevent fluid overload.

5. Follow institutional requirements for continuous IV infusions.

6. Consult a pediatric text or drug reference to determine the safe dosage range.

SELF-TEST 5   Parenteral Medication Calculations

In these practice problems, determine whether the dose is safe, calculate the amount needed, and state how the order should be administered. Answers are given at the end of this chapter. Follow the steps used in the examples.

1. Infant: 6 months; weight, 8 kg
    Order: cefuroxime 200 mg IV q6h in 10 mL D5¼NS
    Literature: The safe dose is 50 to 100 mg/kg/24h given q6–8h
                   Concentration for IV use: 50 mg/mL over 30 minutes
    Supply: 750-mg vial of powder. Directions: Dilute with 8 mL sterile water for injection
                   to make 90 mg/mL; stable for 3 days if refrigerated.

2. Child: 3 years; weight, 15 kg
    Order: Bactrim (as TMP/SMX) 75 mg IV q12h in 75 mL D5W over 1 hr
    Literature: Safe dose for a child is 8 to 10 mg/kg/24h given q12h
                   Concentration for IV use: 1 mL in 15 to 25 mL (supply is a liquid)
    Supply: Vial labeled 80 mg/5 mL

SELF-TEST 5   Parenteral Medication Calculations (Continued)

3. Child: 12 years; weight, 40 kg
   Order: tobramycin 100 mg IV q8h in 50 mL D5⅓NS
   Literature: The safe dose is 3 to 5 mg/kg/24h given q8h
   Concentration for IV use: 2 mg/mL over 15 to 30 minutes
   Supply: vial 80 mg/2 mL

4. Child: 5 years; weight, 18 kg
   Order: cefotaxime 900 mg IV q6h in 25 mL D5⅓NS
   Literature: The safe dose is 50 to 200 mg/kg/24h given q6h
   Concentration for IV use: 50 mg/mL; give over 30 minutes
   Supply: 1 g powder. Directions: Dilute with 10 mL sterile water for injection to make
   95 mg/mL; stable in the refrigerator 10 days.

5. Infant: 3 months; weight, 6 kg
   Order: nafcillin 150 mg IV q8h in 10 mL D5⅓NS
   Literature: The safe dose is 100 to 200 mg/kg/24h given q6h
   Concentration for IV use: 6 mg/mL over 30 to 60 minutes
   Supply: 500-mg vial of powder. Directions: Add 1.7 mL sterile water for injection to
   make 500 mg/2 mL; stable for 48 hr if refrigerated.

6. Child: 8 years; weight, 30 kg
   Order: morphine 2.5 mg IV q4h
   Literature: 0.05 to 0.1 mg/kg/q4h IV. Dilute 2 to 10 mg in at least 5 mL NS. Administer
   over 4 to 5 minutes.
   Supply: morphine injection 1 mg/mL

7. Child: 6 years; weight, 25 kg
   Order: Decadron 4 mg IV bid
   Literature: 0.08 to 0.3 mg/kg/day divided q6–12h. Give undiluted IVP over 30 seconds
   or less.
   Supply: Decadron 4 mg/mL injection

8. Child: 12 years; weight, 45 kg
   Order: Benadryl 25 mg IV q4–6h
   Literature: 12.5 to 25 mg IV q4–6 h; maximum dose, 300 mg/24 hr
   Give undiluted IVP over 1 minute.
   Supply: 50 mg/mL injection

9. Infant: 15 lb
   Order: digoxin maintenance dose IV 50 mcg/day
   Literature: 6 to 7.5 mcg/kg/day. Give undiluted or diluted in 4 mL D5W or NS over
   5 minutes.
   Supply: 0.1 mg/mL injection

10. Child: 9 years; weight, 80 lb
   Order: SoluMedrol IV 60 mg bid
   Literature: 0.5 to 1.7 mg/kg/day divided q12h. Give each 500 mg over 2 to 3 minutes.
   Supply: SoluMedrol 40 mg/mL

CRITICAL THINKING: TEST YOUR CLINICAL SAVVY

You are working in a pediatric unit and taking care of 5-year-old Georgia Smith. Although she usually has a sweet disposition, she has her moments when she will not do anything she doesn't want to do. She is receiving IV fluids continuously and is ordered an oral medication three times a day that has an aftertaste. Each time the medication is brought to her, she refuses to take it.

a. What are techniques to help her take the medication?
b. Are there other alternatives you could use regarding the medication? How would you implement any of these alternatives?
c. Are there strategies to suggest to the family to promote easier compliance?
d. Besides reducing the possibility of fluid overload, what are some other reasons IV infusion pumps are used with children?

Another patient, 14-year-old Sean McBrady, is unable to swallow pills.

a. What are some alternatives to the medication?
b. Are there contraindications to any of the medication alternatives?
c. What are some ways to get children to swallow pills?
d. What would you suggest to the family to promote easier administration?

| **Infants and Children Dosage Problems**

Name: _____

Here is a mix of oral and parenteral pediatric orders. For each problem, determine the safe dose and calculate the amount to be given. If you experience any difficulty, review the content. Answers are given on page 442.

1. Newborn: weight, 4 kg
 Order: vitamin K 1 mg IM × 1 dose
 Literature: Prophylaxis and treatment: 0.5 to 1 mg/dose IM, subcutaneous, IV × 1
 Supply: vial 10 mg/mL

2. Infant: 1 yr; 10 kg
 Order: augmentin 125 mg po q8h
 Literature: Safe dose amoxicillin–clavulanic acid: 20 to 40 mg/kg/24 hours given q8h po
 Supply: 125 mg/5 mL

3. Infant: 10 mo; 10 kg
 Order: benzathine penicillin 500,000 units IM × 1 dose
 Literature: Safe dose 50,000 units/kg × 1 IM. Maximum, 2.4 milliunits
 Supply: vial labeled 600,000 units/mL

4. Infant: 3.6 kg
 Order: gentamicin 9 mg IV q8h in 10 mL D5¼NS
 Literature: Safe dose is 2.5 mg/kg/dose q8h
 Concentration for IV 2 mg/mL given over 15 to 30 min
 Supply: vial 40 mg/mL

5. Infant: 6.7 kg
 Order: Colace Syrup 10 mg po bid
 Literature: Infants and children under 3: 10 to 40 mg/day
 Supply: 20 mg/5 mL

6. Infant: 5.5 kg
 Order: vancomycin 54 mg IV q8h in 12 mL D5¼NS
 Literature: Safe dose is 10 mg/kg q8h IV
 Concentration for IV 5 mg/mL; infuse over 1 hour
 Supply: 500 mg powder
 Directions: Add 10 mL sterile water for injection to give 50 mg/mL; stable in the refrigerator 14 days.

7. Infant: 6.7 kg
 Order: chloral hydrate 350 mg po prior to electroencephalogram
 Literature: Hypnotic for children: 25 to 50 mg/kg/dose po not to exceed 100 mg/kg.
 Supply: 500 mg/5 mL

8. Child: 12 years; height, 60 in; weight, 40 kg; BSA, 1.32
 Order: methotrexate 10 mg po 1–2×/week
 Literature: 7.5–30 mg/m² 1–2×/week
 Supply: 2.5-mg tablet

9. Child: 8 yr; 24 kg
 Order: Fortaz 2 g IVPB q8h in 50 mL D5⅓NS
 Literature: Safe dose is 2 to 6 g/24 hours given q8–12h IV
 Concentration for IV 50 mg/mL over 15 to 30 minutes
 Supply: 2-g vial of powder
 Dilute initially with 10 mL sterile water for injection.

10. Child: 35 lb
 Order: meperidine HCl 20 mg IV stat
 Literature: Children: usual dose 1 to 1.5 mg/kg/dose q 3–4h prn. Maximum dose, 100 mg.
 Supply: 50 mg/mL

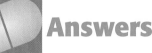 **Answers**

Self-Test 1 Converting Pounds to Kilograms

1. 13.64 kg (calculator)

2. $\dfrac{5 \text{ oz}}{16 \text{ oz}} = 0.3125$ lb (calculator)

Weight = 15.3125 lb
Change to kilograms.

$\dfrac{15.3125}{2.2} = 6.96$ kg (calculator)

3. $\frac{1}{4}$ lb = 0.25 lb
Weight = 7.25 lb
Change to kilograms.

$\dfrac{7.25}{2.2} = 3.3$ kg (calculator)

4. 10 kg (calculator)

5. $\dfrac{8 \text{ oz}}{16} = 0.5$ lb

Weight = 54.5 lb.
Change to kilograms.

$\dfrac{54.5 \text{ lb}}{2.2} = 24.77$ kg

6. $\dfrac{5 \text{ oz}}{16} = 0.3125$ lb

Weight = 4.3125 lb.

$\dfrac{4.3125}{2.2} = 1.96$ kg (calculator)

7. $\dfrac{75 \text{ lb}}{2.2} = 34.09$ kg (calculator)

8. $\dfrac{3 \text{ oz}}{16} = 0.1875$ lb

Weight = 12.1875 lb.

$\dfrac{12.1875}{2.2} = 5.54$ kg

9. $\dfrac{66 \text{ lb}}{2.2} = 30$ kg

10. $\frac{1}{2}$ lb = 0.5 lb
Weight = 10.5 lb.
$\dfrac{10.5}{2.2} = 4.77$ kg

Self-Test 2 Dosage Calculations

1. Step 1. $\dfrac{20}{2.2} = 9.09$ kg

Step 2. Low range   9.09 kg
                  $\times$ 20 mg
                  181.8 mg/day

       High Range   9.09 kg
                  $\times$ 40 mg
                  363.6 mg/day

Step 3. 60 mg $\times$ 3 doses = 180 mg/day
        The order is safe, although on the low side.

Step 4.

Formula Method	*Ratio Method*	*Proportion Method*

$$\frac{60\text{mg}}{125\text{mg}} \times 5 \text{ mL} = 2.4 \text{ mL}$$

5 mL : 125 mg : : x : 60 mg

$$\frac{5 \text{ mL}}{125 \text{ mg}} = \frac{x}{60 \text{ mg}}$$

$$60 \times 5 = 125x$$

$$\frac{300}{125} = x$$

Give 2.4 mL po q8h.

2.4 mL

2. Step 1. 29 lb = 13.18 kg (calculator)

Step 2.   40 mg
         × 13.18 kg
         527.27 mg (calculator) = safe dose

Step 3.   175 mg
         ×   3 doses
         525 mg = child's dose. Order is safe.

Step 4.

Formula Method	*Ratio Method*	*Proportion Method*

$$\frac{D}{H} \times S = A$$

$$\frac{\overset{7}{\cancel{175}} \text{ mg}}{\underset{\underset{1}{25}}{\cancel{125}} \text{ mg}} \times \overset{1}{\cancel{5}} \text{ mL} = 7$$

5 mL : 125 mg : : x : 175 mg

$$\frac{5 \text{ mL}}{125 \text{ mg}} = \frac{x}{175 \text{ mg}}$$

$$5 \times 175 = 125x$$

$$\frac{875}{125} = x$$

Give 7 mL po q8h.

7 mL = x

3. a. It was not necessary to use a rule. The literature was clear. Children 6 to 12 years should receive 600 mg divided into three doses, which equals 200 mg/dose. The ordered dose is safe.

b.

Formula Method	*Ratio Method*	*Proportion Method*

$$\frac{D}{H} \times S = A$$

$$\frac{200}{125} \times 5 = \frac{1000}{125} \overset{8.0 \text{ mL}}{\overline{)1000.}}$$

5 mL : 125 mg : : x : 200 mg

$$\frac{5 \text{ mL}}{125 \text{ mg}} = \frac{x}{200 \text{ mg}}$$

$$5 \times 200 = 125x$$

$$\frac{1000}{125} = x$$

Give 8 mL po tid.

8 mL = x

4. Tylenol 80 mg seems low. Literature says a child of 6 years should receive four chewable tablets. This would be 320 mg. Check with the physician.

5. **a.** The literature states that children under 6 months can receive 1 to 2.5 mg IM three to four times a day. The individual dose for the infant is 1 mg. This is safe, but the physician wrote q3–4h prn for the time. This would allow six to eight doses per 24 hours. The nurse can give the first dose but should clarify the times with the doctor.

b.

Formula Method	*Ratio Method*	*Proportion Method*

$\frac{D}{H} \times S = A$

$\frac{1 \ \text{mg}}{5 \ \text{mg}} \times 1 \ \text{mL} = 0.2 \ \text{mL IM}$

$1 \ \text{mL} : 5 \ \text{mg} :: x : 1 \ \text{mg}$

$\frac{1 \ \text{mL}}{5 \ \text{mg}} = \frac{x}{1 \ \text{mg}}$

$$1 = 5x$$

$$\frac{1}{5} = x$$

Give 0.2 mL IM.

$$0.2 \ \text{mL} = x$$

6. Step 1. 14 kg

   Step 2.
   $$\begin{array}{r} 14 \ \text{kg} \\ \times 1.1 \ \text{mg/kg} \\ \hline 15.4 \ \text{mg} \end{array}$$

   Step 3. The dose is safe. It does not exceed 100 mg/dose.

   Step 4. Calculate using both supplies.

Formula Method	*Ratio Method*	*Proportion Method*

$\frac{\overset{3}{15} \ \text{mg}}{\underset{2}{10} \ \text{mg}} \times 1 \ \text{mL} = 1.5 \ \text{mL}$

$1 \ \text{mL} : 10 \ \text{mg} :: x : 15 \ \text{mg}$

$\frac{1 \ \text{mL}}{10 \ \text{mg}} = \frac{x}{15 \ \text{mg}}$

$$15 = 10x$$

$$\frac{15}{10} = 1.5 \ \text{mL}$$

$\frac{\overset{3}{15} \ \text{mg}}{\underset{5}{25} \ \text{mg}} \times 1 \ \text{mL} = 0.6 \ \text{mL}$

$1 \ \text{mL} : 25 \ \text{mg} :: x : 15 \ \text{mg}$

$\frac{1 \ \text{mL}}{25 \ \text{mg}} = \frac{x}{15 \ \text{mg}}$

$$15 = 25x$$

$$0.6 \ \text{mL} = x$$

Give the 0.6-mL dose subcutaneously because it is less liquid to inject.

7. Step 1. 30 kg

Step 2. 30 kg
$$\frac{\times 1.25 \text{ mg/kg}}{37.5 \text{ mg}}$$

Step 3. 25
$$\frac{\times 4 \ (q6h)}{100 \ \text{mg/day}}$$

The dose does not exceed 300 mg/day.
However, the dose ordered is less than the recommended dose. Check with the physician.

Step 4.

Formula Method	*Ratio Method*	*Proportion Method*
$\dfrac{\overset{1}{25} \text{ mg}}{\underset{2}{50} \text{ mg}} \times 1 \text{ mL} = 0.5 \text{ mL}$	1 mL : 50 mg :: x : 25 mg	$\dfrac{1 \text{ mL}}{50 \text{ mg}} = \dfrac{x}{25 \text{ mg}}$

$$25 = 50x$$
$$x = 0.5 \text{ mL}$$

8. a. 48 lb = 21.82 kg (calculator)

For children more than 20 kg, the dose is 250 to 500 mg every 6 hours. The dose is safe.

b.

Formula Method	*Ratio Method*	*Proportion Method*
$\dfrac{\overset{2}{250} \text{ mg}}{\underset{1}{125} \text{ mg}} \times 5 \text{ mL} = 10 \text{ mL}$	5 mL : 125 mg :: x : 250 mg	$\dfrac{5 \text{ mL}}{125 \text{ mg}} = \dfrac{x}{250 \text{ mg}}$

$$1250 = 125x$$

Give 10 mL PO q6h. $10 \text{ mL} = x$

9. a. 30 kg
$$\frac{\times 10 \text{ mg/kg}}{300 \text{ mg}}$$

The literature states not more than 500 mg/dose. The dose is safe.

b.

Formula Method	*Ratio Method*	*Proportion Method*
$\dfrac{\overset{3}{300} \text{ mg}}{\underset{1}{100} \text{ mg}} \times 5 \text{ mL} = 15 \text{ mL}$	5 mL : 100 mg :: x : 300 mg	$\dfrac{5 \text{ mL}}{100 \text{ mg}} = \dfrac{x}{300 \text{ mg}}$

$$1500 = 100x$$

Give 15 mL × 1 dose. $15 \text{ mL} = x$

10. a. $\frac{8 \text{ oz}}{16} = 0.5$ lb

$\frac{12.5 \text{ lb}}{2.2} = 5.68$ kg

5.68 kg	5.68 kg
× 4 mg/kg	× 8 mg/kg
22.72 mg	45.44 mg

The dose (60 mg) is too high. Check with the physician.

Self-Test 3 Determining BSA

1. 0.54 m²   **3.** 1.1 m² (adult nomogram)

2. 0.51 m²   **4.** 0.255 m²

Self-Test 4 Use of the Nomogram

1. Step 1. Find the BSA in m² = 0.94.

Step 2. Determine safe dose.

Low Dose	High Dose
100 mg	200 mg
× 0.94	× 0.94
94 mg	188 mg

The safe dose is 94 to 188 mg over 24 hr.

Step 3. Is the order safe?

$50 \text{ mg q8h} = 50 \text{ mg} \times 3 = 150 \text{ mg/24 hr}$

The dose is safe.

Step 4. Order is 50 mg; supply is 50 mg. Give 1 tablet q8h.

2. Step 1. Find the BSA in m² = 1.29.

Step 2. The safe dose is

10 mg
× 1.29
12.9 mg

Step 3. Is the order safe? Yes; 12.5 mg is below the maximum.

Step 4.

Formula Method

$\frac{D}{H} \times S = A$

$\frac{\overset{5}{\cancel{12.5 \text{ mg}}}}{\underset{1}{\cancel{2.5 \text{ mg}}}} \times 1 \text{ tablet} = 5 \text{ tablets}$

Give 5 tablets po q week.

Ratio Method

1 tablet : 2.5 mg : : x : 12.5 mg

Proportion Method

$\frac{1 \text{ tablet}}{2.5 \text{ mg}} = \frac{x}{12.5 \text{ mg}}$

$12.5 = 2.5x$

5 tablets = x

3. Step 1. Find the BSA in m² = 0.46.

Step 2. The safe dose is 6.30 mg/m²/24 hr.

Low Dose	*High Dose*
6 mg	30 mg
× 0.46	× 0.46
2.76 mg	13.8 mg

The safe dose is 2.8 mg to 13.8 mg over 24 hr.

Step 3. Order is 5 mg × 12 hr = 10 mg. The dose is safe.

Step 4. Order is 5 mg; supply is 5 mg/5 mL. Give 5 mL PO q12h.

4. Step 1. Find the BSA in m² = 1.1

Step 2. Determine the safe dose.

$$\begin{array}{r} 5 \text{ mg} \\ \underline{\times\ 1.1} \\ 5.5 \text{ mg} \end{array}$$

Step 3. Is the order safe?

Yes. The order is 5 mg.

Step 4.

Formula Method

$$\frac{\overset{2}{\cancel{5\text{ mg}}}}{\underset{1}{\cancel{2.5\text{ mg}}}} \times 1 \text{ capsule} = 2 \text{ capsules}$$

Give 2 capsules po × 1.

Ratio Method

1 capsule : 2.5 mg : : x : 5 mg

Proportion Method

$$\frac{1 \text{ capsule}}{2.5 \text{ mg}} = \frac{x}{5 \text{ mg}}$$

$$5 = 2.5x$$

2 capsules = x

5. Step 1. Find the BSA in m² = 1.4

Step 2. Determine the safe dose.

$$\begin{array}{r} 900 \text{ mg} \\ \underline{\times\ 1.4} \\ 1260 \text{ mg/day} \end{array}$$

Step 3. 250 mg × 5 = 1250 mg/day. The order is safe.

Step 4. Calculate using both dosage supplies.

Formula Method

$$\frac{\overset{5}{\cancel{250\text{ mg}}}}{\underset{4}{\cancel{200\text{ mg}}}} \times 1 \text{ tablet} = 1.25 \text{ tablet}$$

Ratio Method

1 tablet : 200 mg : : x : 250 mg

Proportion Method

$$\frac{1 \text{ tablet}}{200 \text{ mg}} = \frac{x}{250 \text{ mg}}$$

$$250 = 200x$$

1.25 tablet

$$\frac{\overset{5}{\cancel{250\text{ mg}}}}{\underset{6}{\cancel{300\text{ mg}}}} \times 1 \text{ tablet} = 0.83 \text{ tablet}$$

1 tablet : 300 mg : : x : 250 mg

$$\frac{1 \text{ tablet}}{300 \text{ mg}} = \frac{x}{250 \text{ mg}}$$

$$250 = 300x$$

0.83 tablet

Use 200-mg tablets to give 1.25 tablets.

Self-Test 5 Parenteral Medication Calculations

1. Step 1.   The safe dose is 50 to 100 mg/kg/24 h.

Low Range	*High Range*
50 mg	100 mg
× 8 kg	× 8 kg
400 mg/24 hr	800 mg/24 hr

Order is 200 mg q6h (4 doses).

200 mg × 4 = 800 mg/24 h. Dose is safe.

Step 2.   Minimum safe dilution is 50 mg/mL.

$$\frac{4\ mL}{50 \overline{)200\ mg}}\ \text{is the minimum dilution}$$

A total of 10 mL is safe.

Step 3.   Dilute 750 mg with 8 mL sterile water to make 90 mg/mL.

Formula Method

$$\frac{D}{H} \times S = A$$

$$\frac{200\ mg}{90\ mg} \times 1\ mL = 2.2\ mL\ \text{(calculator)}$$

Ratio Method

1 mL : 90 mg : : x : 200 mg

Proportion Method

$$\frac{1\ mL}{90\ mg} = \frac{x}{200\ mg}$$

$$200 = 90x$$

$$2.2\ mL$$

Withdraw 2.2 mL of the drug into a syringe. Label the remainder and store in the refrigerator.

Step 4.   Add about 5 mL D5$\frac{1}{4}$NS to the Buretrol.

Add the 2.2 mL of drug. Add more D5$\frac{1}{4}$NS to make 10 mL.

Step 5.   Set the pump at 20. This means 20 mL/hr. The pump will deliver 10 mL in 30 minutes.

Step 6.   When the IV is finished, add a 20-mL flush of D5$\frac{1}{4}$NS to clear the tubing of medication.

2. Step 1.   The safe dose is 8 to 10 mg/kg/24 hours given q12h.

Low Range	*High Range*
8 mg	10 mg
× 15 kg	× 15 kg
120 mg/24 hr	150 mg/24 hr

Order is 75 mg q12h (two doses) = 150 mg/24h. The dose is safe.

Step 2.   The minimum safe dilution is 1 mL in 15 to 25 mL. The drug comes as a liquid, 80 mg/5 mL.

Formula Method

$$\frac{D}{H} \times S = A$$

$$\frac{75\ mg}{80\ mg} \times 5\ mL = 4.7\ mL\ \text{(calculator)}$$

$$375 = 80x$$
$$47\ mL$$

Ratio Method

5 mL : 80 mg : : x : 75 mg

Proportion Method

$$\frac{5\ mL}{80\ mg} = \frac{x}{75\ mg}$$

$$375 = 80x$$
$$47\ mL$$

Step 4

Formula Method	Ratio Method	Proportion Method
$\frac{\overset{1}{\cancel{25}} \text{ mg}}{\underset{2}{\cancel{50}} \text{ mg}} \times 1 \text{ mL} = 0.5 \text{ mL}$	$1 \text{ mL} : 50 \text{ mg} :: x : 25 \text{ mg}$	$\frac{1 \text{ mL}}{50 \text{ mg}} = \frac{x}{25 \text{ mg}}$

$$25 = 50x$$
$$0.5 \text{ mL}$$

Step 5. Give 0.5 mL undiluted IVP over 1 minute.

9. Step 1. $\frac{15}{2.2} = 6.82$ kg

Step 2. Determine the safe dose.

$$\begin{array}{cc} 6 \text{ mcg/kg} & 7.5 \text{ mcg/kg} \\ \times 6.82 \text{ kg} & \times 6.82 \text{ kg} \\ \hline 40.92 \text{ mcg/day} & 51.15 \text{ mcg/day} \end{array}$$

Step 3. The dose is safe (50 mcg/day).

Step 4. Calculate the dose.

0.1 mg = 100 mcg/1 mL

Formula Method	Ratio Method	Proportion Method
$\frac{\overset{1}{\cancel{50}} \text{ mcg}}{\underset{2}{\cancel{100}} \text{ mcg}} \times 1 \text{ mL} = 0.5 \text{ mL}$	$1 \text{ mL} : 100 \text{ mcg} :: x : 50 \text{ mg}$	$\frac{1 \text{ mL}}{100 \text{ mcg}} = \frac{x}{50 \text{ mcg}}$

$$50 = 100x$$
$$0.5 \text{ mL} = x$$

Step 5. Give 0.5 mL undiluted or diluted in 4 mL D5W or NS over 5 minutes.

10. Step 1. $\frac{80 \text{ lb}}{2.2} = 36.36$ kg

Step 2. Determine the safe dose.

$$\begin{array}{cc} 0.5 \text{ mg/kg} & 1.7 \text{ mg/kg} \\ \times 36.36 \text{ kg} & \times 36.36 \text{ kg} \\ \hline 18.18 \text{ mg/day} & 61.81 \text{ mg/day} \end{array}$$

Step 3. 60 mg bid = 60 mg × 2 = 120 mg/day

The dose is too high. Contact the physician.

Dimensional Analysis

A fourth method of dosage calculation is called *dimensional analysis.* This method is often used in mathematics and science, especially chemistry calculations. Students that I work with say that once you master dimensional analysis, then you use it all the time, and it is simpler and less erroneous than the other methods.

The dimensional analysis method uses similar terminology as other calculation methods. There are several ways to set up the dimensional analysis equation. To be consistent with the rest of this book, we will start with a desired dose. A supply or "available" amount is used. The entire equation is set up with a numerator and denominator, and then the equation is solved.

Oral Solid Medication Equation and Calculation

Let's start with a simple oral solid medication equation and calculation:

Example Order: Zyprexa 7.5 mg po every day

Supply: Zyprexa 5-mg scored tablets (Fig. 11-1)

Write the desired dose first in the numerator:

$\dfrac{7.5 \text{ mg}}{}$

Then write the available dose as a fraction:

$\dfrac{1 \text{ tablet}}{5 \text{ mg}}$

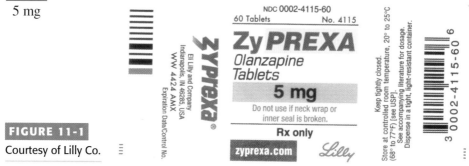

FIGURE 11-1
Courtesy of Lilly Co.

Now let's combine both of these:

$$\frac{7.5 \text{ mg}}{} \quad \frac{1 \text{ tablet}}{5 \text{ mg}}$$

Using the basic rules of reducing fractions (review Chapter 1 if necessary), the "mg" would cancel each other. Reduce the number if possible. Divide both numbers by 5.

$$\frac{\overset{1.5}{\cancel{7.5}} \; \cancel{\text{mg}}}{} \quad \frac{1 \text{ tablet}}{\underset{1}{\cancel{5}} \; \cancel{\text{mg}}}$$

The setup should now look like this:

$$\frac{1.5}{} \quad \frac{1 \text{ tablet}}{1}$$

Multiply the numerators, multiply the denominators, and then divide the product of the numerators by the product of the denominators. In this example, the numbers in the numerator are $1.5 \times 1 = 1.5$. The only number in the denominator is 1. Divide and divide by 1 to get: 1.5 or $1\frac{1}{2}$ tablets.

$$\frac{1.5}{} \quad \frac{1 \text{ tablet}}{1} \quad \frac{1.5 \times 1}{1} = 1.5 \text{ or } 1\frac{1}{2} \text{ tablets}$$

Give $1\frac{1}{2}$ tablets po every day.

Example

Order: Depakote 500 mg po every day

Supply: See Figure 11-2.

The dose desired is 500 mg. The supply is 1 tablet = 250 mg.

The equation would look like

$$\frac{500 \text{ mg}}{} \quad \frac{1 \text{ tablet}}{250 \text{ mg}}$$

Cancel the "mg." Reduce the fraction. Solve.

$$\frac{\overset{2}{\cancel{500}} \; \cancel{\text{mg}}}{} \quad \frac{1 \text{ tablet}}{\underset{1}{\cancel{250}} \; \cancel{\text{mg}}} \qquad \frac{2 \times 1}{1} = 2 \text{ tablets}$$

Give 2 tablets po every day.

FIGURE 11-2

Courtesy of Abbott Laboratories.

Oral Liquid Medication Equation and Calculation

Follow the same basic rules of setting up the equation, using the liquid medication available or the supply dose.

Example

Order: Zithromax 150 mg po every day × 4 days

Supply: See Figure 11-3.

The equation is

$$\frac{150 \text{ mg}}{} \left| \frac{5 \text{ mL}}{200 \text{ mg}} \right.$$

Cancel the "mg." Reduce the fraction by dividing both numbers by 50. Solve.

$$\frac{\overset{3}{\cancel{150}} \ \cancel{mg}}{} \left| \frac{5 \text{ mL}}{\underset{4}{\cancel{200}} \ \cancel{mg}} \right| \frac{3 \times 5}{4} = \frac{15}{4} = 3.75 \text{ mL}$$

> **Learning Aid**
>
> Notice the equation continues until the problem is solved. This helps to decrease errors.
>
>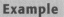

Give 3.75 mL po every day × 4 days.

Parenteral Liquid Medication Equation and Calculation

Follow the same rules as with oral liquid.

Example

Order: Versed 2.5 mg IV q3–4h prn

Supply: See Figure 11-4.

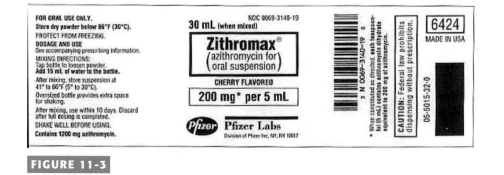

FIGURE 11-3

Courtesy of Pfizer Labs.

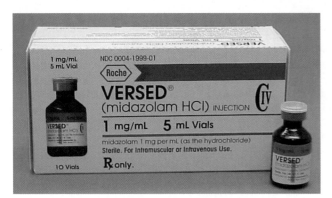

The equation is

$$\frac{2.5\ mg\ |\ 1\ mL}{|\ 1\ mg}$$

Cancel the "mg." The fraction is already reduced. Solve.

$$\frac{2.5\ \cancel{mg}\ |\ 1\ mL\ |\ 2.5 \times 1}{|\ 1\ \cancel{mg}\ |\quad 1} = 2.5\ or\ 2\tfrac{1}{2}\ mL$$

Give $2\tfrac{1}{2}$ mL IV q3–4h prn. Follow dilution and administration guidelines.

▶ Insulin Equation and Calculation

Follow the same basic setup. Insulin is very easy to calculate with dimensional analysis, because the equation is self-explanatory.

Example Order: regular insulin 10 units subcutaneous now

Supply: See Figure 11-5.

The equation is

$$\frac{10\ units\ |}{|} = 10\ units$$

Use an insulin syringe.

Give 10 units subcutaneous.

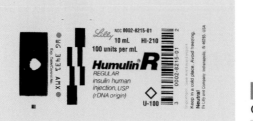

STEPS TO SETTING UP A DIMENSIONAL ANALYSIS PROBLEM

1. Identify the desired dose. Place it in the numerator.
2. Identify the supply or available dose.
3. Identify what you are solving for (this is stated in the problem). Circle this measurement system.
4. Combine steps 1 and 2. Set up the problem so that the measurement systems that you do not need for the answer will cancel. This should leave the measurement system desired on the top.
5. If possible, reduce the fraction. Cancel out any measurement systems.
6. Multiply the numbers in the numerator. Multiply the numbers in the denominator.
7. Divide the numerator by the denominator.

SELF-TEST 1 | **Calculation of Medications**

Solve these problems using dimensional analysis. Answers are given at the end of the chapter. The answers include how to set up the problem and how to solve it.

1. Order: Xanax 0.5 mg po bid
    Supply: Xanax 0.25-mg tablets

2. Order: penicillin 800,000 units po q4h × 10 days
    Supply: 1 tablet equals 400,000 units

3. Order: Zithromax 400 mg po every day × 4 days
    Supply: Zithromax 200 mg/5 mL

4. Order: prednisone 10 mg po tid
    Supply: tablets labeled 2.5 mg

5. Order: Lasix 60 mg po every day
    Supply: scored tablets labeled 40 mg

6. Order: Demerol 75 mg IV q4–6h prn
    Supply: Demerol 50 mg/mL

7. Order: digoxin 0.5 mg IV q4h × 3 doses
    Supply: digoxin 0.25 mg/mL

8. Order: heparin 1500 units subcutaneous bid
    Supply: heparin 5000 units/mL

9. Order: morphine 15 mg IV q4h prn
    Supply: morphine 10 mg/mL

10. Order: Solu Medrol 80 mg IV every day
    Supply: Solu Medrol 125 mg/2 mL

▶ Dimensional Analysis Method with Equivalency Conversions

If the dosage desired and the dosage available are not in the same measurement system, then an added step is needed to accomplish this. The use of a conversion factor will convert the equation so that only one measurement system is in the equation.

Conversion factor is a term used in dimensional analysis. It is simply the equivalents necessary to convert between systems of measurement. A conversion factor is a ratio of units that equals 1.

Example **Metric conversion factors**

$$\frac{1 \text{ g}}{1000 \text{ mg}} \quad \text{or} \quad \frac{1000 \text{ mg}}{1 \text{ g}}$$

$$\frac{1 \text{ mg}}{1000 \text{ mcg}} \quad \text{or} \quad \frac{1000 \text{ mcg}}{1 \text{ mg}}$$

Each of these equals 1.

Metric apothecary conversion factors

$$\frac{60 \text{ mg (or 65 mg with aspirin and Tylenol)}}{1 \text{ gr}} \quad \text{or} \quad \frac{1 \text{ gr}}{60 \text{ mg (or 65 mg)}}$$

Each of these equal 1.

Metric/household conversion factors

$$\frac{1 \text{ tbsp}}{15 \text{ mL}} \quad \text{or} \quad \frac{15 \text{ mL}}{1 \text{ tbsp}}$$

$$\frac{1 \text{ tsp}}{5 \text{ mL}} \quad \text{or} \quad \frac{5 \text{ mL}}{1 \text{ tsp}}$$

$$\frac{1 \text{ kg}}{2.2 \text{ lb}} \quad \text{or} \quad \frac{2.2 \text{ lb}}{1 \text{ kg}}$$

$$\frac{16 \text{ oz}}{1 \text{ lb}} \quad \text{or} \quad \frac{1 \text{ lb}}{16 \text{ oz}}$$

Each of these equal 1.

Example Order: Synthroid 150 mcg po every day

Supply: See Figure 11-6. Use 0.075 mg for this example.

$$\frac{150 \text{ mcg}}{} \left| \frac{1 \text{ tablet}}{0.075 \text{ mg}} \right.$$

We need to add a conversion factor so that the answer is in mcg. 1 mg = 1000 mcg, so we include this in the equation.

$$\frac{150 \text{ mcg}}{} \left| \frac{1 \text{ tablet}}{0.075 \text{ mg}} \right| \frac{1 \text{ mg}}{1000 \text{ mcg}}$$

We solve in the same way. Cancel the measurement systems. Reduce the fraction.

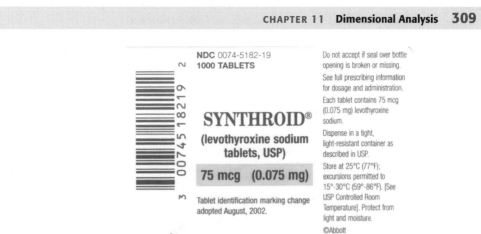

NDC 0074-5182-19
1000 TABLETS

SYNTHROID®
(levothyroxine sodium tablets, USP)

75 mcg   (0.075 mg)

Tablet identification marking change adopted August, 2002.

Do not accept if seal over bottle opening is broken or missing.
See full prescribing information for dosage and administration.
Each tablet contains 75 mcg (0.075 mg) levothyroxine sodium.
Dispense in a tight, light-resistant container as described in USP.
Store at 25°C (77°F); excursions permitted to 15°-30°C (59°-86°F). [See USP Controlled Room Temperature]. Protect from light and moisture.
©Abbott
Abbott Laboratories
North Chicago, IL 60064, U.S.A.

℞ only   02-8660-R2

FIGURE 11-6

Courtesy of Abbott Laboratories.

$$\frac{\overset{3}{\cancel{150}}\ \text{mcg}}{} \left| \frac{1\ \text{tablet}}{0.075\ \text{mg}} \right| \frac{1\ \text{mg}}{\underset{20}{\cancel{1000}}\ \text{mcg}} \left| \frac{3\times 1\times 1}{0.075\times 20} = \frac{3}{1.5} = 2 \text{ or } 2 \text{ tablets}\right.$$

Give 2 tablets po every day.

Learning Aid

Divide 50 into 150 and 1000 to reduce the fraction.

Example

Order: Romazicon 200 mcg IV over 15 seconds for reversal of anesthesia

Supply: See Figure 11-7.

$$\frac{200\ \text{mcg}}{} \left| \frac{5\ \text{mL}}{0.5\ \text{mg}} \right| \frac{1\ \text{mg}}{1000\ \text{mcg}}$$

Learning Aid

Divide 200 into 200 and 1000.

Reduce and solve.

$$\frac{\overset{1}{\cancel{200}}\ \text{mcg}}{} \left| \frac{5\ \text{mL}}{0.5\ \text{mg}} \right| \frac{1\ \text{mg}}{\underset{5}{\cancel{1000}}\ \text{mcg}} \left| \frac{1\times 5\times 1}{0.5\times 5} = \frac{5}{2.5} = 2 \text{ mL}\right.$$

Give 2 mL IV over 15 seconds.

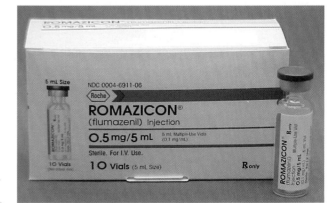

FIGURE 11-7

Reprinted with permission of Roche Laboratories, Inc. All rights reserved.

Follow institutional requirements for dilution and administration of IV drugs.

Remember to place the same unit of measurement opposite in the equation. In this example, "mg" is placed on opposite sides in the fraction and "mcg" is placed on opposite sides. These both cancel each other, leaving "mL" as the remaining unit of measurement.

An advantage to dimensional analysis is that any conversion factor can be placed within the equation. This helps to reduce errors committed in accidentally leaving out any conversions.

We'll add this step to our other steps in setting up a dimensional analysis problem.

STEPS TO SETTING UP A DIMENSIONAL ANALYSIS PROBLEM

1. Identify the desired dose. Place it in the numerator.
2. Identify the supply or available dose.
3. Identify what you are solving for (this is stated in the problem). Circle this measurement system.
4. **Identify any conversions needed. Add the conversion factors to the equation. Add these to the equation so that like measurement systems will cancel each other.**
5. Combine steps 1 and 2. Set up the problem so that the measurement systems that you do not need for the answer will cancel. This should leave the measurement system desired on the top.
6. If possible, reduce the fraction. Cancel out any measurement systems.
7. Multiply the numbers in the numerator. Multiply the numbers in the denominator.
8. Divide the numerator by the denominator.

SELF-TEST 2 Calculation of Medications Involving Equivalencies

Solve these problems using dimensional analysis. Answers are given at the end of the chapter. The answers include how to set up the problem and how to solve it.

1. Order: ibuprofen 0.8 g po bid
   Supply: 400-mg tablets

2. Order: Synthroid 0.3 mg po every day
   Supply: 300-mcg scored tablets

3. Order: codeine ½ gr po q4h prn
   Supply: 30-mg tablets

4. Order: Augmentin 500 mg
   Supply: Augmentin 250 mg/5 mL
   How many tsp?

5. Order: Tegretol 100 mg po qid
   Supply: 100 mg/5 mL
   How many tsp?

6. Order: vitamin B12 1 mg IM every week
   Supply: 1000 mcg/mL

(continued)

SELF-TEST 2   **Calculation of Medications Involving Equivalencies (Continued)**

7. Order: ampicillin 500 mg IM q6h
   Supply: 1 g/mL

8. Order: epinephrine 0.4 mg subcutaneous × 1
   Supply: 1-mL ampule 1:1000 (Remember, 1:1000 = 1 g in 1000 mL)

9. Order: lidocaine 30 mg subcutaneous
   Supply: ampule labeled 2% (Remember, 2% = 2 g in 1000 mL)

10. Order: atropine gr 1/150 IM × 1
    Supply: atropine 0.4 mg/mL

Dimensional Analysis Method with Weight-Based Calculations

Medications that are calculated based on weight will add another step in the dimensional analysis method. The ordered dose will need to be multiplied by the weight or BSA.

Example

Order: Lasix 1 mg/kg IV bid for 12-year-old weighing 30 kg

Supply: See Figure 11-8.

Desired dose: 1 mg/kg

Set up the problem so that "kg" is in the denominator.

$$\frac{1 \text{ mg}}{\text{kg}}$$

Now add the supplied dose.

$$\frac{1 \text{ mg}}{\text{kg}} \; \frac{1 \text{ mL}}{10 \text{ mg}}$$

Add the patient's weight in kg.

$$\frac{1 \text{ mg}}{\text{kg}} \; \frac{1 \text{ mL}}{10 \text{ mg}} \; \frac{30 \text{ kg}}{}$$

Proceed with the rest of the steps. Cancel out "mg" and "kg." Reduce the fraction. Multiply the numerator. Multiply the denominator. Divide the numerator by the denominator.

$$\frac{1 \text{ mg}}{\text{kg}} \; \frac{1 \text{ mL}}{10 \text{ mg}} \; \frac{\overset{3}{30} \text{ kg}}{} \; \frac{1 \times 1 \times 3}{1} = 3 \text{ mL}$$

Give 3 mL IV bid.

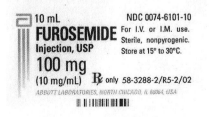

FIGURE 11-8
Courtesy of Abbott Laboratories.

Follow institutional requirements for dilution and administration of IV drugs.

If the patient's weight is given in pounds, then use the conversion factor

$$\frac{1\ kg}{2.2\ lb}$$

to convert pounds to kilograms.

Example

Order: Demerol 1.5 mg/kg IM q3–4h for pediatric patient weighing 75 lb

Supply: See Figure 11-9.

Set up the equation.

$$\frac{1.5\ mg}{kg}\ \Big|\ \frac{1\ mL}{50\ mg}\ \Big|\ \frac{75\ lb}{}\ \Big|\ \frac{1\ kg}{2.2\ lb}$$

Cancel "mg," "kg," and "lb." Reduce the fraction. Solve.

$$\frac{1.5\ mg}{kg}\ \Big|\ \frac{1\ mL}{50\ mg}\ \Big|\ \frac{\overset{3}{75}\ lb}{}\ \Big|\ \frac{1\ kg}{2.2\ lb}\ \Big|\ \frac{1.5\times1\times3\times1}{2\times2.2}=\frac{4.5}{4.4}=1.02\ or\ 1\ mL$$

Give 1 mL IM q3–4h.

Calculation of Medications Based on BSA

Calculation of medications based on BSA is set up in a similar way as weight-based medications.

Example

Order: acyclovir 500 mg/m^2 infused IV over 1 hour; BSA, 1.1 m^2

Supply: reconstituted vial with concentration of 50 mg/mL

$$\frac{500\ mg}{m^2}\ \Big|\ \frac{1\ mL}{50\ mg}\ \Big|\ 1.1\ m^2$$

Cancel out the "mg" and the "m^2." Reduce the fraction. Solve.

$$\frac{\overset{10}{500}\ mg}{m^2}\ \Big|\ \frac{1\ mL}{50\ mg}\ \Big|\ 1.1\ m^2\ \Big|\ \frac{10\times1\times1.1}{1}=11\ mL$$

Give 11 mL IV over 1 hour.

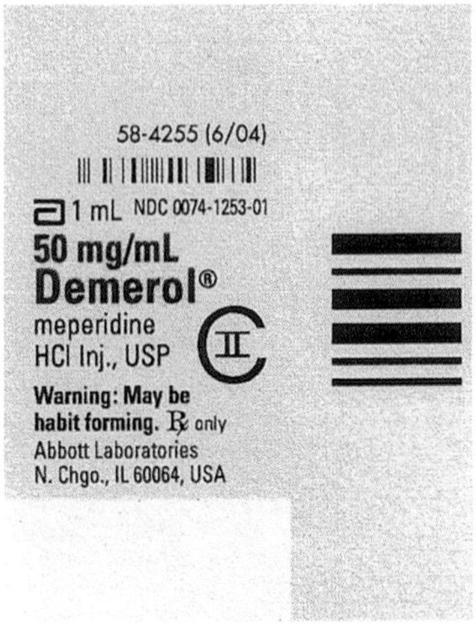

58-4255 (6/04)
1 mL NDC 0074-1253-01
50 mg/mL
Demerol®
meperidine
HCl Inj., USP
Warning: May be habit forming. ℞ only
Abbott Laboratories
N. Chgo., IL 60064, USA

FIGURE 11-9
Courtesy of Abbott Laboratories.

If the weight-based medication is ordered in several doses, then add another step to the equation with the number of doses ordered. The solution will then be the amount of drug per dose.

Example Order: hydrocortisone IM 10 mg/m²/day in 3 divided doses; BSA, 2.0 m²

Available: vial of 25 mg/mL

In this example, we will use $\dfrac{\text{day}}{3 \text{ doses}}$

so that the answer will be in the amount of drug for each dose.

Set up the equation.

$$\frac{10 \text{ mg}}{\text{m}^2/\text{day}} \bigg| \frac{1 \text{ mL}}{25 \text{ mg}} \bigg| \frac{2.0 \text{ m}^2}{} \bigg| \frac{\text{day}}{3 \text{ doses}}$$

Cancel "m²," "mg," "day." Reduce the fraction. Solve.

$$\frac{\overset{2}{\cancel{10}} \text{ }\cancel{\text{mg}}}{\cancel{\text{m}^2}/\cancel{\text{day}}} \bigg| \frac{1\,\text{mL}}{\underset{5}{\cancel{25}}\text{ }\cancel{\text{mg}}} \bigg| \frac{2.0\text{ }\cancel{\text{m}^2}}{} \bigg| \frac{\cancel{\text{day}}}{3\,\text{doses}} \bigg| \frac{2 \times 1 \times 2}{5 \times 3} = \frac{4}{15} = 0.27 \text{ mL/dose}$$

Give 0.27 mL IM per dose.

SELF-TEST 3 **Calculation of Medications Using Weight or BSA**

Solve these problems using dimensional analysis. Answers are given at the end of the chapter. The answers include how to set up the problem and how to solve it.

1. Order: Lasix 1 mg/kg IV; weight, 70 kg
   Supply: Lasix 10 mg/mL

2. Order: Augmentin 10 mg/kg po bid; weight, 30 kg
   Supply: Augmentin 125 mg/5 mL

3. Order: Keflex 25 mg/kg/day in 4 divided doses; weight, 50 lb
   Supply: Keflex 250 mg/5 mL
   How much per dose?

4. Order: Decadron 0.4 mg/kg/day in 4 divided doses; weight, 25 lb
   Supply: Decadron 4 mg/mL
   How much per dose?

5. Order: methotrexate 10 mg/m²/dose q week; BSA, 1.29 m²
   Supply: methotrexate 2.5-mg tablets

Dimensional Analysis Method with Reconstitution of Medications

These are set up with the same method as parenteral calculations. Follow the reconstitution directions and use the result as the dosage available.

Example Order: Rocephin 1 g IV q12h

Supply: Reconstitute with 9.6 mL sterile water to yield 100 mg/mL (Fig. 11-10).

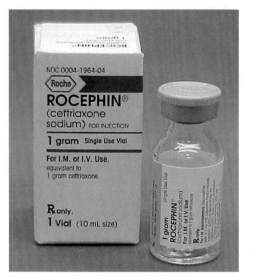

$$\frac{1\ g}{} \left| \frac{1\ mL}{100\ mg} \right| \frac{1000\ mg}{1\ g}$$

> **Learning Aid**
>
> Remember to use conversion factors when needed to change to the same measurement system.

Cancel "mg" and "g." Reduce the fraction. Solve.

$$\frac{1\ \cancel{g}}{} \left| \frac{1\ \textcircled{mL}}{\cancel{100}\ \cancel{mg}} \right| \frac{\overset{10}{\cancel{1000}}\ \cancel{mg}}{1\ \cancel{g}} \left| \frac{1\times1\times10}{1\times1} = 10\ mL \right.$$

Follow institutional requirements for dilution and administration of IV drugs.

SELF-TEST 4 | **Reconstitution**

Solve these problems using dimensional analysis. Answers are given at the end of the chapter. The answers include how to set up the problem and how to solve it.

1. Order: Monocid 0.5 g IM q12h
   Supply: 1-g vial of powder. Follow reconstitution directions to yield solution 250 mg/mL.

2. Order: penicillin 1 million units IM q6h
   Supply: 5-million-unit vial. Follow reconstitution directions to yield solution 1 million units/mL.

3. Order: Ancef 0.3 g IM
   Supply: 500 mg powder. Follow reconstitution directions to yield solution 225 mg/mL.

4. Order: Unasyn 1500 mg IV q8h
   Supply: Unasyn 1.5-g vial. Follow reconstitution directions to yield solution 1.5 g/5 mL.

5. Order: Fortaz 0.25 g
   Supply: Fortaz vial. Follow reconstitution directions to yield solution 500 mg/mL.

Dimensional Analysis Method with Calculation of Intravenous Fluids

Example

Order: D5W 1000 mL over 10 hr

To calculate mL/hr set up the equation:

$$\dfrac{1000 \text{ mL}}{10 \text{ hour}}$$

Reduce the fraction.

$$\dfrac{\overset{100}{\cancel{1000}} \, \cancel{\text{mL}}}{\underset{1}{\cancel{10}} \, \cancel{\text{hr}}} \; \Big| \; \dfrac{100}{1} = 100 \text{ mL/hr}$$

If an infusion pump is used, then the rate will be 100 mL/hr.

If using gravity flow tubing, then the equation will include the drop or tubing factor and the "hour" must be converted to "minutes." The conversion factor

$$\dfrac{1 \text{ hour}}{60 \text{ minutes}}$$

is used.

Example

Order: D5W 1000 mL over 10 hr

Supply: Drop factor of 20 gtts/mL

$$\dfrac{1000 \text{ mL}}{10 \text{ hr}} \; \Big| \; \dfrac{20 \text{ gtts}}{\text{mL}} \; \Big| \; \dfrac{1 \text{ hr}}{60 \text{ min}}$$

Cancel the "mL" and the "hr." Reduce the fraction. Solve.

$$\dfrac{\overset{100}{\cancel{1000}} \, \cancel{\text{mL}}}{\underset{1}{\cancel{10}} \, \cancel{\text{hr}}} \; \Big| \; \dfrac{\overset{1}{\cancel{20}} \, \cancel{\text{gtts}}}{\cancel{\text{mL}}} \; \Big| \; \dfrac{1 \, \cancel{\text{hr}}}{\underset{3}{\cancel{60}} \, \cancel{\text{min}}} \; \Big| \; \dfrac{100 \times 1 \times 1}{1 \times 3} = \dfrac{100}{3} = 33.3 \text{ or } 33 \text{ gtts/min}$$

SELF-TEST 5   Basic IV Calculations and Drop Factors

Solve these problems using dimensional analysis. Answers are given at the end of the chapter. The answers include how to set up the problem and how to solve it.

1. Order: D5½ NS 1000 mL over 8 hr
   How many mL/hr?

2. Order: D5W 500 mL over 5 hr
   How many mL/hr?

3. Order: NS 250 mL over 5 hr
   How many mL/hr?

4. Order: whole blood 500 mL over 4 hr
   How many mL/hr?

5. Order: NS 250 mL over 2 hr; drop factor, 20 gtts/mL
   How many gtts/minute?

(continued)

SELF-TEST 5	Basic IV Calculations and Drop Factors (Continued)

6. Order: D5W 100 mL over 30 min; drop factor, 15 gtts/mL
   How many gtts/minute?

7. Order: NS 500 mL over 4 hr; drop factor, 60 gtts/mL
   How many gtts/minute?

8. Order: D5W 300 mL over 90 minutes; drop factor 60 gtts/mL
   How many gtts/minute?

9. Order: NS 1000 mL over 8 hr; drop factor, 20 gtts/mL
   How many gtts/minute?

10. Order: ½ NS 500 mL over 4 hr; drop factor, 10 gtts/mL
    How many gtts/minute?

Dimensional Analysis Method with Advanced Intravenous Calculations

Medications that are administered with continuous IV infusion can be calculated with the dimensional analysis method. Infusion pumps are always used.

Calculating mL/hr

Example   Order: heparin 1200 units/hr per infusion pump

How many mL/hr? (Infusion pumps are set in mL/hr)

Supply: See Figure 11-11. Heparin 25,000 units in 500 mL ½ NS

Set up the equation.

$$\frac{1200 \text{ units}}{\text{hr}} \left| \frac{500 \text{ mL}}{25000 \text{ units}} \right.$$

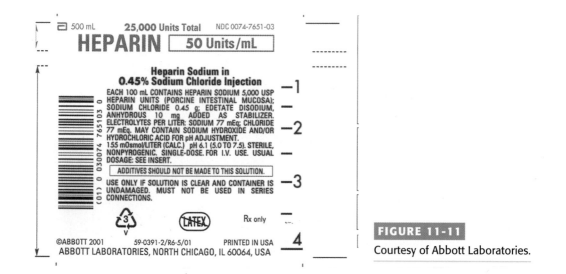

FIGURE 11-11
Courtesy of Abbott Laboratories.

Cancel "units." Reduce the fraction. Solve.

$$\frac{1200 \ \cancel{units}}{\cancel{hr}} \ \left| \ \frac{\overset{1}{\cancel{500}} \ \cancel{mL}}{\underset{50}{\cancel{25000}} \ \cancel{units}} \ \right| \ \frac{1200}{50} = 24 \ mL/hr$$

Set pump at 24 mL/hr.

Example

Order: aminophylline 30 mg/hr per infusion pump

How many mL/hr?

Supply: See Figure 11-12. Aminophylline 500 mg/500 mL D5W

Set up the equation.

$$\frac{30 \ mg}{hr} \ \left| \ \frac{500 \ mL}{500 \ mg} \right.$$

Cancel "mg." Reduce the fraction. Solve.

$$\frac{30 \ \cancel{mg}}{\cancel{hr}} \ \left| \ \frac{\overset{1}{\cancel{500}} \ \cancel{mL}}{\underset{1}{\cancel{500}} \ \cancel{mg}} \ \right| \ \frac{30}{1} = 30 \ mL/hr$$

Set the infusion pump at 30 mL/hour.

Calculating mg/hr or Units/hr

Dimensional analysis can be used to determine how much of a given drug is infusing per an infusion pump.

Example

Order: heparin 10 mL/hr per infusion pump

How many units infusing per hour?

Supply: heparin 25,000 units/500 mL ½ NS.

Set up the equation.

$$\frac{10 \ mL}{hr} \ \left| \ \frac{25,000 \ units}{500 \ mL} \right.$$

Cancel "mL." Reduce the fraction. Solve.

$$\frac{10 \ \cancel{mL}}{\cancel{hr}} \ \left| \ \frac{\overset{50}{\cancel{25,000}} \ \cancel{units}}{\underset{1}{\cancel{500}} \ \cancel{mL}} \ \right| \ \frac{10 \times 50}{1} = 500 \ units/hr$$

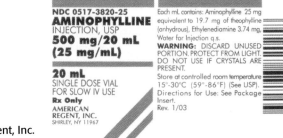

FIGURE 11-12
Courtesy of American Regent, Inc.

Example

Order: calcium gluconate 25 mL/hr

How many grams are infusing per hour?

Supply: calcium gluconate 1 g in 100 mL D5W.

Set up the equation.

$$\frac{25 \text{ mL}}{\text{hr}} \left| \frac{1 \text{ g}}{100 \text{ mL}} \right.$$

Cancel "mL." Reduce the fraction. Solve.

$$\frac{\overset{1}{\cancel{25}} \ \cancel{\text{mL}}}{\cancel{\text{hr}}} \left| \frac{1 \ \cancel{\text{g}}}{\underset{4}{\cancel{100}} \ \cancel{\text{mL}}} \right| \frac{1}{4} = \frac{1}{4} \text{ or } 0.25 \text{ g/hr}$$

Calculating mL/hr for Drugs Ordered in mg or mcg/min

Vasoactive drugs are ordered in dosages per minute. Use the conversion factor

$$\frac{60 \text{ min}}{1 \text{ hr}}$$

Example

Order: procainamide 3 mg/min per infusion pump

How many mL/hr?

Available: See Figure 11-13. Procainamide 1 g/250 mL D5W

Set up the equation. Use the conversion factor $\frac{1 \text{ g}}{1000 \text{ mg}}$. Use $\frac{60 \text{ min}}{1 \text{ hr}}$ because the order is in minutes but the answer will be in hours.

$$\frac{3 \text{ mg}}{\text{min}} \left| \frac{250 \text{ mL}}{1 \text{ g}} \right| \frac{1 \text{ g}}{1000 \text{ mg}} \left| \frac{60 \text{ min}}{\text{hr}} \right.$$

Cancel "mg," "g," and "min." Reduce the fraction. Solve.

$$\frac{3 \ \cancel{\text{mg}}}{\cancel{\text{min}}} \left| \frac{\overset{1}{\cancel{250}} \ \text{mL}}{1 \ \cancel{\text{g}}} \right| \frac{1 \ \cancel{\text{g}}}{\underset{4}{\cancel{1000}} \ \cancel{\text{mg}}} \left| \frac{60 \ \cancel{\text{min}}}{\cancel{\text{hr}}} \right| \frac{3 \times 1 \times 1 \times 60}{1 \times 4} = \frac{180}{4} = 45 \text{ mL/hr}$$

Set the infusion pump at 45 mL/hr to deliver 3 mg/min.

Example

Order: nitroglycerine 30 mcg/min per infusion pump

How many mL/hr?

2 mL Multiple-dose
PROCAINAMIDE
HCl Injection, USP ℞ only
ABBOTT LABS., N. CHGO., IL 60064, USA

NDC 0074-1903-01
1 gram/2 mL TOTAL
(500 mg/mL)
58-3873-2/R3-10/02

Supply: nitroglycerine 50 mg in 250 mL D5W

Set up the equation. Use the conversion factor $\dfrac{1 \text{ mg}}{1000 \text{ mcg}}$.

$$\dfrac{30 \text{ mcg}}{\text{min}} \; \left| \; \dfrac{250 \text{ mL}}{50 \text{ mg}} \; \right| \; \dfrac{1 \text{ mg}}{1000 \text{ mcg}} \; \left| \; \dfrac{60 \text{ min}}{\text{hr}} \right.$$

Cancel "mcg," "mg," and "min." Reduce the fraction. Solve.

$$\dfrac{30 \; \cancel{\text{mcg}}}{\cancel{\text{min}}} \; \left| \; \dfrac{\overset{1}{\cancel{250}} \; \cancel{(\text{mL})}}{\underset{10}{\cancel{50}} \; \cancel{\text{mg}}} \; \right| \; \dfrac{1 \; \cancel{\text{mg}}}{\underset{4}{\cancel{1000}} \; \cancel{\text{mcg}}} \; \left| \; \dfrac{\overset{12}{\cancel{60}} \; \cancel{\text{min}}}{\cancel{(\text{hr})}} \right. \; \left| \; \dfrac{30 \times 1 \times 1 \times 12}{10 \times 4} = \dfrac{360}{40} = 9 \text{ mL/hr} \right.$$

Set the infusion pump at 9 mL/hr to deliver 30 mcg/minute.

Calculating mL/hr for Drugs Ordered in mcg/kg/min

Vasoactive drugs such as dobutamine, dopamine, nipride, and others are ordered in dosages per kilogram per minute. Convert pounds to kilograms using the conversion factor. Use the conversion factor $\dfrac{60 \text{ min}}{1 \text{ hr}}$ to convert minutes to hours.

Example

Order: Infuse dopamine at 2 mcg/kg/min per infusion pump.

How many mL/hr?

Available: dopamine 800 mg/500 mL D5W; weight, 70 kg (Fig. 11-14). (Label represents a single dose; this will be mixed in 500 mL.)

Set up the equation. Use the conversion factor $\dfrac{1 \text{ mg}}{1000 \text{ mcg}}$.

$$\dfrac{2 \text{ mcg}}{\text{kg/min}} \; \left| \; \dfrac{500 \text{ mL}}{800 \text{ mg}} \; \right| \; \dfrac{1 \text{ mg}}{1000 \text{ mcg}} \; \left| \; 70 \text{ kg} \; \right| \; \dfrac{60 \text{ min}}{\text{hr}}$$

Cancel "mcg," "mg," "kg," and "min." Reduce the fraction. Solve.

$$\dfrac{2 \; \cancel{\text{mcg}}}{\cancel{\text{kg}} / \cancel{\text{min}}} \; \left| \; \dfrac{\overset{1}{\cancel{500}} \; \cancel{(\text{mL})}}{\cancel{800} \; \cancel{\text{mg}}} \; \right| \; \dfrac{1 \; \cancel{\text{mg}}}{\underset{2}{\cancel{1000}} \; \cancel{\text{mcg}}} \; \left| \; 7\cancel{0} \; \cancel{\text{kg}} \; \right| \; \dfrac{6\cancel{0} \; \cancel{\text{min}}}{\cancel{(\text{hr})}} \; \left| \; \dfrac{2 \times 1 \times 1 \times 7 \times 6}{8 \times 2} \right.$$

$$= \dfrac{84}{16} = 5.25 \text{ or } 5 \text{ mL/hr}$$

Set the infusion pump at 5 mL/hr to deliver 2 mcg/kg/min for a 70-kg patient.

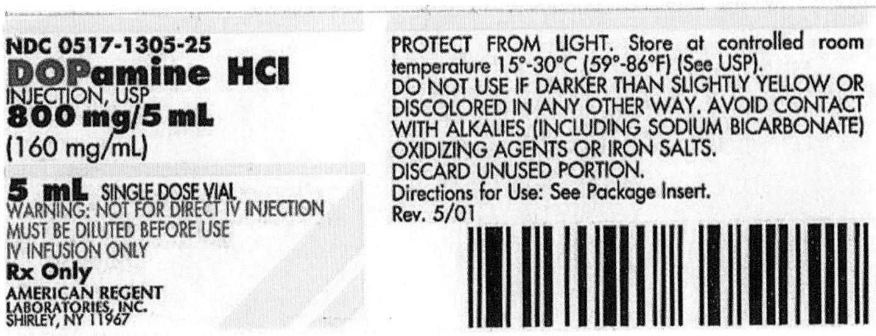

NDC 0517-1305-25
DOPamine HCl
INJECTION, USP
800 mg/5 mL
(160 mg/mL)

5 mL SINGLE DOSE VIAL
WARNING: NOT FOR DIRECT IV INJECTION
MUST BE DILUTED BEFORE USE
IV INFUSION ONLY
Rx Only
AMERICAN REGENT
LABORATORIES, INC.
SHIRLEY, NY 11967

PROTECT FROM LIGHT. Store at controlled room temperature 15°-30°C (59°-86°F) (See USP).
DO NOT USE IF DARKER THAN SLIGHTLY YELLOW OR DISCOLORED IN ANY OTHER WAY. AVOID CONTACT WITH ALKALIES (INCLUDING SODIUM BICARBONATE) OXIDIZING AGENTS OR IRON SALTS.
DISCARD UNUSED PORTION.
Directions for Use: See Package Insert.
Rev. 5/01

FIGURE 11-14
Courtesy of American Regent Laboratories, Inc.

SELF-TEST 6   Advanced IV Calculations

Solve these problems using dimensional analysis. Answers are given at the end of the chapter. The answers include how to set up the problem and how to solve it.

1. Order: Infuse heparin at 1000 units/hr via infusion pump
   Supply: heparin 25,000 units in 250 mL D5W IV
   How many mL/hr?

2. Order: Infuse insulin at 20 units/hr via infusion pump
   Supply: insulin 125 units in 250 mL NS IV
   How many mL/hr?

3. Order: Infuse aminophylline at 50 mg/hr via infusion pump
   Supply: aminophylline 250 mg in 250 mL D5W
   How many mL/hr?

4. Order: Infuse heparin at 40 mL/hr
   Supply: heparin 25,000 units in 500 mL D5W
   How many units are infusing per hour?

5. Order: Infuse aminophylline at 60 mL/hr
   Supply: aminophylline 500 mg/250 mL D5W
   How many mg are infusing per hour?

6. Order: Infuse Bretylium 2 mg/min via infusion pump
   Supply: Bretylium 1 g/500 mL D5W
   How many mL/hr?

7. Order: lidocaine 3 mg/min via infusion pump
   Supply: lidocaine 2 g/500 mL D5W
   How many mL/hr?

8. Order: nitroglycerine 20 mcg/min via infusion pump
   Supply: nitroglycerin 50 mg/250 mL D5W
   How many mL/hr?

9. Order: isuprel 5 mcg/min via infusion pump
   Supply: isuprel 2 mg/250 mL D5W
   How many mL/hr?

10. Order: dopamine 5 mcg/kg/min via infusion pump
    Supply: dopamine 200 mg/250 mL D5W; weight, 70 kg
    How many mL/hr?

11. Order: Pitocin 5 milliunits/min via infusion pump
    Supply: Pitocin 15 units/250 mL NS
    Solve using the same equation used for questions 8 and 9. Use the equivalency
    1 unit = 1000 milliunits.
    How many mL/hr?

12. Order: nipride 2 mcg/kg/min via infusion pump
    Supply: nipride 50 mg/250 mL D5W; weight, 110 lb
    How many mL/hr?

Solve these problems using the dimensional analysis method. Set up the equation first, then cancel out any like measurement systems, reduce the fraction, and solve. Answers are given on page 446.

1. Order: augmentin 500 mg q8h
   Supply: 125 mg/5 mL

2. Order: heparin 5000 units subcutaneous bid
   Supply: heparin 10,000 units/mL

3. Order: Lasix 20 mg IV bid
   Supply: Lasix 40 mg/4 mL

4. Order: Halcion 0.25 mg po at bedtime
   Supply: Halcion 0.125 mg/tablet

5. Order: Tylenol elixir 650 mg po q4h
   Supply: Tylenol elixir 325 mg/5 mL

6. Order: calcium gluconate 0.5 g IV × 1
   Supply: calcium gluconate 10%

7. Order: digoxin 125 mcg IV every day
   Supply: digoxin 0.25 mg/mL

8. Order: amoxicillin 375 mg q6h
   Supply: amoxicillin 125 mg/5 mL
   How many tsp?

9. Order: nitroglycerine 1/150 gr SL × 3
   Supply: 0.4-mg tablets

10. Order: Tylenol 5 gr q3–4h prn
    Supply: Tylenol elixir 325 mg/5 mL

11. Order: prednisone 40 mg/m^2 × 1 dose; BSA, 0.44 m^2
    What is the calculated dose?

12. Order: morphine 0.1 to 0.2 mg/kg IM; weight, 32 lb
    Supply: 10 mg/mL

13. Order: cefazolin 0.44 g IM q12h
    Supply: cefazolin vial
    Follow reconstitution directions to yield solution 330 mg/1 mL

14. Order: penicillin 1 million units
    Supply: penicillin vial
    Follow reconstitution directions to yield solution 500,000 units/1 mL.

15. Order: D5W 500 mL over 6 hr
    How many mL/hr?

(continued)

16. Order: NS 1000 mL over 16 hr
How many mL/hr?

17. Order: D5W 1000 mL over 10 hr
Drop factor is 60 gtt/mL. How many gtts/minute?

18. Order: D5W 250 mL over 2 hr
Drop factor is 15 gtts/mL. How many gtts/minute?

19. Order: regular insulin 5 units/hr via infusion pump
Supply: regular insulin 125 units/125 mL NS
How many mL/hr?

20. Order: heparin 1500 units/hr via infusion pump
Supply: heparin 25,000 units/500 mL D5W
How many mL/hr?

21. Order: heparin 30 mL/hr via infusion pump
Supply: heparin 25,000 units/250 mL D5W
How many units infusing per hour?

22. Order: nitroglycerine 15 mcg/min per infusion pump
Supply: nitroglycerine 50 mg/250 mL D5W
How many mL/hr?

23. Order: procainamide 2 mg/min per infusion pump
Supply: procainamide 2 g/500 mL D5W
How many mL/hr?

24. Order: dobutamine 10 mcg/kg/min per infusion pump
Supply: dobutamine 500 mg/500 mL D5W; weight, 100 kg
How many mL/hr?

25. Order: nipride 5 mcg/kg/min per infusion pump
Supply: nipride 50 mg/250 mL D5W; weight, 220 lb
How many mL/hr?

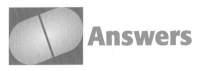 **Answers**

Self-Test 1 Calculation of Medications

1. $\dfrac{0.5 \text{ mg}}{} \left| \dfrac{1 \text{ tablet}}{0.25 \text{ mg}} \right.$

$\dfrac{\overset{2}{\cancel{0.5}} \text{ } \cancel{\text{mg}}}{} \left| \dfrac{1 \text{ } \boxed{\text{tablet}}}{\underset{1}{\cancel{0.25}} \text{ } \cancel{\text{mg}}} \right| \dfrac{2 \times 1}{} = 2 \text{ tablets}$

2. $\dfrac{800,000 \text{ units}}{} \left| \dfrac{1 \text{ tablet}}{400,000 \text{ units}} \right.$

$\dfrac{\overset{2}{\cancel{800,000}} \text{ } \cancel{\text{units}}}{} \left| \dfrac{1 \text{ } \boxed{\text{tablet}}}{\underset{1}{\cancel{400,000}} \text{ } \cancel{\text{units}}} \right| \dfrac{2 \times 1}{} = 2 \text{ tablets}$

3. $\dfrac{400 \text{ mg}}{} \left| \dfrac{5 \text{ } \boxed{\text{mL}}}{200 \text{ mg}} \right.$

$\dfrac{\overset{2}{\cancel{400}} \text{ } \cancel{\text{mg}}}{} \left| \dfrac{5 \text{ mL}}{\underset{1}{\cancel{200}} \text{ } \cancel{\text{mg}}} \right| \dfrac{2 \times 5}{} = 10 \text{ mL}$

4. $\dfrac{10 \text{ mg}}{} \left| \dfrac{1 \text{ tablet}}{2.5 \text{ mg}} \right.$

$\dfrac{\overset{4}{\cancel{10}} \text{ } \cancel{\text{mg}}}{} \left| \dfrac{1 \text{ } \boxed{\text{tablet}}}{\underset{1}{\cancel{2.5}} \text{ } \cancel{\text{mg}}} \right| \dfrac{4 \times 1}{} = 4 \text{ tablets}$

5. $\dfrac{60 \text{ mg}}{} \left| \dfrac{1 \text{ tablet}}{40 \text{ mg}} \right.$

$\dfrac{\overset{3}{\cancel{60}} \text{ } \cancel{\text{mg}}}{} \left| \dfrac{1 \text{ } \boxed{\text{tablet}}}{\underset{2}{\cancel{40}} \text{ } \cancel{\text{mg}}} \right| \dfrac{3 \times 1}{2} = \dfrac{3}{2} = 1.5 \text{ or } 1\frac{1}{2} \text{ tablets}$

6. $\dfrac{75 \text{ mg}}{} \left| \dfrac{1 \text{ mL}}{50 \text{ mg}} \right.$

$\dfrac{\overset{3}{\cancel{75}} \text{ } \cancel{\text{mg}}}{} \left| \dfrac{1 \text{ } \boxed{\text{mL}}}{\underset{2}{\cancel{50}} \text{ } \cancel{\text{mg}}} \right| \dfrac{3 \times 1}{2} = \dfrac{3}{2} = 1.5 \text{ mL}$

7. $\dfrac{0.5 \text{ mg}}{} \bigg| \dfrac{1 \text{ mL}}{0.25 \text{ mg}}$

$$\dfrac{\overset{2}{\cancel{0.5}} \text{ mg}}{} \bigg| \dfrac{1 \text{ mL}}{\underset{1}{\cancel{0.25}} \text{ mg}} \bigg| \dfrac{2 \times 1}{1} = 2 \text{ mL}$$

8. $\dfrac{1500 \text{ units}}{} \bigg| \dfrac{1 \text{ mL}}{5000 \text{ units}}$

$$\dfrac{\overset{3}{\cancel{1500}} \text{ units}}{} \bigg| \dfrac{1 \text{ mL}}{\underset{10}{\cancel{5000}} \text{ units}} \bigg| \dfrac{3 \times 1}{10} = \dfrac{3}{10} \text{ or } 0.3 \text{ mL}$$

9. $\dfrac{15 \text{ mg}}{} \bigg| \dfrac{1 \text{ mL}}{10 \text{ mg}}$

$$\dfrac{\overset{3}{\cancel{15}} \text{ mg}}{} \bigg| \dfrac{1 \text{ mL}}{\underset{2}{\cancel{10}} \text{ mg}} \bigg| \dfrac{3 \times 1}{2} = \dfrac{3}{2} = 1.5 \text{ mL}$$

10. $\dfrac{80 \text{ mg}}{} \bigg| \dfrac{2 \text{ mL}}{125 \text{ mg}}$

$$\dfrac{\overset{16}{\cancel{80}} \text{ mg}}{} \bigg| \dfrac{2 \text{ mL}}{\underset{25}{\cancel{125}} \text{ mg}} \bigg| \dfrac{16 \times 2}{25} = \dfrac{32}{25} = 1.28 \text{ or } 1.3 \text{ mL}$$

Self-Test 2 Calculation of Medications Involving Equivalencies

1. $\dfrac{0.8 \text{ g}}{} \bigg| \dfrac{1 \text{ tablet}}{400 \text{ mg}} \bigg| \dfrac{1000 \text{ mg}}{1 \text{ g}}$

$$\dfrac{0.8 \cancel{\text{ g}}}{} \bigg| \dfrac{1 \text{ tablet}}{\cancel{400} \text{ mg}} \bigg| \dfrac{\cancel{1000} \text{ mg}}{1 \cancel{\text{ g}}} \bigg| \dfrac{0.8 \times 1 \times 10}{4 \times 1} = \dfrac{8}{4} = 2 \text{ tablets}$$

2. $\dfrac{0.3 \text{ mg}}{} \bigg| \dfrac{1 \text{ tablet}}{300 \text{ mcg}} \bigg| \dfrac{1000 \text{ mcg}}{1 \text{ mg}}$

$$\dfrac{0.3 \cancel{\text{ mg}}}{} \bigg| \dfrac{1 \text{ tablet}}{\cancel{300} \text{ mcg}} \bigg| \dfrac{\cancel{1000} \text{ mcg}}{1 \cancel{\text{ mg}}} \bigg| \dfrac{0.3 \times 1 \times 10}{3 \times 1} = \dfrac{3}{3} = 1 \text{ tablet}$$

3. $\dfrac{\frac{1}{2} \text{ gr}}{} \bigg| \dfrac{1 \text{ tablet}}{30 \text{ mg}} \bigg| \dfrac{60 \text{ mg}}{1 \text{ gr}}$

$$\dfrac{\frac{1}{2} \cancel{\text{ gr}}}{} \bigg| \dfrac{1 \text{ tablet}}{\underset{1}{\cancel{30}} \text{ mg}} \bigg| \dfrac{\overset{2}{\cancel{60}} \text{ mg}}{1 \cancel{\text{ gr}}} \bigg| \dfrac{\frac{1}{2} \times 1 \times 2}{1} = \dfrac{2}{2} = 1 \text{ tablet}$$

4. $\dfrac{500\ \text{mg}}{} \bigg| \dfrac{5\ \text{mL}}{250\ \text{mg}} \bigg| \dfrac{1\ \text{tsp}}{5\ \text{mL}}$

$$\frac{\overset{2}{\cancel{500}}\ \text{mg} \bigg| \cancel{5}\ \cancel{\text{mL}} \bigg| 1\ \textcircled{tsp}}{\underset{1}{\cancel{250}}\ \text{mg} \bigg| \underset{1}{\cancel{5}}\ \cancel{\text{mL}}} \bigg| \frac{2 \times 1}{} = 2\ \text{tsp}$$

5. $\dfrac{100\ \text{mg}}{} \bigg| \dfrac{5\ \text{mL}}{100\ \text{mg}} \bigg| \dfrac{1\ \text{tsp}}{5\ \text{mL}}$

$$\frac{\overset{1}{\cancel{100}}\ \text{mg} \bigg| \cancel{5}\ \cancel{\text{mL}} \bigg| 1\ \textcircled{tsp}}{\underset{1}{\cancel{100}}\ \text{mg} \bigg| \underset{1}{\cancel{5}}\ \cancel{\text{mL}}} = 1\ \text{tsp}$$

6. $\dfrac{1\ \text{mg}}{} \bigg| \dfrac{1\ \text{mL}}{1000\ \text{mcg}} \bigg| \dfrac{1000\ \text{mcg}}{1\ \text{mg}}$

$$\frac{1\ \text{mg} \bigg| \cancel{1}\ \textcircled{mL} \bigg| \overset{1}{\cancel{1000}}\ \cancel{\text{mcg}}}{\underset{1}{\cancel{1000}}\ \cancel{\text{mcg}} \bigg| \cancel{1}\ \cancel{\text{mg}}} = 1\ \text{mL}$$

7. $\dfrac{500\ \text{mg}}{} \bigg| \dfrac{1\ \text{mL}}{1\ \text{g}} \bigg| \dfrac{1\ \text{g}}{1000\ \text{mg}}$

$$\frac{\overset{1}{\cancel{500}}\ \text{mg} \bigg| 1\ \textcircled{mL} \bigg| \cancel{1}\ \cancel{\text{g}}}{\cancel{1}\ \cancel{\text{g}} \bigg| \underset{2}{\cancel{1000}}\ \text{mg}} = \frac{1}{2}\ \text{or}\ 0.5\ \text{mL}$$

8. $1:1000 = 1\ \text{g in } 1000\ \text{mL}$

$$\frac{0.4\ \text{mg}}{} \bigg| \frac{1000\ \text{mL}}{1\ \text{g}} \bigg| \frac{1\ \text{g}}{1000\ \text{mg}}$$

$$\frac{0.4\ \text{mg} \bigg| \overset{1}{\cancel{1000}}\ \textcircled{mL} \bigg| \cancel{1}\ \cancel{\text{g}}}{\cancel{1}\ \cancel{\text{g}} \bigg| \underset{1}{\cancel{1000}}\ \cancel{\text{mg}}} = 0.4\ \text{mL}$$

9. $2\% = 2\ \text{g in } 100\ \text{mL}$

$$\frac{30\ \text{mg}}{} \bigg| \frac{100\ \text{mL}}{2\ \text{g}} \bigg| \frac{1\ \text{g}}{1000\ \text{mg}}$$

$$\frac{30\ \cancel{\text{mg}} \bigg| \overset{1}{\cancel{100}}\ \textcircled{mL} \bigg| \overset{1}{\cancel{1}}\ \cancel{\text{g}}}{\underset{2}{\cancel{2}}\ \cancel{\text{g}} \bigg| \underset{10}{\cancel{1000}}\ \cancel{\text{mg}}} = \frac{30}{10 \times 2} = \frac{30}{20} = 1.5\ \text{mL}$$

10. $\dfrac{^1\!/_{150}\ \text{gr}}{} \bigg| \dfrac{1\ \text{mL}}{0.4\ \text{mg}} \bigg| \dfrac{60\ \text{mg}}{1\ \text{gr}}$

$$\frac{^1\!/_{150}\ \cancel{\text{gr}} \bigg| 1\ \textcircled{mL} \bigg| 60\ \cancel{\text{mg}}}{0.4\ \cancel{\text{mg}} \bigg| 1\ \cancel{\text{gr}}} = \frac{^1\!/_{150} \times 60}{0.4} = \frac{0.4}{0.4} = 1\ \text{mL}$$

> **Example**   Nalbuphine is contraindicated if hypersensitivity to the drug exists or if the patient has dependency on other opioids. Use cautiously in head trauma, increased intracranial pressure (ICP), severe respiratory disease, undiagnosed abdominal pain, and pregnancy (depressed respirations in newborn). Safety is not established in children.

Interactions and Incompatibilities

When more than one drug is administered at a time, unexpected or nontherapeutic responses may occur. Some interactions are desirable. For example, naloxone (Narcan) is a narcotic antagonist that reverses the effects of a morphine overdose. Other interactions, however, are undesirable. For example, aspirin should not be taken with an oral anticoagulant because the possibility of an adverse effect (eg, increased bleeding) increases.

Some drugs may be incompatible and should not be mixed. This information is especially important when medications are combined for injection in IV administration. Chemical incompatibility is usually indicated by a visible sign such as precipitation or color change. Physical incompatibility can occur without any visible sign; therefore, the nurse should check a suitable reference before combining drugs. A good rule of thumb is: When in doubt, do not mix.

COMMON DRUGS AND DRUG CLASSIFICATIONS THAT CAUSE UNEXPECTED OR NONTHERAPEUTIC RESPONSES

Refer to a drug handbook for specific interactions.

MAO inhibitors, anticonvulsants, lithium

Tricyclic antidepressants, antifungals, methotrexate

Alcohol, barbiturates, NSAIDs

Aluminum, beta blockers, oral contraceptives

Aminoglycosides, cimetidine, phenothiazines

Antacids, clonidine, phenytoin

Anticoagulants, cyclosporine, probenecid

Heparin, digoxin, rifampin

Coumadin, erythromycin, theophylline

ASA, isoniazid

Interactions also may occur between drugs and certain foods. Calcium present in dairy products interferes with the absorption of tetracycline. Foods high in vitamin B_6 can decrease the effect of an antiparkinsonian drug. Foods high in tyramine, such as wine and cheese, can precipitate a hypertensive crisis in patients taking monoamine oxidase (MAO) inhibitors. Grapefruit juice interferes with the absorption of multiple drugs.

Cigarette smoke can increase liver metabolism of drugs and decrease drug effectiveness. Even individuals who are passively exposed to cigarette smoke may require higher doses of medication.

> **Example**   Nalbuphine produces additive CNS depression with alcohol, antihistamines, and sedative/hypnotics. It can produce withdrawal in patients dependent on opioids and can diminish the analgesic effect. Exercise care when giving to patients receiving MAO inhibitors. Severe reactions are possible.

Nursing Implications

The nurse needs this information to administer the drug safely and to assess, manage, and teach the patient. This can include whether the drug should be taken with or without food, any specific vital signs to monitor, and lab values affected by the drug or that need to be ordered to check the drug's effectiveness or toxicity.

| **Example** | Some nursing implications related to nalbuphine include the following: assess pain before and 1 hour following the dose; assess BP, pulse, respirations before and periodically after the dose; assess for dependency and tolerance. |

Signs of Effectiveness

Few drug references actually list this heading, yet the nurse is expected to evaluate the drug regimen, and to record and report observations. Knowledge of the drug's class, its action, and its use leads to an understanding of expected therapeutic outcomes.

For example, ampicillin sodium is a broad-spectrum antibiotic that is used for urinary, respiratory, and other infections. Signs of effectiveness might include normal temperature, the laboratory report of the WBC count indicating a normal result, clear urine, no pain on urination, no WBC in urine, decreased pus in an infected wound, wound healing, a patient who is more alert and interested in surroundings, and improved appetite.

| **Example** | Nalbuphine: relief of pain, sedation |

Patient Teaching

The patient has a right to know the name and dose of the drug, why the drug is ordered, and what effects to expect or watch for. In addition, the patient who is to take a drug at home needs specific information. This is a professional responsibility shared by the physician or health care provider, the nurse, and the pharmacist.

Pharmacokinetics

When a drug is taken orally, it is absorbed through the villi of the small intestine, distributed to the cells by the bloodstream, metabolized to a greater or lesser extent, and then excreted from the body. Pharmacokinetics includes absorption, distribution, biotransformation, and excretion.

Absorption

Absorption of an oral drug depends on the degree of stomach acidity, the time it takes for the stomach to empty, whether food is present, the amount of contact with villi in the small intestine, and blood flow to the villi.

Absorption of a drug may be affected in many ways. Enteric-coated (EC) tablets are not meant to dissolve in the acidic stomach. They ordinarily pass through the stomach to the duodenum. When an antacid is administered with an EC tablet, the pH of the stomach is raised and the tablet may dissolve prematurely. The drug may become less potent or it may irritate the gastric lining. Timed-release EC capsules that dissolve prematurely can deliver a huge dose of drug, causing adverse effects.

Laxatives increase gastrointestinal movement and decrease the time a drug is in contact with the villi of the small intestine, where most absorption occurs. The presence of food in the stomach can impair absorption. Penicillin is a good example of a drug that should be taken on an empty stomach. Foods that contain calcium, such as milk and cheese, form a complex with some drugs and inhibit absorption.

Distribution

Distribution is the movement of a drug through body fluids, chiefly the bloodstream, to cells. Drugs do not travel freely in the blood. Most travel attached to plasma proteins, especially albumin. Drugs that are free can attach to cells, on which they produce an effect.

When more than one drug is present in the bloodstream, they may compete for protein binding sites. One drug may displace another. The displaced drug is now free to act with the cells, and its effect will be more pronounced. Aspirin is a common drug for displacement; it should not be given with oral anticoagulants, which are 99% bound to albumin. Aspirin displaces the anticoagulant; more is free to act at the cellular level, and the toxic effect of bleeding may occur.

Biotransformation

This refers to the chemical change of a drug to a form that can be excreted. Most biotransformation occurs in the liver. Because oral drugs are carried first to the liver, this process begins when the drug is absorbed. Here, too, one drug can interfere with the effects of another. Barbiturates increase the liver enzyme activity. Because drugs are metabolized more quickly, their effect is reduced. Conversely, acetaminophen (Tylenol) will block the breakdown of penicillin in the liver, thereby increasing its activity.

Excretion

Excretion refers to the removal of a drug from the body. The major organ of excretion is the kidney. Drug interactions may also occur at this level. For example, probenecid inhibits the excretion of penicillin and increases its length of action. Furosemide (Lasix), a diuretic, blocks the excretion of aspirin and can lead to adverse effects by aspirin.

Drug interactions are not necessarily harmful. For example, narcotic antagonists are used to reverse the adverse effects of general anesthetics. This action is termed *antagonism. Synergism* is a term used when a second drug increases the intensity or prolongs the effect of a first drug. For example, a narcotic and a minor tranquilizer produce more pain relief than the narcotic alone. The nurse administering medications needs to be aware of possible interactions and evaluate the patient's response.

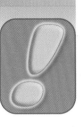

Clinical Alert!

Cultural Considerations

- Drug metabolism and side effects can vary among different cultures, races, and ethnic groups.

- Pharmacoanthropology deals with differences in drug responses among racial and ethnic groups. Ethnocultural perception deals with various cultural perceptions and beliefs of illness, disease, and drug therapy.

- Assessment of different personal beliefs of client and family is essential to drug administration.

- Communication must meet the cultural needs and respect the culture and cultural practices of the client and family.

To minimize adverse interactions, the nurse should know the patient's drug profile, give as low a dose as possible, know the actions and adverse effects of the drugs administered, and monitor the patient. Some drug interactions may take several weeks to develop.

Tolerance

When a pain or sleeping medication is given frequently, the liver enzymes become skilled in biotransforming more quickly. Less drug is available, thus the drug is less effective in relieving pain or aiding sleep. Some nurses call this reaction "addiction," because the patient complains that the drug is not working and asks for more. In fact, it is a physiologic response. The patient requires more of the drug or a drug with a different molecular structure.

Cumulation

When biotransformation or excretion is inhibited, as can occur in liver or kidney disease, the drug accumulates in the body and an adverse effect can occur. Cumulation can also result from taking too much drug or from taking a drug too frequently.

Other factors that affect drug action include

- Weight: Larger individuals need a higher dose.

- Age: Extremes of life respond more strongly. The liver and kidneys of infants are not well developed; in the elderly, systems are less efficient.

- Pathologic conditions: especially of liver and kidneys.

- Hypersensitivity to a drug: allergic reaction.

- Psychological and emotional state: Depression or anxiety can decrease or increase body metabolism and affect drug action.

Adverse reactions may occur in any system or organ. Drug knowledge will enhance the nurse's observational skills and will lead to responsible and appropriate intervention.

Half-Life

Half-life of a drug correlates roughly with its duration of action and gives an indication of how often the drug may be given to continue therapeutic effect. For example, piroxicam has a half-life of 48 to 72 hours and is given po as a single dose once a day. Carisoprodol has a half-life of 4 to 6 hours and is administered three to four times daily.

Clinical Alert!

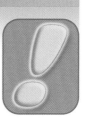

Herbs, Herbs, Herbs

- Herbal therapy is one of the oldest forms of medication. Use is worldwide. More and more people are taking herbal medications.

- However, herbal therapies and other alternative medications are not subject to FDA regulations.

- Clients should consult with their health care provider before beginning herbal therapy, when taking any herbal therapy, when experiencing any side effects from the products, and before discontinuing herbal therapy.

- The Office of Alternative Medicine is under the auspices of the National Institutes of Health and studies alternative medicine and therapies (see www.nccam.nih.gov).

- The Dietary Supplement Health and Education Act of 1994 clarified regulations for herbal remedies (see http://vm.cfsan.fda.gov/~dms/dietsupp.html).

- Health care providers need to be aware of potential drug interactions between herbal therapy and conventional drugs (prescription or over the counter).

Legal Considerations

There are two types of law that affect nursing practice—criminal and civil.

Criminal Law

Criminal law relates to offenses against the general public that are detrimental to society as a whole. Criminal actions are prosecuted by governmental authorities. If the defendant is judged guilty, the penalty may be a fine, imprisonment, or both.

Nurses must know the scope of nursing practice in the state in which they function. They should be familiar with government regulations—federal, state, and local—that affect nursing. The policies and procedures of the agency in which they practice also have legal status. Failure to follow guidelines, or lack of knowledge, can lead to liability.

Criminal charges include unlawful use, possession, or administration of a controlled substance. The Comprehensive Drug Abuse, Prevention and Control Act of 1970 classified drugs that are subject to abuse into one of five schedules according to their medical usefulness and abuse potential.

Schedule I drugs have no valid use and are not available for prescription use (eg, LSD).

Schedule II drugs have a valid medical use and are available for prescriptions but exhibit a high abuse potential. Misuse can lead to physical and psychological dependence. Labels for these drugs are marked with the symbol Ⓘ. An order for a narcotic in a hospital setting might be valid for 3 days. When the 3 days have elapsed, the order must be rewritten. A nurse who administers a controlled drug after the order has expired commits a medication error.

Schedule III, IV, and *V* drugs are classified as having less abuse potential than schedule II drugs, but they can cause some physical and psychological dependence. Note that Ⓘ, Ⓘ, and Ⓥ identify these drugs. A few examples of these drugs are Percodan, Fiorinal, diazepam (Valium), and Tylenol #3 (Tylenol with codeine).

Schedule II, III, IV, and V drugs are kept locked on nursing units. A locked narcotic cabinet or cart is used, and a record is kept for each narcotic administered. The Pyxis® system is being used in many hospitals, which is a computerized locked cabinet that dispenses controlled substances (Fig. 12-1). Controlled drugs are counted each shift, and discrepancies are reported. Government and institutional policies specify how these drugs are stored and protected.

Nurses who become impaired (unable to function) because of alcohol or drug abuse leave themselves open to criminal action, as well as to disciplinary action by the state board of nursing. Many states have laws requiring mandatory reporting of impaired nurses.

Civil Law

Civil law is concerned with the legal rights and duties of private persons. When an individual believes that a wrong was committed against him or her personally, that individual can sue for damages in the form of money.

The legal wrong is called a *tort*. *Malpractice* refers to negligence on the part of the nurse. There are four elements of negligence:

1. A claim that the nurse owed the patient a special duty of care—that is, a nurse–patient relationship existed

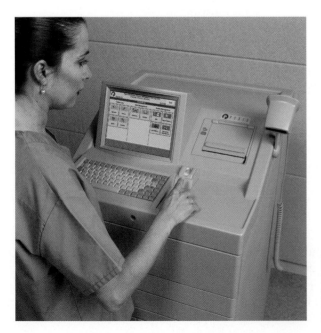

FIGURE 12-1

Pyxis Controlled Medication System. (With permission from Roach, S. [2004]. *Introductory clinical pharmacology* [7th ed.]. Philadelphia: Lippincott Williams & Wilkins, p. 18.)

2. A claim that the nurse was required to meet a specific standard of care in carrying out the action or function. To prove or disprove this element, both sides bring in expert witnesses to testify.

3. A claim that the nurse failed to meet the required standard

4. A claim that harm or injury resulted for which compensation is sought

The nurse–patient relationship is a legal status that is created the moment a nurse actually provides nursing care to another person.

For administration of medications, *a nurse is required by law to exercise the degree of skill and care that a reasonably prudent nurse with similar training and experience, practicing in the same community, would exercise under the same or similar circumstances.* When a nursing student performs duties that are customarily performed by a registered nurse, the courts have held the nursing student to the higher standard of care of the registered nurse.

Mistakes in administering medications are among the most common causes of malpractice. Liability may result from administering the wrong dose, giving a medication to the wrong patient, giving a drug at the wrong time, or failing to administer a drug at the right time or in the proper manner.

A frequent cause of medication errors is misreading the physician's order or failing to check with the physician when the order is questionable. Faulty technique in administering medications, especially injections that result in injury to the patient, is another common medication error.

Not all malpractice is a result of negligence. Malpractice claims are also founded on the daily interaction between the nurse and the patient; consequently, the nurse's personality plays a major role in fostering or preventing malpractice claims. All nurses should be familiar with the principles of psychology. The surest way to prevent claims is to recognize the patient as a human being who has emotional as well as physical needs, and to respond to these needs in a humane and competent manner.

Should an error occur, primary consideration must be given to the patient. The nurse notifies the physician and the immediate nursing supervisor; students notify the instructor. Error-in-medication forms are filled out and appropriate action is taken under the direction of the physician or health care provider.

To prevent malpractice claims, the nurse must render, as consistently as possible, the best possible care to patients. Every nurse involved in direct care should regard prevention of malpractice claims as an integral part of daily nursing responsibilities for two fundamental reasons:

1. Such measures result in higher-quality care.

2. All affirmative measures taken to minimize malpractice will minimize the nurse's exposure to personal liability.

How can liability claims be avoided? First and foremost are the three checks and five rights (see pp. 341–342). Accurate dosage calculation is also a safeguard against medication errors and potential liability claims. Other safeguards include:

- Know and follow institutional policies and procedures.

- Look up what you do not know.

- Do not leave medicines at the bedside.

- Chart carefully.

- Listen to the patient: "I never took that before," and the like.

- Check.

- *Double-check* when a dose seems high. Most oral tablet doses range from $\frac{1}{2}$ to 2 tablets.

- Most injections are less than 3 mL.

- Label any powder you dilute. Label any IV bag you use.

- When necessary, seek advice from competent professionals.

- Do not administer drugs poured by another nurse.

- Keep drug knowledge up to date. Attend continuing education programs and update nursing skills.

It is possible to render high-quality nursing care and never commit a medication error. Safe effective drug therapy is a combination of knowledge, skill, carefulness, and caring.

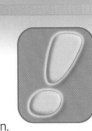

Clinical Alert!

Medication Errors

- Prevent them.
- Don't make them.
- Don't be in a hurry.
- If you do make them, learn from your mistakes and don't make them again.

Reporting

- It is the nurse's legal and ethical responsibility to report medication errors.
- Follow institutional policy in reporting and documenting medication errors.
- The FDA maintains a confidential database for medication errors: 1-800-23-ERROR. The FDA Medication Error web site is www.fda.gov/cder/drug/MedErrors.
- The National Coordinating Council for Medication Error Reporting and Prevention (NCCMERP) provides assistance on medication errors and promoting medication safety: 1-800-822-8772. Web site: www.nccmerp.org.

▶ Ethical Principles in Drug Administration

A moral as well as legal dimension is involved in the administration of medications. Nurses are responsible for their actions.

The American Nurses Association Code of Ethics contains several statements that apply to drug therapy. Briefly stated, they are the following:

1. The nurse provides services with respect for the human dignity and the uniqueness of the patient.
2. The nurse safeguards the patient's right to privacy.
3. The nurse acts to safeguard the patient from incompetent, unethical, or illegal practice.
4. The nurse assumes responsibility and accountability for nursing judgments and actions.
5. The nurse maintains competence in nursing.

Several principles can be used as guides when an ethical decision must be made. These principles are autonomy, truthfulness, beneficence, nonmaleficence, confidentiality, justice, and fidelity.

Autonomy

Autonomy is self-determination. It is a form of personal liberty in which an individual has the freedom to decide, knows the facts and understands them, and acts without outside force, deceit, or constraints. For the patient, this implies a right to be informed about drug therapy and a right to refuse medication. For the nurse, autonomy brings a responsibility to discuss drug information with the patient and to accept the patient's right to refuse. Autonomy also gives the nurse the right to refuse to participate in any drug therapy deemed to be unethical or unsafe for the patient.

Truthfulness

The nurse has the obligation not to lie. Telling the truth, however, is not the same as telling the *whole* truth. Ethically it is sometimes difficult to decide what may be concealed and what must be revealed.

In drug research the patient has a right to informed consent—to be told the truth before signing as a participant. Double-blind studies are used in determining effectiveness. Patients are randomly assigned to an experimental group that receives the drug or to a control group that receives a placebo (a preparation devoid of pharmacologic effect). Neither the patient nor the nurse knows to which group he or she is assigned. The patient must receive full disclosure of risks and benefits, and understand the research design to participate freely.

Beneficence

This principle holds that the nurse should act in the best interests of the patient. Actions are limited by the respect due to the freedom of the patient and the right of the patient to self-determination. Conflict can arise when the nurse decides what is best for the patient and violates the patient's rights.

Nonmaleficence

This principle holds that the nurse must not inflict harm on the patient and must prevent harm whenever possible. In drug therapy every medication has the risk of inducing some undesirable side and/or adverse effect. Chemotherapy may reduce the size of a tumor but may cause nausea, vomiting, decreased white cell count, and so forth. The nurse anticipates the untoward effects of drugs that may occur and acts to minimize them.

Confidentiality

Confidentiality is respect for information learned from professional involvement with patients. A patient's drug therapy and responses should be discussed only with those individuals who have a right to know— that is, other professionals caring for the patient. The extent to which the family or significant others have a right to know depends on the specific situation and wishes of the patient. These varying interests may cause conflict.

Justice

Justice refers to the patient's right to receive the right drug, the right dose, by the right route, at the right time. In addition, the patient has a right to the nurse's careful assessment, management, and evaluation of drug therapy, and to those nursing actions that promote the patient's safety and well-being. The nurse's obligation is to maintain a high standard of care.

Fidelity

A nurse should keep promises made to the patient. Statements such as "I'll be right back" and "I'll check the chart and let you know" create a covenant that should be respected.

▶ Specific Points That May Be Helpful in Giving Medications

Three Checks and Five Rights

The nurse always observes the three checks and five rights of medication administration.

Three Checks When Preparing Medications

Read the label

- ✓ When reaching for the container or unit dose package
- ✓ Immediately before pouring or opening the medication, or preparing the unit dose
- ✓ When replacing the container or before giving the unit dose to the patient

Oral Medications—Tablets and Capsules

- Administer irritating oral drugs with meals or a snack to decrease gastric irritation.

- If the patient is nauseous or vomiting, withhold oral medications and notify the physician or the immediate superior. Be sure to chart this action.

- Break a tablet only if it is scored.

- Never open capsules or break EC tablets. If the patient cannot swallow them, ask the physician to order a liquid, or check with the pharmacist.

- Check tablets in a stock container. Are they the same size? Same color? If not, return them to the pharmacy.

- Hydrophilic capsules are not medications. They are labeled DO NOT EAT and are placed in stock containers of tablets and capsules to absorb dampness and to maintain the drug in a solid state.

Liquid Medications

- Read labels three times: (1) when removing the drug from storage, (2) when calculating the dose, and (3) after pouring the drug.

- Quiet and concentration are needed to pour drugs. Follow a routine in pouring. *Methodology is the best safeguard in preventing error.*

- Never return any poured drug to a stock bottle once the drug has been taken from the preparation room.

- Never combine medications from two stock bottles. Return both bottles to the pharmacy. It is the responsibility of the pharmacists to combine drugs.

- Some liquid medications require dilution. Check references for directions.

- Some liquids may have to be administered through a straw. For example, liquid iron preparations discolor and should not come in contact with teeth.

- Liquids are poured at eye level using a medicine cup. Measure at the *center* of the meniscus. Pour with the label up to prevent soiling.

- After the patient has taken a liquid antacid, add 5 to 10 mL water to the cup, mix, and have patient drink it as well. Antacids are thick and medication often remains in the cup.

- The nurse who pours medications is responsible for administering and charting.

- Do not give drugs that another nurse has poured.

- Aqueous or water-based solutions do not need to be shaken before pouring.

Giving Medications

- Follow the universal safeguards in administration of medication (see Chapter 13).

- *Always* check the patient's ID band before administering medications. If the patient does not have an ID band, have a responsible person identify the patient for you and obtain an ID band for the patient.

- Listen to the patient's comments and act on them—for example, "Not mine" or "Never took this before." Check carefully, then return to the patient with the result of your investigation. Failure to do this will result in loss of the patient's trust and confidence, and may result in a medication error.

- If a patient refuses a drug, find out why. Then implement nursing action to correct the situation. Chart the reason for refusal and notify the physician who wrote the order.

- Watch to make sure the patient takes the drugs. Stay until oral drugs are swallowed.

- Keep drugs within view at all times.

- Never leave any drug at the bedside stand unless hospital policy permits this. If a medication is left, inform the patient why the drug is ordered, how to take it, and what to expect. Check to determine whether the drug was taken and record findings.

Charting

Charting is commonly called the "sixth right" of medication administration. The always-quoted axiom is still true: "If it's not charted, it's not done."

- Chart medications after administration.
- Chart single doses, stat doses, and prn medications immediately, and note the *exact time* when administered.
- Chart any nursing actions done prior to administering drugs (*ie,* apical heart rate [with digoxin] or blood pressure [with antihypertensives]). The safest place is on the medication administration record where the drug is documented.
- If the drug was refused, or the drug withheld (not given), write the reason on the nurse's notes and/or medication administration record, and notify the health care provider who ordered the medication. Also, note the time the health care provider was notified, and any response.

Evaluation

- Check for the expected effect of the drug. Did side effects or adverse effects occur? Perform indicated nursing actions. Record observations.

Clinical Alert!

Age-Specific Considerations

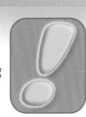

- Neonatal clients—The nurse needs to consider organ function immaturity, the importance of weight, and the precision of dosage calculation (rounding to the nearest one hundredth).
- Pediatric clients—The nurse needs to remember the principles of atraumatic care and the developmental stage considerations.
- Geriatric clients—The nurse needs to take into account decreasing organ function (especially liver and kidney), circulatory changes leading to decreased perfusion, and physical limitations (poor eyesight, decreased coordination, decreased ability to chew and/or swallow).

Error in Medication

- Report an error immediately to the charge nurse and the physician or health care provider.
- Primary concern must be given to the patient.
- Error-in-medication forms should be filled out. Follow the physician's directions in caring for the patient.

CRITICAL THINKING: TEST YOUR CLINICAL SAVVY

Mr. T is a patient who is receiving a drug that is in a drug study.

a. What is your ethical responsibility as a nurse administering this drug?

b. What is an appropriate response if the patient asks, "Is it safe to take this drug?" What should you do if the patient refuses to take the drug?

c. You are in agreement with the patient that he should not take the experimental drug. What are your ethical responsibilities? What are your legal responsibilities?

Mr. T discovers from the Internet that the drug he is taking is an experimental drug and that another drug with similar actions has been released by the FDA and is available by prescription.

d. How do you respond to the information that he has acquired? What are some questions that the patient should ask regarding information acquired over the Internet?

e. What are some responses if he asks you if he should continue to take the experimental drug, or discontinue his participation in the drug study and obtain a prescription for the similar drug?

f. What are the reasons you can give Mr. T regarding the benefits of participating in a drug study?

SELF-TEST 1   Basic Information

Give the information requested. Answers are given at the end of the chapter.

1. List at least ten kinds of information the nurse needs to know to give drugs safely.

   _____   _____

   _____   _____

   _____   _____

   _____   _____

   _____   _____

2. List the five pregnancy categories used to identify the safety of drugs for the fetus and briefly define each.

   _____

   _____

   _____

   _____

   _____

3. Name the major organ for these drug activities.

   a. Absorption _____   **c.** Biotransformation _____

   b. Distribution _____   **d.** Excretion _____

4. Define

   a. Tolerance _____

   _____

   _____

   b. Cumulation _____

   _____

   _____

5. List the four elements of negligence.

   _____ ,

   _____ ,

   _____ , and

   _____

6. What is the standard by which a tort is judged?

   _____

   _____

   _____

(continued)

SELF-TEST 1   Basic Information (Continued)

7. List at least five positive actions to avoid liability.

_____

_____

_____

_____

_____

8. List and briefly describe five ethical principles in drug therapy.

_____

_____

_____

_____

_____

9. What are the seven elements of a correct medication order?

_____

_____

_____

_____

_____

_____

10. What action should a nurse take when an order is not clear?

_____

PROFICIENCY TEST 1 | **Basic Drug Information**

Name: _____

Choose the correct answer. Answers are given on page 450.

1. Two drugs are given for different reasons, but drug Y interferes with the excretion of drug X. The effect of drug X would be

   a. Increased
   b. Decreased
   c. Unchanged
   d. Stopped

2. Major biotransformation of drugs occurs in the

   a. Lungs
   b. Kidney
   c. Liver
   d. Urine

3. Toxicity to a drug is more likely to occur when

   a. Elimination of the drug is rapid
   b. The drug is bound to the plasma protein albumin
   c. The drug will not dissolve in the lipid layer of the cell
   d. The drug is free in the blood circulation

4. The term USP after a drug name indicates that the drug

   a. Is made only in the United States
   b. Meets official standards in the United States
   c. Cannot be made by any other pharmaceutical company
   d. Is registered by the US Public Health Service

5. When an order is written to be administered "as needed" it is called a

   a. Standing order
   b. prn order
   c. Single order
   d. stat order

6. Signs of effectiveness of a drug are based on what information?

   a. Action and use
   b. Untoward effects
   c. Generic and trade names
   d. Drug interaction

7. Drug classification is an aid in understanding

   a. Use of the drug
   b. Drug idiosyncrasy
   c. The trade name
   d. The generic name

(continued)

PROFICIENCY TEST 1   **Basic Drug Information (Continued)**

8. Names of many drugs include

    a. Several generic, several trade names
    b. Several generic, one trade name
    c. One generic, one trade name
    d. One generic, several trade names

9. Which pregnancy category is considered safe for the fetus?

    a. A
    b. B
    c. C
    d. D

10. What is the primary purpose of EC medications?

    a. Improve taste
    b. Delay absorption
    c. Code the drug for identification
    d. Make the drug easier to swallow

11. Which of the following drug preparations does *not* have to be shaken before pouring?

    a. Magma
    b. Gel
    c. Suspension
    d. Aqueous solution

12. Most oral drugs are absorbed in the

    a. Mouth
    b. Stomach
    c. Small intestine
    d. Large intestine

13. Nursing legal responsibilities associated with controlled substances include

    a. Storage in a locked place
    b. Assessing vital signs
    c. Evaluating psychological response
    d. Establishing automatic 24-hour stop orders

14. Characteristics of a schedule II drug include

    a. Accepted medical use with a high abuse potential
    b. Medically accepted drug with low-dependence possibility
    c. No accepted use in patient care
    d. Unlimited renewals

15. The responsibilities of the nurse regarding medication in the hospital include

    a. Prescribing drugs
    b. Teaching patients
    c. Regulating automatic expiration times of drugs
    d. Preparing solutions

(continued)

16. Under what condition does a nurse have a right to refuse to administer a drug?

    a. The pharmacist ordered the drug.
    b. The drug is manufactured by two different companies.
    c. The drug is prescribed by a licensed physician.
    d. The dose is within the range given in the *PDR*.

17. When administering medication in the hospital, the nurse should

    a. Chart medications before administering them
    b. Chart only those drugs that she or he personally gave the patient
    c. Chart all medications given for the day at one time
    d. Determine the best method for giving the drugs

18. Which of the following illustrates a medication error?

    a. Administering a 10 AM dose at 10:20 AM
    b. Giving 2 tablets of gantrisin 500 mg when 1 g is ordered
    c. Pouring 5 mL of cough syrup when 1 tsp is ordered
    d. Giving digoxin IM when digoxin po 0.25 mg is ordered

19. A nurse reads a medication order that is not clear. What action is indicated?

    a. Ask the charge nurse to explain the order.
    b. Ask a doctor at the nurses' station for help.
    c. Check the *PDR* on the unit.
    d. Check with the doctor who wrote the order.

20. Which nursing action is illegal?

    a. Pouring medication from one stock bottle into another
    b. Counting control drugs in the narcotic cabinet or Pyxis each shift
    c. Labeling a vial of powder after dissolving it
    d. Refusing to carry out an order that is confusing

Answers

Self-Test I Basic Information

1. Generic/trade name, class, pregnancy category, dose and route, action, use, side/adverse effects, contraindications/precautions, interactions/incompatibilities, nursing implications, evaluation of effectiveness, patient teaching

2. **A.** No risk to fetus
   B. No adverse effects in animals, but no human studies
   C. Animals show adverse effects; calculated risk to fetus
   D. Fetal risk exists
   X. Absolute fetal abnormality

3. **a.** Small intestines
   b. Blood
   c. Liver
   d. Kidney

4. **a.** Repeated administration of a drug increases microsomal enzyme activity in the liver. The drug is broken down more quickly and its effectiveness is decreased.
   b. Biotransformation is inhibited and the drug level remains high. Adverse effects are more likely to occur.

5. A claim that a nurse–patient relationship existed
   The nurse was required to meet a standard of care
   A claim that the nurse failed to meet that standard
   A claim that this resulted in injury

6. Whether the nurse exercised the degree of skill and care that a reasonably prudent nurse with similar training and experience, practicing in the same community, would exercise under the same or similar circumstances

7. Know policies and practices of the institution.
   Research unfamiliar drugs.
   Do not leave medicines at the bedside.
   Chart carefully.
   Listen to the patient's complaints.
   Check yourself (eg, read labels three times).
   Label anything you dilute.
   Keep up to date.

8. Autonomy: freedom to decide based on knowledge with no constraint
   Truthfulness: truth telling that can create a dilemma. Is it absolute or is there a beneficent deceit?
   Beneficence: obligation to help others
   Nonmaleficence: do no harm
   Confidentiality: keep secrets
   Justice: rights of an individual
   Fidelity: keep promises

9. Patient's name and room, date, name of drug, dose, route, times of administration, doctor's or health care provider's signature

10. The nurse does not administer the drug and checks with the physician or health care provider who wrote the order.

Administration Procedures

Throughout this text we have calculated dosages and studied information related to drug therapy. Finally we arrive at the "how to" chapter—methods of administering drugs orally, parenterally, and topically. The adages "practice makes perfect" and "one picture is worth a thousand words" apply. Learning to administer medications is a skilled activity that requires practice, with supervision, to ensure correct technique. A medication administration skill book and a pharmacology textbook are also recommended.

Every institution has a standard procedure for administering medications, which depends on the way the drugs are dispensed—unit-dose, multidose containers, or a combination of the two. Institutional procedure may call for the use of medication tickets, for a mobile cart with medication sheets, or for the use of a computer printout.

Whatever the procedure is, follow it carefully. Do not look for shortcuts. *Methodology*—a step-by-step attention to detail—is the best safeguard to ensure the patient's five rights. Research has proved time after time that most medication errors occur because the nurse violated procedural guidelines.

▶ Universal or Standard Precautions Applied to Administration of Medications

When administering drugs, there is a risk of potential exposure to hepatitis A virus (HAV), hepatitis B virus (HBV), hepatitis C virus (HCV), Hepatitis D virus (HDV), Hepatitis E virus (HEV), and the human immunodeficiency virus (HIV) through contact of the nurse's skin or mucous membranes with patient blood, body fluids, or tissues. The Centers for Disease Control and Prevention (CDC) in Atlanta recommend that *universal precautions be employed in caring for all patients and when handling equipment contaminated with blood or blood-streaked body fluids.* In 1996, the term *standard precautions* replaced *universal precautions.* These two terms are interchangeable (see web site: www.cdc.gov).

The following points based on CDC guidelines are offered to aid in determining appropriate safeguards in giving medications. These points are *dependent on the type of contact you have with patients.*

General Safeguards in Administering Medications

1. Oral medications: Handwashing is adequate unless there is a possibility of exposure to blood or body secretions.

2. Injections: Handwashing and gloves are required. Carefully dispose of used sharps in a puncture-proof container. Hold the sharp away from you. Never take your eyes from the sharp during the disposal process! Do not recap needles.

3. Heparin locks, IV catheters, and IV needles: Wear gloves when inserting or removing IV needles and catheters. The use of a clamp is recommended to hold contaminated IV needles and catheters being carried to a puncture-proof container. There are some IV catheter needles that have a protective device to help prevent needlesticks.

4. Secondary administration sets or IVPB sets: Handwashing is adequate after removing this equipment from the main IV tubing because there is no direct exposure to blood or body secretions. Place used needles in a puncture-proof container.

5. Application of medication to mucous membranes: Wear gloves (see the following guidelines for using gowns, masks, and protective eyewear).

6. Applications to skin: Exercise nursing judgment. Handwashing may be sufficient protection when applying such drug forms as transdermal patches. Use gloves when the patient's skin is not intact. Use gloves when applying lotions, ointments, or creams to areas with a rash or skin lesions.

Hands

1. Wash hands before preparing medications and after administering medications to each patient.

2. Wash hands *after* removing gloves, gowns, masks, and protective eyewear; and *before* leaving the room of any patient for whom they are used.

3. Wash hands immediately when soiled with patient blood or body fluids.

4. Wash hands *after* handling equipment soiled with blood or body fluids.

Gloves

1. Wear gloves for any direct ("hands-on") contact with a patient's blood, bodily fluids, or secretions while administering medications.

2. Wear gloves when handling materials or equipment contaminated with blood or body fluids.

3. When gloves are used, they must be changed on completion of procedures for each patient *and* between patients.

Gowns

When administering medications, gowns are required *only* if the nurse's clothing may become contaminated with a patient's blood or body fluids.

Masks, Protective Eyewear, and Face Shields

1. Masks are required when caring for a patient on *strict* or *respiratory* isolation procedures.

2. Masks and protective eyewear or face shields are required when a medication procedure may cause blood or body fluids to splash directly onto the nurse's face, eyes, or mucous membranes.

3. Masks and protective eyewear must be worn during a medication procedure that is known to cause aerosolization of fluids containing chemicals or body fluids.

Management of Used Needles and Sharps

1. All used needles, syringes, sharps, stylets, butterfly needles, and IV catheters must be placed in appropriate, labeled, puncture-proof containers.

2. Do not break, bend, or recap needles after use. Immediately place needles into a puncture-proof container.

3.   Exercise caution in removing heparin locks, IV catheters, and IV needles. Gloves should be worn. The use of a clamp is advisable to hold the used IV needle being transported to a puncture-proof container. *Do not remove the IV needle from the IV tubing by hand. Use a clamp or use the needle unlocking device on the sharps container.* There are IV catheter needles that have a protective device to prevent needlesticks.

4.   If *reusable* needles and syringes are used, the needle should be separated from the syringe with a clamp. *Never manipulate a used needle by hand.* Place the needle and syringe in appropriate puncture-proof containers for sterilization. *It is strongly recommended that disposable needles and syringes be used.*

5.   Never take your eyes from the sharps container as you dispose of the sharp.

Needleless Systems

Needleless systems are being used to reduce the risk of needlesticks and blood-borne pathogens. These devices are used in several ways. Some syringes have a needle that retracts into the syringe after it is used. There are needleless adapters for syringes to withdraw medication from vials (Fig. 13-1). Needleless systems are available for IV tubing (Fig. 13-2) and for use at the patient's IV site. The needleless equipment is disposed into sharp containers.

Management of Materials Other Than Needles and Sharps

Paper cups, plastic cups, and other equipment not contaminated with blood or body fluids may be discarded according to routine hospital procedures. In cases of *strict* or *respiratory* isolation precautions, follow the protocol established by the institution.

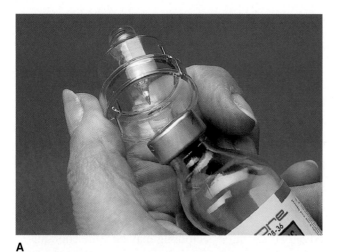

A

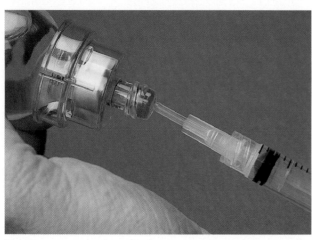

B

FIGURE 13-1

(**A**) Needleless system adapter for vial. (**B**) Use syringe (without needle) to withdraw medication.

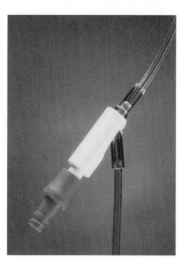

FIGURE 13-2
Needleless system for IV tubing.

Management of Nurse Exposed to Blood or Body Fluids

The nurse who is exposed to blood or blood-streaked body fluids of any patient through a personal needle-stick or injury, or through a skin laceration should immediately squeeze the area if this is indicated, wash the area with soap and copious water, and apply acceptable antiseptic. If mucous membrane exposure occurs, flush the exposed areas with copious amounts of warm water. The protocol established by the health care institution for management of needlestick injury or accidental exposure to blood or body fluids should be followed.

Systems of Administration

In an institutional setting, medications may be administered using tickets, the mobile cart, a locked medication cabinet near the patient's bedside, or computer printouts.

The ticket system is used when drugs are dispensed in multidose containers. Drugs are prepared in a medication room and are carried on a tray to the patient. When unit-dose packaging is available, drugs are placed in individual patient drawers on a mobile cart. The cart is wheeled into the patient's room and medications are prepared at the bedside for administration.

Ticket System

With this system, a medication order is transferred to three places: a medication ticket, the patient's medication sheet, and the patient's Kardex file, which contains the nursing care plan.

Tickets for all patients are kept in a central location. The nurse sorts them according to time of administration. Each ticket is compared with the Kardex entry. If there is a discrepancy, the nurse checks the original order on the patient's chart. After all tickets are verified, the nurse enters the medication room or unlocks the medication cart.

The nurse separates the first patient's tickets and places them together in a pile, one on top of another, so that only one ticket is visible at a time. The nurse reads the ticket, locates the medication, and verifies the label with the ticket (first check).

The nurse compares the dose on the ticket with the label, and calculates and pours the amount of drug (second check).

Before discarding the unit-dose packet or returning the container to the shelf, the nurse reads the order and the label again, and verifies the poured dose (third check).

The nurse places the medication on a tray with the ticket in front to identify it (Fig. 13-3). The nurse then dispenses the medication to the patient, identifying the patient by ID band and keeping the medications in sight. Any required nursing assessment is completed. The nurse administers the drugs, then takes the medication tray to the next patient and follows the same procedure. After medications are given, the nurse takes the medication tickets and charts the medications on each patient's chart. If a stat medication is given and charted, the ticket is destroyed.

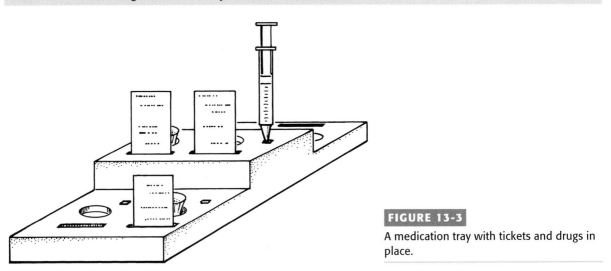

FIGURE 13-3

A medication tray with tickets and drugs in place.

There are several disadvantages to this system. Every order must be transcribed to three different places. Each time the order is rewritten, an error is possible. Tickets may be lost or misplaced. An error may occur in choosing the stock. The tickets may become mixed, so that the wrong patient receives a medication. Medications that require assessment must be tagged in some way to identify them. It is time-consuming to locate the chart of each patient.

This system is rarely used because of the unit-dose system and medication carts.

Mobile Cart System

Compared with the ticket system, the mobile cart system has many advantages. The pharmacist dispenses unit-dose medications directly to the patient's drawer. Each drawer is labeled with the patient's name. The cart contains all the equipment the nurse might require to administer medications.

When a drug is ordered, the nurse transcribes the order to one place—the patient's medication sheet found in a medication book on the cart. This book contains the medication sheets for every patient on the unit.

When it is time to administer medications, the nurse washes his or her hands and rolls the cart to the bedside of the first patient, greets the patient by name, unlocks the cart, and opens the medication book to the first patient's medication sheet.

The nurse checks the sheet for special nursing actions required before giving medication. The nurse carries out the orders, records the results, and decides to withhold or to administer the medication.

The nurse places the patient's drawer on the top of the cart. The nurse reads each medication order, starting with the first medication listed. When a dose is to be given, the nurse chooses the unit dose from the drawer and compares the label with the order (first check; Fig. 13-4).

The nurse computes the dose after comparing the order with the unit measure, opens or prepares the unit dose, and pours the amount (second check).

The nurse labels the unit dose, reads the order again, and verifies the dose (third check). After preparing all the patient's medications, the nurse reads the name on the medicine sheet, checks the patient's ID band, and administers the drugs. The nurse remains with the patient until the medications are taken, provides any comfort measures, washes his or her hands, and returns to the cart to chart the drugs administered. The nurse replaces the patient's drawer and rolls the cart to the next patient. When all medications have been administered, the nurse returns the mobile cart to its designated area.

This system has several advantages. There are two professionals involved in checking the medication in the drawer—the pharmacist and the nurse. All the medication sheets are together on the cart. This is time saving. Nursing assessment can be carried out and results charted before any medication is poured. The drugs can be signed for immediately after administration.

Note, however, that with both systems, the nurse checks the label three times—when choosing the drug, when calculating and pouring the dose, and before replacing the stock.

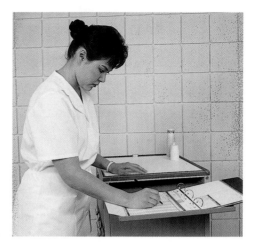

FIGURE 13-4

The nurse compares the medication with the order. (With permission from Roach, S. [2004]. *Introductory clinical pharmacology* [7th ed.]. Philadelphia: Lippincott Williams & Wilkins, p. 16.)

A variation of the mobile cart system is having the medications locked in a cabinet at or near the patient's bedside. This is similar in that the pharmacy fills the cabinet with the unit-dose medications. Medications sheets are in the patient chart, which is in the cabinet. Medications are prepared in the same manner, utilizing the three checks and five rights. Having the medications and the patient chart closer to the patient helps save time for the nurse and patient.

Computer Printouts

Institutions may have computerized medication procedures. Doctors input orders directly on the computer. The order is received in the pharmacy, where it is added to the patient's drug profile. The nursing unit receives the computer printout listing the medications and times of administration. The printout replaces the medication administration record (MAR).

There are several advantages to this system. Neither the nurse nor the pharmacist has to interpret the doctor's handwriting. The nurse does not have to transfer the written orders to an MAR, thus reducing the chance for error and saving time. Moreover, a computer check will identify possible interactions among the patient's medications and alert the nurse and the pharmacist.

Figure 13-5 is an example of a computerized MAR. The patient's name, ID number, room, date of admission, age, diagnosis, gender, and attending physician are printed at the top. The administration period for this record covers 24 hours using military time.

Clinical Alert!

Medication Errors

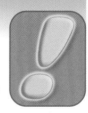

- Medication errors can cause unnecessary side effects, adverse effects, illnesses, and sometimes death.

- An FDA study between 1993 and 1998 indicated 5366 medication errors, with 469 of these errors being fatal.

- The most common types of errors? Administering an improper dose, administering the wrong drug, or using the wrong route of administration.

- Medication errors are preventable. As a nurse, the way to prevent medication errors is to follow the five rights of medication administration and the three checks of medication identification. Information on medication errors can be found on the FDA web site (www.fda.gov/cder/drug/MedErrors/reports.htm).

McFARLAND MEDICAL CENTER
MEDICATION ADMINISTRATION RECORD

Patient Name	Room No.	Hospital Number	Diagnosis	
Velder, Chelsea	1401	204452896	CHF	
Allergies	Admitted	Age	Sex	Physician
Penicillin	6/25/01	50	F	Richardson

DOSAGE ADMINISTRATION PERIOD: 6/26/01-6/27/01

	0601-1400	1401-2200	2201-0600
Aspirin 325 mg PO daily	0900		
Kefzol i Gm. Q 6 h IVPB	0800 1400	2000	0200
Lopressor 50 mg. PO BID	0900	2100	
Morphine Sulfate 4-6 mg. IV q 2-3 h prn pain			
Tylenol gr X q. 4 h prn temp > 101			

Signature   Initials   Signature   Initials   Signature   Initials

_____ (   )   _____ (   )   _____ (   )

FIGURE 13-5

A sample 24-hour computerized medication record. Scheduled drugs are listed at the top of the sheet and PRN orders at the bottom. Military time is used. The nurse initials the boxes to indicate the drug was administered and signs at the bottom of the sheet.

Routes of Administration

Oral Route

Regardless of the system used to pour the medications, the procedure for administering drugs contains specific steps. The nurse greets the patient verbally and checks his ID band. The patient is assisted to a sitting position. He should be alert and able to swallow. Oral solids are given first, together with a full glass of water whenever possible, followed by oral liquid medications. Before leaving, the nurse watches to be sure the patient has swallowed all the drugs. The paper and plastic cups may be discarded according to routine hospital procedure, unless the patient is on strict or respiratory isolation. For this, special isolation bags are utilized. The nurse makes the patient comfortable, washes his or her hands, and charts the doses given. The oral route is the least expensive, the safest, and the easiest to take.

Special considerations for oral administration include the following:

- Check expiration dates on all labels. Do not administer expired drugs.

- Check patients for allergies to drugs. This should be a routine procedure.

- Some drugs are best taken on an empty stomach; others may be taken with food.

- The nurse should be aware of foods or fluids that may be ingested with the drug, and those that are contraindicated.

- If the patient is NPO (nothing by mouth), check with the doctor to determine whether oral medication can be administered with a small amount of water. The doctor may not wish to withhold certain drugs (eg, an anticonvulsant for a patient with epilepsy).

- Solid stock medications are poured first into the container lid and then into a paper cup, using medical asepsis. The medication is not touched. Several solids may be combined in the cup, but each medication should first be poured into a separate cup until the third check is completed. Unit-dose medications should be checked three times before the package container is discarded.

- Medical asepsis is followed to break a scored tablet. This means that clean, not sterile, technique is required. One method is to place the tablet in a paper towel, fold the towel over and, with thumbs and index fingers in apposition, break the tablet along the score line. Tablets that are not scored should not be broken.

- If the patient has difficulty swallowing solids, first determine whether the medication is available in a liquid form. Enteric- and film-coated tablets should not be crushed. Ordinarily, capsules should not be opened. Check with the pharmacist for alternative forms. If a capsule can be opened, mix the drug with a small amount of applesauce, custard, or other vehicle that will make the medication more palatable and easy to swallow.

- If a medication can be crushed, it is best to use a "pill crusher," with the medication placed between two paper cups. If using a mortar and pestle, be sure they are cleaned before and after crushing so there is no residue. If no equipment is available, place the tablet in a paper towel and use the edge of a bottle or other hard surface to crush the drug. A crushed drug may be mixed with water or semi-solids, such as applesauce or custard, for ease in swallowing.

- The nurse should be knowledgeable about food–drug and drug–drug interactions, and should act to safeguard the patient.

Special Considerations for Liquid Medications

- Failure to shake some liquid medications can result in a wrong dose. The drug settles to the bottom and only the weak diluent is poured. Shake magmas, gels, and suspensions before pouring.

- Pour liquids at eye level, with the thumb indicating the meniscus. When pouring liquids, the label should be face up so it will not become stained. Before recapping, wipe the lip of the bottle with a paper towel.

- Note the presence of an unusual color change or precipitate in a liquid. If such a change is present, do not use it. Send the container to the pharmacy with a note indicating your observation.

- Check references to determine how to disguise liquids that are distasteful or irritating. Two possibilities are to mix them with juice or administer them through a straw after diluting well. Liquid iron preparations stain the teeth and are taken through a straw placed in the back of the mouth. Tinctures are always diluted.

- Liquid cough mixtures are not diluted. They have a secondary soothing (demulcent) effect on the mucous membranes in addition to their antitussive action.

Parenteral Route

Medications may be given by IM, subcutaneous, IVPB, or IV routes, or intradermally. The parenteral route is used when a drug cannot be given orally, when it is necessary to obtain a rapid systemic effect, or when a drug would be rendered ineffective or destroyed by the oral route. Aseptic technique is used with parenteral routes.

Choosing the Site

The following areas should be avoided: bony prominences, large blood vessels, nerves, sensitive areas, bruises, hardened areas, abrasions, and inflamed areas. The site for IM injections should be able to accept 3 mL; rotate sites when repeated injections are given.

Preparation of the Skin

Cleanse the site with an alcohol pad while using a circular motion from the center out. Grasp the area firmly between the thumb and forefinger and insert the needle with a dartlike motion (Fig. 13-6). If the area is obese, the skin may be spread rather than pinched together.

Syringes for Injection

The most common syringe used for injections is a standard 3-mL size, marked in minims and in milliliters to the nearest tenth. The precision (tuberculin) syringe is marked in half minims and milliliters to the nearest

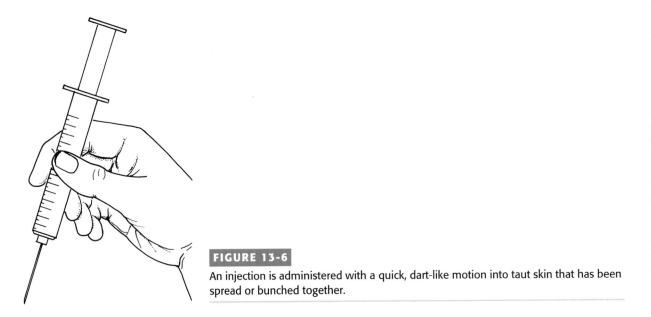

FIGURE 13-6
An injection is administered with a quick, dart-like motion into taut skin that has been spread or bunched together.

hundredth. There are two insulin syringes: a regular 1-mL size marked to 100 units, and a 0.5-mL size (low-dose) insulin syringe marked to 50 units.

Needles for Injections

Needles are chosen for their gauge and their length. *Gauge* is the diameter of the needle opening. The principle is: The higher the gauge number, the finer the needle.

The 28-gauge needle on the insulin syringe is the finest needle currently available for routine injections. Numbers 25, 26, and 28 are used for subcutaneous injections for adults, and for IM injections for children and emaciated patients. Numbers 23 and 22 are used for IM injections, 20 and 21 for IV therapy, and 16 and 18 for blood transfusions. Needle lengths vary from $\frac{5}{16}$ to 2 in. The appropriate length is determined by the route.

Angle of Insertion

INTRAMUSCULAR. For an IM injection, the syringe should be held at a right angle to the skin and the injection given at a 90-degree angle (Fig. 13-7).

SUBCUTANEOUS. For subcutaneous injections, the syringe should be held at a 45-degree angle when the needle is inserted. Some subcutaneous injections may be administered at a 90-degree angle if the subcutaneous layer of fat is thick and the needle is short. Care must be exercised to reach the correct site. When in doubt, use the 45-degree angle. Intramuscular sites have a good blood supply and absorption is rapid. Subcutaneous sites have a poor blood supply and absorption is prolonged (Fig. 13-7).

INTRADERMAL. A 26-gauge or other fine needle is used for skin testing for allergies and tuberculosis (Fig. 13-7).

Preparing the Dose

Ordinarily, to prevent incompatibility of drugs, only one medication should be drawn up in a syringe. When two drugs are given in one syringe, follow the procedure for mixing after determining that the drugs are compatible.

ADDING AIR TO A SYRINGE
Some nurses add 0.1 to 0.2 mL air to the syringe after obtaining the dose and before giving the injection. The air bubble rises to the top of the barrel and is injected last. The air acts as a seal to prevent medication from oozing into the skin from the injection tract and it empties the needle of medication. This procedure is required in giving a Z-tract injection; otherwise, it is optional. Institutional policy should be followed.

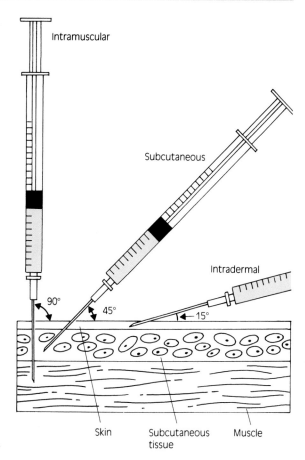

FIGURE 13-7

Comparison of angles of intersection for intramuscular, subcutaneous, and intradermal injections.

DRUGS THAT ARE LIQUIDS IN VIALS

1. Cleanse the top of the vial with an alcohol sponge.

2. Draw the amount of air equivalent to the amount of solution desired into the syringe (Fig. 13-8A).

3. Inject the needle through the rubber diaphragm into the vial.

4. Expel air from the syringe into the vial. This increases the pressure in the vial and makes it easier to withdraw medication.

5. Invert the vial and draw up the desired amount into the syringe (Fig. 13-8B).

6. Withdraw the needle quickly from the vial.

7. The rubber diaphragm will seal.

DRUGS THAT ARE POWDERS IN VIALS

1. Cleanse the top of the vial with an alcohol sponge.

2. Draw up the amount of calculated diluent from a vial of distilled water or normal saline for injection. Follow pharmaceutical directions if another solvent is indicated.

3. Add the diluent to the powder and roll the vial between your hands to dissolve the powder.

4. Label the vial with the solution made, your initials, and the date and time.

5. Cleanse the top of the vial again.

6. Draw up the amount of air equivalent to the amount of solution desired into the syringe.

7. Inject the needle through the rubber diaphragm into the vial.

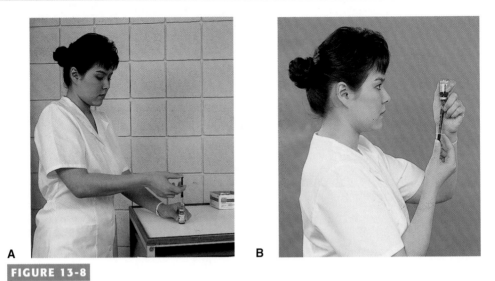

A   B

FIGURE 13-8

(**A**) Injecting air into the vial. (**B**) Invert the vial and draw up the desired amount of medication into the syringe.

8. Expel the air into the vial. This increases pressure in the vial and makes it easier to remove medication. Invert the vial and draw up the desired amount of medication into the syringe.

9. Check directions for storage of any remaining drug.

   Note: When the whole amount of powder contained in a vial is needed for an IVPB medication, a reconstitution device may be used to dilute the powder without using a syringe.

DRUGS IN GLASS AMPULES

1. Tap the top of the ampule with your finger to clear out any drug.

2. Place an opened alcohol pad around the neck of the ampule.

3. Hold the ampule sideways.

4. Place thumbs above and index fingers below the ampule neck.

5. Press down with thumbs to break the ampule.

6. Invert the ampule, insert the syringe needle, and withdraw the dose (Fig. 13-9). *Important: Do not add air before removing the dose.* This will cause medication to spray from the ampule.

UNIT-DOSE CARTRIDGE AND HOLDER

Insert the cartridge into the metal or plastic holder and screw it into place. Move the plunger forward until it engages the shaft of the cartridge. Twist the plunger until it is locked into the cartridge. The holder is reusable. Place the cartridge in a sharps container after use.

UNIT-DOSE PREFILLED SYRINGES

The medication is in the syringe. Some prefilled syringes are simple and require no action other than removing the needle cover; others are packaged for compactness, and directions are given to prepare the syringe for use. These syringes are disposable.

MIXING TWO MEDICATIONS IN ONE SYRINGE

General Principles

1. Determine that the drugs are compatible by consulting a standard reference.

2. When in doubt about compatibility, prepare medications separately and administer into different injection sites.

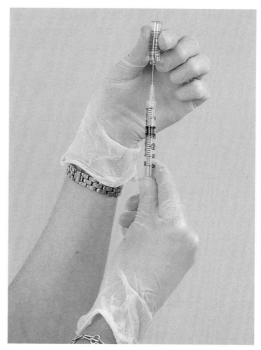

FIGURE 13-9

Invert the ampule for withdrawal. (© B. Proud.)

3. When medications are in a vial and an ampule, draw up the medication from the vial first then add the medication from the ampule. Discard the ampule in a sharps container.

4. When preparing two types of insulin in one syringe, the vial containing *regular insulin must be drawn first* into the syringe. Regular insulin has not been adulterated with protein as have other insulins such as protamine zinc insulin.

Method

1. Clean both vials with an alcohol pad.

2. Choose one vial as the *primary*. For example, with vials of a narcotic and a nonnarcotic, the narcotic is the primary. With two insulins, regular insulin is the primary.

3. Inject air into the *second* vial equal to the medication to be withdrawn. Do not permit the needle to touch the medication.

4. Inject air into the *primary* vial equal to the amount to be withdrawn and withdraw medication in the usual way. Be sure there are no air bubbles.

5. Insert the needle into the *second* vial. To avoid pushing the primary medication into the second vial, do not touch the plunger while doing this.

6. *Slowly* withdraw the needed amount of drug from the second vial. The two medications are now combined.

7. Remove the needle from the second vial and cap it. Note: Some authorities suggest that the needle be changed after withdrawing medication from the primary vial. Because this may result in air bubbles, be careful withdrawing the second medication to obtain an accurate dose.

Identifying the Injection Site—Adults

INTRAMUSCULAR

Common sites are the dorsogluteal, ventrogluteal, vastus lateralis, and deltoid muscles.

Dorsogluteal Site The dorsogluteal site is composed of the thick gluteal muscles of the buttocks.
Position: The patient may be prone or in a side-lying position with both buttocks fully exposed.

Location of injection site: The area must be chosen very carefully to avoid striking the sciatic nerve, major blood vessels, or bone. The landmarks of the buttocks are the crest of the posterior ilium as the superior boundary and the inferior gluteal fold as the lower boundary. The exact site can be identified in either of two ways:

1. *Diagonal landmark* (Fig. 13-10): Find the posterior superior iliac spine and the greater trochanter of the femur. Draw an imaginary diagonal line between these two points, and give the injection lateral and superior to that line 1 to 2 inches below the iliac crest to avoid hitting the iliac bone. Should you hit the bone, withdraw the needle slightly and continue the procedure. This method is preferred because all the landmarks are bony prominences.

2. *Quadrant landmark* (Fig. 13-11): Divide the buttocks into imaginary quadrants. The vertical line extends from the crest of the ilium to the gluteal fold. The horizontal line extends from the medial fold of the buttock to the lateral aspect of the buttock. Locate the upper aspect of the upper outer quadrant. The injection should be given in this area, 1 to 2 inches below the crest of the ilium, to avoid hitting bone. The crest of the ilium must be palpated for precise site selection.

Ventrogluteal Site The ventral part of the gluteal muscle has no large nerves or blood vessels and less fat. It is identified by finding the greater trochanter, anterior superior iliac spine, and the iliac crest. The nurse should be standing by the patient's knee. Use the hand opposite to the patient's leg (eg, left leg, right hand). Open an alcohol pad. Place the palm of the hand on the greater trochanter. Point the index finger toward the anterior superior iliac spine. Point the middle finger toward the iliac crest. The injection is given in the center of the triangle between the middle finger and the index finger (Fig. 13-12). Place the alcohol pad over the site. Remove the hand and proceed with the injection in the usual manner. Use the alcohol pad to prep the area from the center out.
Position: The patient may be supine, lying on the side, sitting, or standing.

Vastus Lateralis Site: Lateral Thigh Measure one hand's width below the greater trochanter and one hand's width above the knee (Fig. 13-13). Give the injection in the lateral thigh. Ask the patient to point the big toe to the center of his body. This relaxes the vastus muscle.
Position: The patient may be supine, lying on the side, or standing.

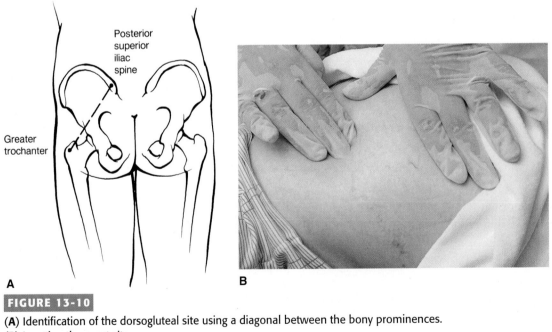

A **B**

FIGURE 13-10

(A) Identification of the dorsogluteal site using a diagonal between the bony prominences.
(B) Locating the exact site.

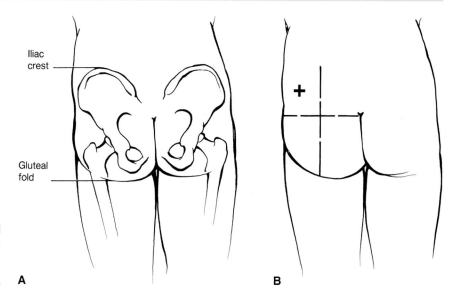

FIGURE 13-11

(**A**) Identification of the dorsogluteal injection site using quadrants. Draw an imaginary line from the iliac crest to the gluteal fold, and from the medial to the lateral buttock. (**B**) The *cross* indicates the injection area.

Deltoid Site The deltoid muscle on the lateral aspect of the upper arm is a small muscle close to the radial and brachial arteries. *It should be used for IM injections only if specifically ordered,* and no more than 2 mL should be injected. The boundaries are the lower edge of the acromion process (shoulder bone) and the axilla (armpit, Fig. 13-14). Give the injection into the lateral arm between these two points, about 2 inches below the acromion process.

Position: The patient may be sitting or lying down.

SUBCUTANEOUS

Common injection sites include the upper arms, anterior thighs, lower abdomen, and upper back (Fig. 13-15). Insulin subcutaneous is administered in the arm, lower abdomen, and thigh. Heparin subcutaneous is given in the lower abdomen. The injection is usually given at a 45-degree angle to avoid reaching muscle. Subcutaneous injections may be given at a 90-degree angle if the subcutaneous layer of fat is thick. No more than 1 mL medication should be injected.

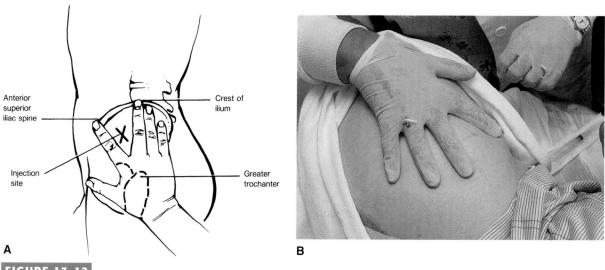

FIGURE 13-12

(**A**) The ventrogluteal site for IM injections; the *cross* indicates the injection site. (**B**) Locating the exact site.

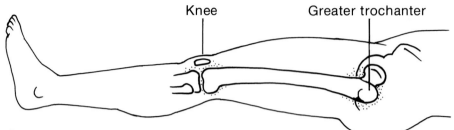

A

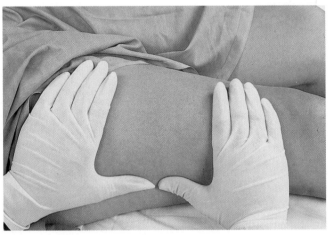

B

FIGURE 13-13

(**A**) Vastus lateralis injection site. (**B**) Locating the site.

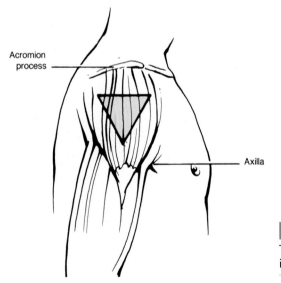

FIGURE 13-14

The deltoid muscle site for IM injections. The *triangle* indicates the injection site.

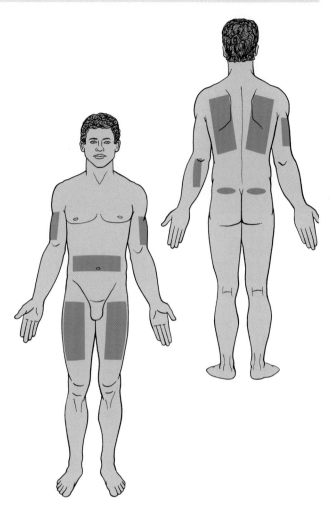

FIGURE 13-15

Sites for subcutaneous injection. The deltoid muscle may be used for subcutaneous injections, or, when ordered, small intramuscular injections.

INTRADERMAL (INTRACUTANEOUS)

The intradermal site is used for skin testing for allergies and diseases such as tuberculosis. Injecting an antigen causes an antigen–antibody sensitivity reaction if the individual is susceptible. If positive, the area will become raised, warm, and reddened.

The site is the inner aspect of the forearm. Prepare the skin with an alcohol pad and allow it to dry. Place your nondominant hand around the arm from below and pull the skin tightly to make the forearm tissue taut. Hold the syringe in your four fingers and thumb, with the bevel (opening) of the needle up, and insert the needle about $\frac{1}{8}$ in almost parallel to the skin (Fig. 13-16A). The needle remains visible under the skin. Inject the solution such that it raises a small wheal (a raised bump or a blister; Fig. 13-16B). Remove the needle and allow the injection site to dry. *Do not massage the skin.* Place the needle and syringe in a sharps container. Make the patient comfortable. Wash your hands. Chart the procedure.

Identifying the Injection Site—Children

The site for the IM injection in the child depends on the age of the child, the child's size, and the volume and density of medication administered. Infants cannot tolerate volumes greater than 0.5 mL in a single site. Older infants or small children can tolerate 1 mL in a single site. Needle gauges range from 21 to 25 gauge.

The preferred site for infants is the vastus lateralis muscle (Fig. 13-17). After the child has been walking for more than a year, the dorsogluteal site can be used; however, usually it is not recommended until the child is 5 years of age. For the older child and adolescent, the same injection sites can be used as in adults.

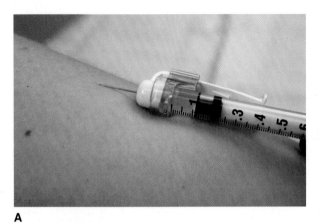 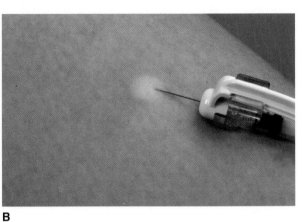

A   **B**

FIGURE 13-16

(**A**) Inserting the needle almost level with the skin. (**B**) Observing for wheal while injecting medication. (Used with permission from Evans-Smith, P. [2005]. *Taylor's clinical nursing skills.* Philadelphia: Lippincott Williams & Wilkins, p. 132.)

Administering Injections

Handwashing and gloves are required.

1. Identify the patient verbally by name.

2. Check the patient's ID band.

3. Perform any assessment before administering the injection (eg, vital signs, apical rate, site integrity).

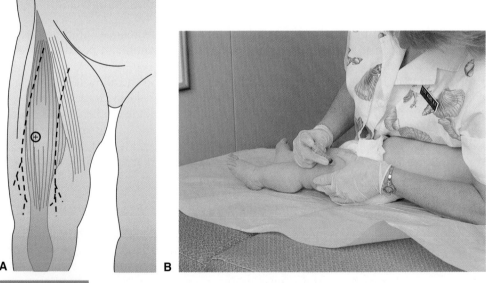

A   **B**

FIGURE 13-17

(**A**) For infants under walking age, use the vastus lateralis muscle for intramuscular injections. (**B**) Technique for administering an intramuscular injection to an infant. Note the way the nurse uses her body to restrain and stabilize the infant. (With permission from Pillitteri, A. [2002]. *Maternal and child health nursing* [4th ed.]. Philadelphia: Lippincott Williams & Wilkins, p. 1102.)

4. Explain the procedure to the patient.

5. Ask the patient where the last injection was given. The sites should be rotated.

6. Prepare the area with an alcohol pad, using a circular motion from the center out.

7. Place the alcohol pad between your fingers or lay it on the patient's skin above the site.

8. Remove the needle cover.

9. Make the skin taut by mounding the tissue between the thumb and index finger or by spreading it firmly.

10. Dart the needle in quickly (Fig. 13-18A).

11. Hold the barrel with your nondominant hand and with your dominant hand pull the plunger back. This is termed *aspiration* and is done to be sure the needle is not in a blood vessel (Fig. 13-18B).

12. If blood enters the syringe, withdraw the needle, discard the needle and syringe into a sharps container, and prepare another injection.

13. If no blood is aspirated, inject the medication slowly (Fig. 13-18C).

14. Remove the needle quickly.

15. Press down on the area with the alcohol pad or a dry gauze pad to inhibit bleeding.

16. *Do not recap the needle.* Dispose of the needle and syringe in a sharps container. Make the patient comfortable. Wash your hands. Chart the medication, documenting the site of injection.

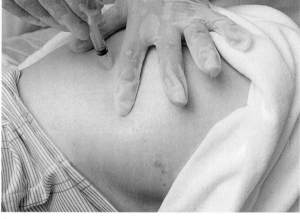

A

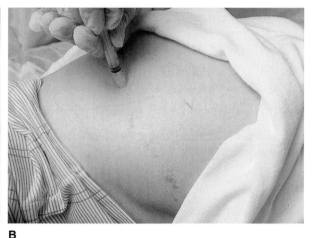

B

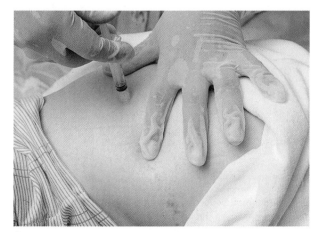

C

FIGURE 13-18

(**A**) Dart the needle into the skin; (**B**) aspirate slowly;
(**C**) inject medication slowly.

Special Injection Techniques

SUBCUTANEOUS HEPARIN

Heparin is an anticoagulant and care must be taken to minimize tissue trauma. Slow bleeding at the site of the injection can cause bruising. Several changes in routine injection technique are indicated. The injection is given with a fine (25-gauge) ½-in needle into the lower abdominal fold at least 2 in from the umbilicus. Gloves should be worn.

1. Change the needle after drawing up the dose to prevent leakage along the tract.

2. Allow the skin to dry after prepping with an alcohol pad.

3. Bunch the tissue with the nondominant hand to a depth of at least ½ in.

4. Inject the needle at a 90-degree angle.

5. *Do not aspirate.* This minimizes tissue damage.

6. Inject the medication slowly.

7. Hold the needle in place for 10 seconds.

8. Remove the needle quickly.

9. *Do not massage the area.* If bleeding is noted, apply pressure with a dry gauze pad or alcohol pad for 1 to 2 minutes.

Z-TRACK TECHNIQUE FOR INTRAMUSCULAR INJECTIONS

Some medications, such as iron dextran (Imferon) and hydroxyzine (Vistazine), are irritating to the tissues and can stain the skin. The Z-track method may be used at the dorsogluteal site to prevent medication seepage into the needle tract and onto the skin.

1. After preparing the medication, change the needle to prevent leakage along the tract.

2. Add 0.2 mL air to the syringe. As medication is injected, the air will rise to the top of the syringe and will be administered last. This will seal off the medication and prevent its leakage to the skin.

3. Prepare the patient and the site in the usual manner.

4. Use the fingers on your nondominant hand to retract the tissue to the side. *Hold this position during the injection* (Fig. 13-19).

5. Inject as usual at a 90-degree angle. Be sure to aspirate before giving this injection (Fig. 13-20).

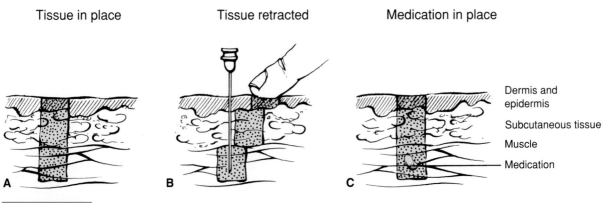

Tissue in place   Tissue retracted   Medication in place

Dermis and epidermis
Subcutaneous tissue
Muscle
Medication

A   B   C

FIGURE 13-19

Z-track technique—dorsogluteal site. The tissue is retracted to one side and held there until the injection in given. When the hand is removed, the tissue closes over the injection tract, preventing medication from rising to the surface.

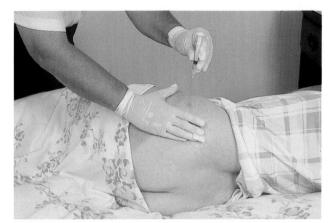

FIGURE 13-20
Displacing tissue in a Z-track manner and darting needle into tissue.

6. Count 10 seconds after giving the injection.

7. Remove the needle quickly.

8. Remove the hand that has been retracting the tissue.

9. *Do not massage the site.*

10. Using an alcohol pad or dry gauze pad, press down on the site to inhibit bleeding.

Application to Skin and Mucous Membrane

Drug preparations are administered for their local effect or to act systematically. To achieve a systemic effect, the drug must be absorbed into the circulation.

Buccal Tablet (Universal Safeguard: Handwashing)

Identify the patient verbally. Check the ID band. Explain the procedure and give the tablet to the patient. The patient should place the tablet between his gum and his cheek. The tablet should not be disturbed as it dissolves. Systemic absorption is rapid across mucous membranes. Doses should be alternated between cheeks to minimize irritation. Withhold food and liquids until the tablet is dissolved.

Ear Drops (Universal Safeguard: Handwashing)

The ear drops will be labeled otic or auric. They should be warmed to body temperature. Greet the patient verbally and check the patient's ID band. Explain the procedure. Place the patient sitting in an upright position, with the head tilted toward his unaffected side or lying on his side with the affected ear up. Be sure the patient is comfortable. With a dropper, draw the medication up. *Straighten the ear canal by pulling the pinna up and back in the adult, or down and back in a child 3 years or younger* (Fig. 13-21).

Place the tip of the dropper at the opening of the canal and instill the medication into the canal (Fig. 13-22). The patient should rest on his unaffected side 10 to 15 minutes. A cotton ball may be placed in the canal if the patient wishes. Make sure the patient is comfortable. Wash hands. Chart the medication.

Clinical Alert!

Ear Drop Administration

- Should the ear pinna be pulled up or down with adults?

- Should the ear pinna be pulled up or down with children?

- Adults are usually taller than children, so the ear pinna is pulled "up" and back for ear drops.

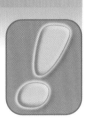

- Children younger than 3 years old are usually smaller than adults, so the ear pinna is pulled "down" and back for ear drops.

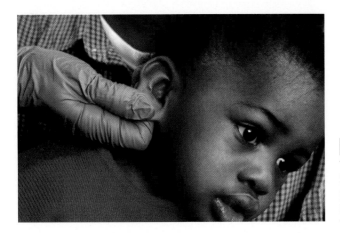

FIGURE 13-21

Technique for administering eardrops in children under 3 years old. (Use with permission from Evans-Smith, P. [2005]. *Taylor's clinical nursing skills.* Philadelphia: Lippincott Williams & Wilkins, p. 173.)

Eye Drops or Ointment (Universal Safeguard: Gloves)

Greet the patient and check his ID band. Explain the procedure. Hand the patient a tissue. The patient may be sitting or lying down. If exudate is present, it may be necessary to cleanse the eyelid with cotton or gauze and either normal saline or distilled water for the eye. Any medication placed in the eye must be labeled "ophthalmic" or "for the eye." Eye medications may come in a monodrop container, in a bottle with a dropper, or as an ophthalmic ointment. Gently draw the lower eyelid down to create a sac (Fig. 13-23). Instruct the patient to look up. Instill the liquid medication into the lower conjunctival sac, taking care not to touch the membrane. The ophthalmic ointment should be placed from the inner to the outer canthus of the eye.

Instruct the patient to close his eyelids gently and rotate his eyes. The patient may use a tissue to wipe away excess medication. After instilling eye drops, have the patient apply gentle pressure with his index finger to the inner canthus for a minute. This action inhibits the medication from entering the tear duct.

Each patient should have individual medication containers to prevent cross-contamination. Provide a safe environment if the medication impairs the patient's vision. Make the patient comfortable. Dispose of the gloves according to institutional procedure. Wash your hands and chart the medication.

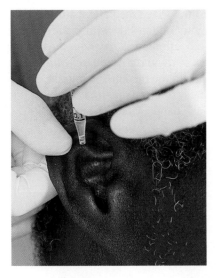

FIGURE 13-22

Straighten the ear canal and instill the medication.

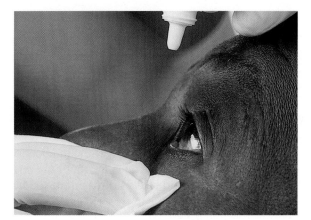

FIGURE 13-23

Applying eye drops: Gently draw the lower eyelid down to create a pocket. Insert the medication into this pocket.

Clinical Alert!

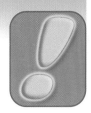

Eye and Ear Abbreviations

- The Joint Commission on Accreditation of Healthcare Organizations (JCAHO) has identified abbreviations that are problematic. Eye and ear medication abbreviations are included. Although not prohibited by JCAHO, the recommendation is to not use the following abbreviations:

- AS (left ear), AD (right ear), AU (both ears). These are often mistaken with the terms for eyes: OS (left eye), OD (right eye), OU (both eyes).

- Recommendations: Write out "left ear," "right ear," or "both ears," as appropriate. Eye abbreviations may still be used; however, qd (every day) is to be written out as "every day" or "daily" so as not to be confused with "OD." For safety, it is suggested that eye abbreviations be written out: "left eye," right eye," "both eyes."

Nasogastric Route (Universal Safeguard: Gloves)

When possible, obtain the medication in liquid form. Before opening capsules or crushing tablets, check with the pharmacist for alternatives. Use a bulb syringe or a 60-mL syringe.

Dilute the medication with water. The fluid mixture should be at room temperature. Greet the patient, check the ID band, and explain the procedure. Elevate the head of the bed when possible. Put on gloves. Insert the syringe into the tube. Remove the clamp on the tube. Check the position of the tube in the stomach by (1) aspirating some stomach contents or (2) placing a stethoscope on the stomach and inserting about 15 mL air. A swishing sound indicates proper placement. A more accurate method is to check stomach contents for acidity using pH paper.

Close off the tube by bending it on itself. Hold the syringe and bent tube in your nondominant hand. Remove the bulb or plunger and leave the syringe in place.

Flush the tube with at least 30 mL warm water to ensure patency. Clamp the tube. Pour the medication into the syringe. Release the tubing and allow the medication to flow in by gravity. *Do not force medication to flow by using pressure on the bulb.* Occasionally, slight pressure may be applied. If the patient shows discomfort, stop the procedure and wait until he or she appears relaxed.

Before all the medication flows in, flush the tube by adding at least 30 mL water to the syringe. Shut the tube by bending it on itself before the syringe completely empties. Clamp the tube and remove the syringe. Make the patient comfortable. If possible, leave the head of the bed elevated. Dispose of gloves according to institutional procedures. Wash your hands. Chart the medication.

Nose Drops (Universal Safeguard: Gloves)

Greet the patient, check the ID band, and explain the procedure. The patient may have to blow his nose gently to clear the nasal passageway. The patient may be sitting or lying down. Have him tilt his head back. In bed, a pillow may be placed under the shoulders to hyperextend the neck. Insert the dropper about one third of the way into each nostril. Do not touch the nostril. Instill the nose drops (Fig. 13-24). Instruct the patient to maintain the position 1 to 2 minutes. If the patient feels the medication flowing down his throat, he may sit up and bend his head down to allow the medication to flow into his sinuses.

The patient should have his own medication container to prevent cross-contamination. Make the patient comfortable. Wash your hands. Chart the medication.

If a nasal spray is ordered, push the tip of the nose up and place the nozzle tip just inside the nares, so the spray will be directed backward when the medication is given.

Rectal Suppository (Universal Safeguard: Gloves)

Greet the patient, check the ID band, and explain the procedure. Encourage the patient to defecate (unless the suppository is ordered for this purpose). Position the patient in the left lateral recumbent position (Fig. 13-25). Moisten the suppository with a water-soluble lubricant. Instruct the patient to breathe slowly and deeply through the mouth. Ask the patient to "bear down" as if having a bowel movement to open the anal sphincter. Using a gloved finger, insert the suppository past the sphincter. You will feel the suppository move into the canal. Wipe away excess lubricant. Encourage the patient to retain the suppository. Make the patient comfortable. Dispose of gloves according to institutional procedure. Wash your hands. Chart the medication.

The patient may insert his or her own suppository if he or she is able and wishes to do so. Provide a glove, lubricant, and suppository. Check to be sure the suppository was inserted and is not in the bed.

Respiratory Inhaler (Universal Safeguard: Handwashing)

An inhaler is a small, pressurized metal container that holds medication. It is accompanied by a mouthpiece. *The following are general directions to teach the patient* (Fig. 13-26):

1. Shake the inhaler well immediately before use.
2. Remove the cap from the mouthpiece.
3. Breathe out fully, expel as much air as you can, and hold your breath.
4. Place the mouthpiece in your mouth and close your lips around it. The metal inhaler should be upright.
5. While breathing in deeply and slowly, fully depress the metal inhaler with your index finger.
6. Remove the inhaler from your mouth and release your finger. Hold your breath for several seconds.
7. Wait 1 minute and shake the inhaler again. Repeat the steps for each inhalation prescribed. (An order might read "Proventil inhaler 2 puffs qid.")
8. Cleanse the mouthpiece and cap by rinsing in warm running water at least once a day. When dry, replace the mouthpiece and cap.

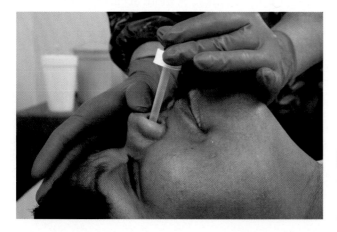

FIGURE 13-24

Administering nose drops. (Used with permission from Evans-Smith, P. [2005]. *Taylor's clinical nursing skills.* Philadelphia: Lippincott Williams & Wilkins, p. 178.)

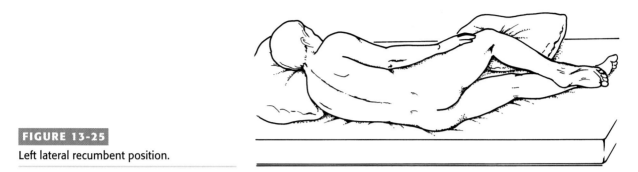

FIGURE 13-25

Left lateral recumbent position.

The inhaler may be left at the bedside stand if the institution's policy permits. Make the patient comfortable, wash your hands, and chart the medication.

Skin Applications (Universal Safeguard: Gloves)

Greet the patient, check the ID band, and explain the procedure. Avoid personal contact with the medication to prevent absorption of the drug. Apply the medication with a tongue blade, glove, gauze pad, or cotton-tipped applicator. Cleanse the area as appropriate before a new application.

Obtain the following information before proceeding, because many kinds of medicines are applied topically:

- Preparation of the skin
- Method of application
- Whether the skin should be covered or uncovered

Drug preparations include the following:

- Powders: Sprinkle on your gloved hands, then apply. Use sparingly to avoid caking. Skin should be dry.
- Lotions: Pat on lightly. Use gloved hand or gauze pad.
- Creams: Rub into skin using gloves.
- Ointments: Use gloved hand or applicator. Apply an even coat and place a dressing on the skin.

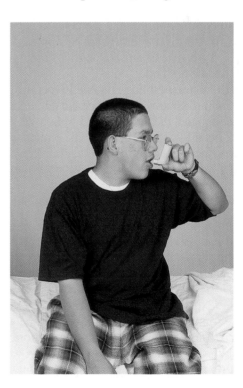

FIGURE 13-26

Many children with asthma use a metered dose inhaler to administer a bronchodilator. (With permission from Pillitteri, A. [2002]. *Maternal and child health nursing* [4th ed.]. Philadelphia: Lippincott Williams & Wilkins, p. 1210.)

Make the patient comfortable. Dispose of gloves according to institutional policy. Wash your hands. Chart the medication.

Nitroglycerin Ointment (Universal Safeguard: Gloves)

Greet the patient, check the ID band, and explain the procedure. Take a baseline blood pressure and record. Don the gloves to protect yourself from contact with the drug, a potent vasodilator. Remove the previous dose and cleanse the skin.

Measure the prescribed dose in inches on the ruled paper that comes with the ointment. Select a nonhairy site on the trunk—chest, upper arm, abdomen, or upper back. If necessary, shave the area. (Seek advice before doing this.) Spread the measured ointment on the skin, using the ruled paper. Apply the ointment in a thin layer about 6×6 in. *Do not rub.* Tape the ruled paper in place over the ointment. Cover the area with plastic wrap and tape the plastic in place. Check the patient's blood pressure within 30 minutes.

If a headache occurs or the blood pressure lowers, have the patient rest until the blood pressure returns to normal. Make the patient comfortable. Dispose of gloves according to institutional procedure. Wash your hands. Chart the medication.

Transdermal Disks, Patches, and Pads (Universal Safeguard: Handwashing)

These products are unit-dose adhesive bandages consisting of a semipermeable membrane that allows medication to be released continuously over time. Some patches are effective for 24 hours, some for 72 hours, and some last as long as 1 week.

The skin should be free of hair and not subject to excessive movement; therefore, avoid distal extremities. The site should be changed with each administration. If the patch loosens with bathing, apply a new pad.

Medications that can be administered by this route include hormones, nitroglycerin, antihypertensive drugs such as clonadine (Catapres), and antimotion sickness drugs such as scopolamine.

Greet the patient, check the ID band, and explain the procedure. Select the site. The skin should be clear and dry with no signs of irritation. Open the packet. Remove the cover from the adhesive transdermal drug. *Do not touch the inside of the pad.* Apply the pad to the skin. Press firmly to be certain all edges are adherent. Make the patient comfortable, wash your hands, and chart the medication.

Sublingual Tablets (Universal Safeguard: Handwashing)

The most common sublingual medication is nitroglycerin, which is prescribed to abort an attack of angina pectoris. If relief is not felt within 5 minutes, a second and then a third tablet may be taken at 5-minute intervals. Tolerance to nitroglycerin is common. If the pain is not relieved within 15 minutes, the physician should be notified.

To administer a sublingual tablet, greet the patient, check the ID band, and explain the procedure. Instruct him to sit down and place the tablet under the tongue. If the patient is unable to place the tablet under the tongue, the nurse should wear a glove to place the tablet. The tablet should not be swallowed or chewed, but allowed to dissolve. The patient should not eat or drink anything because this will interfere with the effectiveness of the medication. Stay with the patient until the pain is relieved. Consult an appropriate text for further information. Wash your hands and chart the medication.

Vaginal Suppository or Tablet (Universal Safeguard: Gloves)

Greet the patient, check the ID band, and explain the procedure. Ask her to void in a bed pan. (If the perineal area has much secretion, it may be necessary to perform perineal care after the patient voids.) Insert the suppository or tablet into the applicator. Assist the patient into a lithotomy position (lying on the back with knees flexed and legs apart) and drape her, leaving the perineal area exposed. Don gloves.

Separate the labia majora and identify the vaginal opening. Insert the applicator down and back and eject the suppository or tablet into the vagina. (The patient may do this procedure herself if she wishes.) Place a pad at the opening to collect secretions. Make the patient comfortable before leaving.

Wash the applicator with soap and water, wrap it in a paper towel, and leave it at the bedside. Dispose of gloves and equipment according to institutional procedure. Chart the medication.

Vaginal Cream or Vaginal Tablet (Universal Safeguard: Gloves)

Vaginal cream may come in a prefilled disposable syringe or in a tube with its own applicator. To fill the applicator, remove the cap from the tube and screw the top of the tube into the barrel of the applicator. Squeeze the tube to fill the barrel to the prescribed dose. Unscrew the tube from the applicator and cap it.

Prepare the patient as described in the previous section. Insert the applicator down and back, and press the plunger to empty the barrel of medication (Fig. 13-27). The patient may do this herself if she wishes. Remove the applicator. Place a pad at the vaginal opening to collect secretions. Make the patient comfortable before leaving. She should remain in bed for a minimum of 20 minutes.

If the applicator is a prefilled unit dose, dispose of it according to institutional policy. If it is reusable, wash it with soap and water, and place it in a clean paper towel on the bedside stand. Dispose of gloves. Chart the medication.

Special Considerations

The basics of medication administration apply to all age groups. However, there are considerations for pediatric and geriatric administration.

Neonatal and Pediatric Considerations

Dosages of medications for neonatal and pediatric administration are briefly covered in Chapter 10. Differences in medication administration are mainly developmental. A nursing pediatric textbook is necessary for specifics and special skills are needed for medication administration.

Here are some suggestions for oral medication administration in children:

- Offer a Popsicle prior to administering an oral medication. This will numb the taste buds.

- Mix the drug with a teaspoon of puréed fruit, ice cream, or syrup. Using essential foodstuffs may cause the child to refuse them later.

- With older children, have them pinch their nostrils closed and drink the medication through a straw. This interferes with the ability to smell.

- Use a specially manufactured medication nipple or pacifier for infants.

For IM administration in children:

- Explain the procedure to the child using terms he or she can easily understand.

- Predetermine the injection site to make sure the muscle is large enough to accommodate the amount and type of medication.

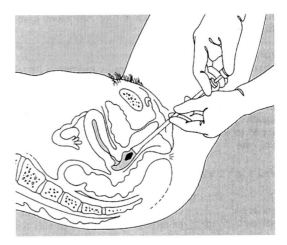

FIGURE 13-27

Vaginal applicator should be inserted down and back. (From Taylor, C., Lillis, C., and LeMone, P. [2001]. *Fundamentals of nursing* [4th ed.]. Philadelphia: Lippincott Williams & Wilkins, p. 627.)

- A local anesthetic such as lidocaine is often injected subcutaneously to reduce the pain of deep needle administration. A topical anesthetic can also be used to the reduce the pain of a needlestick.

- Provide sufficient help in holding the child because a child's behavior is unpredictable.

- Distract the child with conversation or a toy.

- Insert the needle quickly and inject the medication slowly.

- Use a decorative adhesive bandage to cover the injection site.

Geriatric Considerations

In the geriatric client, decreasing organ function (especially liver and kidney), circulatory changes leading to decreased perfusion, and physical limitations (poor eyesight, decreased coordination, decreased ability to chew and/or swallow) need to be considered prior to administering medications.

Here are some suggestions for oral tablet and liquid administration in geriatric clients:

- Offer a Popsicle prior to administering a liquid medication. This will numb the taste buds.

- Mix the crushed tablet (when possible) with a teaspoon of puréed fruit, ice cream, or syrup.

- Clients who are post CVA often have tongue mobility problems and/or a decreased gag reflex. It may be necessary for the nurse to place the tablet or capsule in the client's mouth toward the pharynx and on the unaffected side to promote swallowing. A thorough check of the client's mouth needs to be done to determine whether the tablet or capsule has been swallowed.

Subcutaneous and/or IM administration in geriatric clients:

- Explain the procedure to the client.

- Predetermine the injection site to make sure there is sufficient subcuticular tissue or the muscle is large enough to accommodate the amount and type of medication.

- Distract the client with conversation.

- Insert the needle quickly and inject the medication slowly.

CRITICAL THINKING: TEST YOUR CLINICAL SAVVY

A client in your outpatient clinic is to receive an IM injection. The drug literature states the preferred site is the gluteus maximus or vastus lateralis.

a. When would the deltoid muscle be preferable or used over either of these sites? What are the contraindications for using the deltoid muscle?

b. The client requests the injection in the deltoid. What is your response in light of the recommended site in the drug literature?

c. If a patient is bedridden, which site would you choose for an IM injection and why?

d. Why are gloves necessary when giving IM injections, even though you are not actually touching the injection site?

SELF-TEST 1 | **Universal Safeguards**

Provide the information requested for universal safeguards in administering medications. Answers are given at the end of the chapter.

1. Universal safeguards should be applied when administering medications

   a. To all patients

   b. Only to patients with HIV or hepatitis B virus

2. The type of safeguard to be used by the nurse depends on _____

   _____

3. When administering medications, gloves must be worn when

   _____ and

   _____

4. After administering an injection, the syringe should be placed _____

   _____

5. Five safeguards stressed by the CDC are _____,

   _____, and

   _____.

6. When administering medications, hands must be washed

   a. _____

   b. _____

   c. _____

   d. _____

7. General safeguards while administering medications advise the nurse to use a clamp to

   _____

   _____

8. A gown should be worn to protect the nurse's uniform whenever _____

   _____

9. Protective eyewear should be worn whenever _____

   _____

   _____

10. A mask should be worn when

    _____ or

    _____

SELF-TEST 2	Medication Administration

Supply the following information. Answers are given at the end of the chapter.

1. The primary reason patients should have individual eye medication is to _____
   _____

2. Two methods of checking the positioning of a nasogastric tube are _____
   _____ and
   _____

3. For administration of a rectal suppository, the patient should lie _____
   _____

4. How should each of the following be applied to a patient's skin?
   a. Powders _____
   b. Lotions _____
   c. Creams _____
   d. Ointments _____

5. How many sublingual nitroglycerin tablets may a patient take to relieve pain? _____
   At what time interval? _____

6. Identify these administration procedures as parenteral or non-parenteral.
   a. Subcutaneous injection _____   f. Nitroglycerin ointment _____
   b. Sublingual tablet _____   g. Respiratory inhaler _____
   c. Vaginal suppository _____   h. Nasogastric route _____
   d. Nose drops _____   i. Intradermal _____
   e. IM injection _____   j. Rectal suppository _____

7. How should a vaginal applicator be inserted? _____

8. How should the skin be prepared for an injection? _____
   _____

9. List three reasons for administering medication by injection. _____
   _____
   _____

10. What is the difference in administering ear drops to an adult and a 2-year-old child?
    _____
    _____

Name: _____

Choose the correct answer for each of these questions. There are 33 questions, and each is worth 0.3 credit. Aim to achieve a grade of 90% or better. Review material you find difficult. Answers are given on page 450.

1. The purpose of the medication ticket in the ticket system is to identify the drug from the time the order is written until it is

   a. Transferred to the Kardex
   b. Poured
   c. Administered
   d. Charted

2. Which of the following is an appropriate action regarding medication tickets in the ticket system?

   a. All tickets are checked against the physician's order sheet.
   b. Tickets are made out only for standing orders.
   c. A new ticket is written each time a drug is given.
   d. The ticket is destroyed after charting a stat order.

3. Checking the Kardex before administering medication by ticket will enable the nurse to determine

   a. The name of the physician who ordered the medication
   b. Whether some tickets have been misplaced
   c. Whether a stat medication is to be administered
   d. Whether the patient can have the next prn dose

4. When pouring an oral liquid medication; the nurse should

   a. Place the cup on the tabletop and bend over to get the right level
   b. Hold the cup in the hand and pour to the top of the meniscus
   c. Hold the cup at eye level and pour to the center of the meniscus
   d. Rest the cup on the medication shelf and pour to the meniscus line

5. Which statement is *false* regarding injections from powders?

   a. Read the label twice before drawing up and once after.
   b. Draw up one medication at a time.
   c. Always use sterile water as a diluent.
   d. Pull back on the plunger before injecting the medication.

6. Withdrawing medication from a vial is facilitated if a specific amount of air is injected into the vial beforehand. Which of these statements explains this action?

   a. It creates a partial vacuum in the vial.
   b. It makes the pressure in the vial greater than atmospheric pressure.
   c. It makes the pressure in the vial the same as atmospheric pressure.
   d. It makes the pressure in the vial less than atmospheric pressure.

7. If a patient has difficulty swallowing medications, which oral form of drug may be crushed?

   a. Sugar-coated tablet
   b. Enteric-coated tablet
   c. Buccal tablet
   d. Capsule

(continued)

8. A major advantage in the unit-dose system of drug administration is that

   a. The drug supply is always available
   b. No error is possible
   c. The drugs are less expensive than stock distribution
   d. The pharmacist provides a second professional check

9. When a drug is to be administered sublingually, the patient should be instructed to

   a. Drink a full glass of water when swallowing
   b. Rinse the mouth with water after taking the drug
   c. Chew the tablet and allow the saliva to collect under the tongue
   d. Hold the medication under the tongue until it dissolves

10. Ampules differ from vials in that ampules

   a. Are always glass containers
   b. Contain only one dose
   c. Contain solids as well as liquids
   d. Are not used for injections

11. The Z-track technique for injections can be used to

   a. Administer more than one drug at a single site
   b. Inhibit hematoma formation by promoting drug absorption
   c. Prevent skin discoloration by inhibiting drug seepage
   d. Reduce allergic reactions at the injection site

12. Which action is *correct* when giving a Z-track injection?

   a. The skin is retracted and held to one side while the medication is given.
   b. The skin is massaged after the injection is given.
   c. The plunger is not pulled back after the needle has been inserted.
   d. Medication is injected quickly.

13. Which angle of injection is *correctly* matched with the route of administration?

   a. Intradermal—45-degree angle
   b. IM—90-degree angle
   c. Subcutaneous—30-degree angle
   d. Z track—45-degree angle

14. A patient asks how to put drops in his eye. The nurse instructs the patient to place the drops

   a. Into the lower conjunctival sac
   b. Under the upper lid
   c. Directly on the cornea
   d. In the inner canthus

15. When administering a vaginal suppository, which statement is *false?*

   a. Universal safeguards should be used.
   b. The patient may insert the medication.
   c. The patient should be lying on her back.
   d. The applicator must be kept sterile.

(continued)

16. When applying the next dose of a transdermal medication, the nurse should

   a. Shave the new area and prepare with povidone–iodine
   b. Cleanse the previous area and use a different site
   c. Rotate the use of arms and legs as sites
   d. Allow the previous patch to remain on the skin

17. Which is the muscle of choice to be used when an injection is irritating to the tissues?

   a. Deltoid—subcutaneous
   b. Dorsogluteal—Z track
   c. Ventrogluteal—intradermal
   d. Vastus lateralis—IM

18. Discomfort of an injection is reduced when the needle is inserted

   a. Slowly into loose tissue
   b. Slowly into firm tissue
   c. Rapidly into loose tissue
   d. Rapidly into firm tissue

19. After administering an injection, the nurse should

   a. Immediately recap the needle
   b. Break the needle off the syringe for safety
   c. Place the used syringe in a nearby sharps container
   d. Don gloves to carry the syringe to the utility room

20. Which statement is *incorrect* when administering drugs to mucous membranes?

   a. Eye medications must be labeled *ophthalmic*.
   b. Patients may insert their own rectal suppositories.
   c. Sublingual medications are applied to the space between the teeth and cheek.
   d. Eye medications may be left on the client's bedside stand.

PROFICIENCY TEST 1–PART B   **Administration Procedures**

Decide whether the following actions are correct or incorrect according to the safeguards when administering medications. Explain your choice. Answers are given on page 450.

1. A nurse wears gloves to remove an IV heparin lock from a patient's arm. This action is

   _____

   _____

2. A nurse who has just removed a gown and gloves puts them into the disposal container in the patient's room and leaves the room. This action is

   _____

   _____

3. In the medication room, a nurse puts on gloves to prepare an IV for administration. This action is

   _____

   _____

4. A nurse puts on a mask to administer an oral medication to a patient on respiratory isolation precautions. This action is _____

   _____

5. A nurse applies universal precautions in caring for all patients on the unit. This action is

   _____

6. A nurse wears gloves to place a transdermal pad behind a patient's ear. This action is

   _____

   _____

   _____

7. A nurse puts on gloves and gown to administer 500 mL of a vaginal douche to a lethargic patient. This action is _____

   _____

8. A nurse whose finger has been stuck with a contaminated IV needle carefully washes her hands with soap and water, and applies a band-aid to the site. Because the patient's diagnosis is brain tumor, the nurse decides no further action is necessary. This action is

   _____

9. A nurse giving an injection to a patient makes the judgment *not* to wear gloves. This action is

   _____

   _____

   _____

10. A nurse puts on gloves to administer an oral tablet to an alert patient with a positive HIV blood count. This action is _____

    _____

    _____

(continued)

11. After administering an injection, the nurse carefully caps the needle. This action is

    _____

    _____

12. A nurse wears gloves to apply nitroglycerin ointment to a patient's chest even though there is no break in the skin. This action is _____

    _____

    _____

13. A nurse makes a judgment to omit wearing gloves when administering eye drops because they are too bulky. This action is _____

    _____

    _____

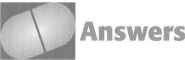 **Answers**

Self-Test 1 Universal Safeguards

1. To *all* patients. There is a risk of potential exposure to hepatitis virus and HIV that may not have been detected by standard laboratory methods.

2. The type of contact the nurse has with the patient

3. When there is any direct "hands-on" contact with patient's blood, bodily fluids, or secretions; when handling materials or equipment contaminated with blood or body fluids

4. In a labeled, puncture-proof container

5. Handwashing, gloves, gowns, masks, and protective eyewear

6. **a.** Before preparing medications and after administering medicines to each patient
   b. After removing gloves, gowns, masks, and protective eyewear, and before leaving each patient

   c. Immediately when soiled with the patient's blood or body fluids
   d. After handling equipment soiled with blood or body fluids

7. Hold contaminated IV needles being carried to a puncture-proof container

8. The nurse's clothing may become contaminated with a patient's blood or body fluids

9. A nurse is in extremely close contact with the patient and there is the possibility of the patient's blood or blood-tinged fluids being splashed or sprayed into the nurse's eyes or mucous membranes.

10. The patient is placed on *strict* or *respiratory* isolation precautions. Carrying out a medication procedure may cause blood or body fluids to splash directly onto the nurse's face

Self-Test 2 Medication Administration

1. Prevent cross-contamination

2. Aspirate stomach contents and check for pH *or* place a stethoscope on the stomach and insert 15 mL air. A swishing sound indicates proper placement.

3. On the left side, left lateral recumbent position

4. **a.** Sprinkle on gloved hands and apply, use sparingly to prevent caking
   b. Pat on lightly with gloved hand or gauze pad
   c. Rub into skin while wearing gloves
   d. Use a gloved hand to apply an even coat and cover with a dressing

5. Three tablets, 5 minutes apart

6. **a.** Parenteral
   b. Non-parenteral
   c. Non-parenteral
   d. Non-parenteral
   e. Parenteral
   f. Non-parenteral
   g. Non-parenteral
   h. Non-parenteral
   i. Parenteral
   j. Non-parenteral

7. Back and up

8. Rub the skin with an alcohol pad in a circular motion from the center of the site out

9. The drug would be destroyed orally, a rapid effect is desired, the patient is unable to take the drug orally

10. In the adult, pull the ear back and up. In a 2-year-old child, pull the ear back and down.

Proficiency Test Answers

Chapter 1

Test 1: Arithmetic

A. a)

$$
\begin{array}{r}
647 \\
\times\ \ 38 \\
\hline
5176 \\
1941\ \ \\
\hline
24586
\end{array}
$$

b)

$$\frac{\overset{1}{\cancel{8}}}{\underset{3}{\cancel{9}}} \times \frac{\overset{\overset{1}{\cancel{4}}}{\cancel{12}}}{\underset{\underset{1}{\cancel{4}}}{\cancel{32}}} = \frac{1}{3}$$

c)

$$
\begin{array}{r}
0.56 \\
\times\ 0.17 \\
\hline
392 \\
56\ \ \\
\hline
0.0952
\end{array}
$$

B. a)

$$
\begin{array}{r}
9.670 = 9.67 \\
82\overline{)793.000} \\
\underline{738}\ \ \ \ \ \\
55\,0\ \ \ \\
\underline{49\,2}\ \ \ \\
5\,80\ \\
\underline{5\,74}\ \\
60
\end{array}
$$

b)

$$5\frac{1}{4} \div \frac{7}{4} = \frac{\overset{3}{\cancel{21}}}{\underset{1}{\cancel{4}}} \times \frac{\overset{1}{\cancel{4}}}{\underset{1}{\cancel{7}}} = 3$$

c)

$$
\begin{array}{r}
20. \\
0.015\overline{)0.300}
\end{array}
$$

C. a)

$$
\frac{1}{18}\begin{array}{r} 0.055 = 0.06 \\ \overline{)1.000} \\ \underline{90}\ \ \\ 100 \\ \underline{90} \\ 100 \end{array}
$$

b)

$$
\frac{3}{8}\begin{array}{r} 0.375 = 0.38 \\ \overline{)3.000} \\ \underline{2\,4}\ \ \ \\ 60\ \\ \underline{56}\ \\ 40 \\ \underline{40} \end{array}
$$

D. a)

$$0.35 = \frac{\overset{7}{\cancel{35}}}{\underset{20}{\cancel{100}}} = \frac{7}{20}$$

b)

$$0.08 = \frac{\overset{2}{\cancel{8}}}{\underset{25}{\cancel{100}}} = \frac{2}{25}$$

E. a) 0.4

b) 0.8

c) 0.83

d) 0.3

F. a)
$$\frac{\frac{5}{20}}{\frac{12}{3}} = \frac{5}{3}$$

$$3\overline{)5.00} = 1.666 = 1.67$$
$$\underline{3}$$
$$20$$
$$\underline{18}$$
$$20$$
$$\underline{18}$$
$$20$$
$$\underline{18}$$

b)
$$\frac{\frac{1}{7}}{\frac{84}{12}} = \frac{1}{12}$$

$$12\overline{)1.00} = 0.083 = 0.08$$
$$\underline{96}$$
$$40$$
$$\underline{36}$$
$$4$$

c)
$$\frac{6}{13}$$

$$13\overline{)6.00} = 0.461 = 0.46$$
$$\underline{5\,2}$$
$$80$$
$$\underline{78}$$
$$20$$
$$\underline{13}$$

G. a) 5.3

b) 0.63

c) 0.924

H. a) $\frac{1}{3}\% =$

$$\frac{\frac{1}{3}}{100} = \frac{1}{3} \div 100 =$$

$$\frac{1}{3} \times \frac{1}{100} = \frac{1}{300}$$

b) Three ways:

1) $0.8\% = \underset{\smile}{00.8} = 0.008 =$

$$\frac{\frac{1}{8}}{\underset{125}{\cancel{1000}}} = \frac{1}{125}$$

2)

$$0.8\% = \frac{0.8}{100}$$

$$0.800\overline{)} = .008 = 0.008 =$$

$$\frac{\frac{1}{8}}{\underset{125}{\cancel{1000}}} = \frac{1}{125}$$

3) $0.8\% = \frac{\frac{8}{10}}{100} = \frac{8}{10} \div 100 = \frac{8}{10} \times \frac{1}{100} = \frac{\frac{1}{8}}{\underset{125}{\cancel{1000}}} = \frac{1}{125}$

I. a) $\frac{32}{128} = \frac{4}{x}$

$$\frac{\overset{1}{\cancel{32}}x}{\underset{1}{\cancel{32}}} = \frac{\overset{4}{\cancel{128}} \times 4}{\underset{1}{\cancel{32}}}$$

$$x = 16$$

b) $8 : 72 :: 5 : x$

$$\frac{\overset{1}{\cancel{8}}}{\underset{1}{\cancel{8}}}x = \frac{\overset{9}{\cancel{72}} \times 5}{\underset{1}{\cancel{8}}}$$

$$x = 45$$

c) $\frac{0.4}{0.12} = \frac{x}{8}$

$$0.12x = 0.4 \times 8$$

$$\frac{\cancel{0.12}}{\cancel{0.12}}x = \frac{0.4 \times 8}{0.12}$$

$$x = \frac{3.2}{0.12}$$

$$0.12\overline{)3.2000} = 26.66 = 26.7$$
$$\underline{2\,4}$$
$$80$$
$$\underline{72}$$
$$80$$
$$\underline{72}$$
$$8$$

$$x = 27$$

Chapter 2

Test 1: Abbreviations

1. Twice a day
2. Do not use hs. Use "at bedtime."
3. When necessary
4. Both eyes (suggested to write out "both eyes")
5. By mouth
6. By rectum
7. Sublingually
8. Swish and swallow
9. Do not use tiw. Use "three times weekly."
10. Milliliter
11. Every 4 hours
12. Do not use cc. Use "milliliter."
13. Do not use sc. Use "subcutaneous."
14. Do not use AU. Use "both ears."
15. Gram
16. After meals
17. Do not use qd. Use "every day."
18. Immediately
19. Every 12 hours
20. Three times a day
21. Left eye (suggested to write out "left eye")
22. Kilogram
23. Every night
24. Every hour
25. Right eye (suggested to write out "right eye")
26. Milliequivalent
27. Before meals
28. Four times a day
29. Milligram
30. Intramuscularly
31. Do not use qod. Use "every other day."
32. Twice a week
33. Nasogastric tube
34. Every 8 hours
35. Liter
36. Microgram
37. Every 6 hours
38. Do not use µg. Use "microgram" or "mcg."
39. Do not use U. Use "unit."
40. Teaspoon
41. Do not use AD. Use "right ear."
42. Grain
43. Intravenously
44. Suspension
45. Tablespoon
46. Intravenous piggyback
47. Minim
48. Gram
49. Every 2 hours
50. Every 3 hours

Test 2: Reading Prescriptions

1. Nembutal one hundred milligrams at the hour of sleep, as needed, by mouth (eg, 10 PM)
2. Propranolol hydrochloride forty milligrams by mouth twice a day (eg, 10 AM, 6 PM)
3. Ampicillin one gram intravenous piggyback every 6 hours (eg, 6 AM, 12 noon, 6 PM, 12 midnight)
4. Demerol fifty milligrams intramuscularly every 4 hours as needed for pain
5. Tylenol three hundred twenty-five milligrams, two tablets by mouth immediately. (Give two tablets of Tylenol. Each tablet is 325 mg.)
6. Pilocarpine drops two in both eyes every 3 hours (eg, 3 AM, 6 AM, 9 AM, 12 noon, 3 PM, 6 PM, 9 PM, 12 midnight)
7. Scopolamine eight-tenths of a milligram subcutaneously immediately
8. Elixir of digoxin twenty-five hundredths of a milligram by mouth every day (eg, 10 AM)
9. Kaochlor thirty milliequivalents by mouth twice a day (eg, 10 AM and 6 PM)
10. Liquaemin sodium six thousand units subcutaneously every 4 hours (eg, 2 AM, 6 AM, 10 AM, 2 PM, 6 PM, 10 PM)
11. Tobramycin seventy milligrams intramuscularly every 8 hours (eg, 6 AM, 2 PM, 10 PM)
12. Prednisone ten milligrams by mouth every other day (eg, even days of the month at 10 AM). You might substitute "odd days of the month."
13. Milk of magnesia one tablespoon by mouth at the hour of sleep every night (eg, 10 PM)
14. Septra one double-strength tablet every day by mouth (eg, 10 AM)
15. Morphine sulfate fifteen milligrams subcutaneously immediately and ten milligrams every 4 hours as needed. The stat time given determines when the next dose can be administered. (Next dose must be *at least 4 hours later.*)

Test 3: Interpreting Written Prescription Orders

1. Colace one hundred milligrams by mouth three times a day (eg, 10 AM, 2 PM, 6 PM)

2. Ativan one milligram intravenous push times one dose now.

3. Ten milliequivalents potassium chloride in one hundred cubic centimeters of normal saline over one hour, times one dose. Should be one hundred "milliliters".

4. Tylenol number three two tablets by mouth every four hours as needed for pain

5. Heparin twenty-five thousand international units in two hundred fifty cubic centimeters dextrose five percent in water at five hundred units per hour. Should write out "international unit." Should write out "500 units." Should write out "mL."

6. Ticlid two hundred fifty milligrams one tablet by mouth twice a day (eg, 10 AM, 6 PM)

7. Lopressor 25 milligrams by mouth twice a day (eg, 10 AM, 6 PM)

8. Benadryl 25 milligrams by mouth every hour of sleep (eg, every night at 10 PM); should write "at bedtime"

Chapter 3

Test 1: Labels and Packaging

1. a. 1. Individually wrapped and labeled drugs

    2. Large stock containers of drugs

   b. 1. Glass container holding a single dose. Container must be broken to reach the drug. Any portion not used must be discarded.

    2. Glass or plastic container with a sealed top that allows medication to be kept sterile

   c. 1. Drug applied to skin or mucous membranes to achieve a local effect. May be absorbed into the circulation and causes a systemic effect.

    2. Drugs given by injection include subcutaneous, IM, IV, and IVPB

   d. 1. Brand or proprietary name of manufacturer. Identified by symbol ®.

    2. Official name of a drug as listed in the USP

   e. 1. Liquid sterile medication ready to administer

    2. Powder or crystals diluted according to specific directions. Date and time of preparation must be written on the label, and the expiration date noted.

2. a. 4	**c.** 2	**e.** 1
b. 2	**d.** 1	

3. 1. g	**4.** i	**7.** j	**9.** c
2. e	**5.** d	**8.** a	**10.** b
3. h	**6.** f		

Test 2: Interpreting a Label

1. Fortaz

2. Ceftazidime

3. Intravenous, intramuscular

4. Varies: 1.8 mL, 3.6 mL, 5.3 mL, 10.6 mL

5. 500 mg, 1 g

6. Reconstitute with sterile water for injection, bacteriostatic water for injection, or 0.5% or 1% lidocaine hydrochloride injection. Dilute with 1.5 mL, approximate available volume 1.8 mL to equal 500 mg (intramuscular route); add 3.0 mL, approximate available volume 3.6 mL to equal 1 g (intramuscular route); add 5.0 mL, approximate available volume 5.3 mL to equal 500 mg (intravenous route); add 10.0 mL, approximate available volume 10.6 mL to equal 1 g (intravenous infusion). Shake well.

7. Powder

8. Protect from light. Maintains satisfactory potency for 24 hours at room temperature or for 7 days under refrigeration. Solutions in sterile water for injection that are frozen immediately after constitution in the original container are stable for 3 months when stored at −20°C. Once thawed, solutions should not be refrozen. Thawed solutions may be stored for up to 8 hours at room temperature or for 4 days in a refrigerator.

9. Not shown

10. 500 mg or 1 g (adults)

11. Federal law prohibits dispensing without prescription. This vial is under reduced pressure. Addition of diluent generates a positive pressure. Color changes do not affect potency.

Chapter 4

Test 1: Exercises in Equivalents and Mixed Conversions

1. 0.1
2. 30
3. 1000
4. 5
5. 15
6. 0.01
7. 1
8. 200
9. 0.03
10. 0.5
11. 30
12. 1/5
13. 15
14. 2.2
15. 1000
16. 0.06
17. 1
18. 16
19. 45
20. 1
21. 100
22. 1
23. 0.6
24. 0.01
25. 1000
26. 0.0005 mg
27. 0.0006 g
28. 0.25 mg
29. 0.001
30. 125
31. 10
32. 1
33. 1000
34. 0.6 mg
35. gr 1/2
36. 120 mg
37. gr 4
38. 0.48 mg
39. gr 17
40. 0.3 mg

Chapter 5

Test 1: Drug Preparations and Equipment

1. Diabetes mellitus, alcoholism
2. Two teaspoons or less
3. Subcutaneous, IM, IVPB, and IV
4. a. The date
   b. The nurse's initials
   c. The dilution made
   d. The time
5. Aseptic technique is required in preparing and administering drugs parenterally (IM, subcutaneous, IV, IVPB).
6. Milk of magnesia
7. Before an oral suspension is poured, the liquid must always be shaken.
8. Aerosol powders, creams, ointments, pastes, suppositories, transdermal medications
9. Ease in administering; prolonged action
10. An ointment is a semisolid preparation in a petroleum or lanolin base for topical use.
11. 1. Pour to a line. Never estimate a dose.
    2. Pour liquids at eye level.
12. a. The natural curve of the surface of a liquid in a container
    b. Diameter or width of a needle. The higher the gauge number, the finer the needle.
13. Route of administration, size and condition of the patient, amount of adipose tissue present at the site
14. 1. When the last number is 5 or more, add 1 to the previous number.
    2. When the last number is 4 or less, drop the number.
15. The equipment used
    3-mL syringe—nearest 10th in milliliters
    precision syringe—nearest 100th in milliliters
    medicine cup—metric, apothecary, or household lines

Chapter 6

Test 1: Calculation of Oral Doses

Formula Method

Ratio Method

Proportion Method

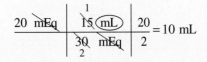

1. $\dfrac{\overset{10}{\cancel{\overset{\cancel{20}\ \cancel{mEq}}{\cancel{30}\ \cancel{mEq}}}}}{\underset{1}{2}} \times \overset{1}{\cancel{15}}\ mL = 10\ mL$

$15\ mL : 30\ mEq :: x : 20\ mEq$

$\dfrac{15\ mL}{30\ mEq} = \dfrac{x}{20\ mEq}$

$\dfrac{300}{30} = x$

$10\ mL = x$

Dimensional Analysis Method

$\dfrac{20\ \cancel{mEq}\ \Big|\ \overset{1}{\cancel{15}}\ \cancel{(mL)}\ \Big|\ 20}{\Big|\ \underset{2}{\cancel{30}}\ \cancel{mEq}\ \Big|\ 2} = 10\ mL$

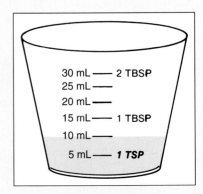

Formula Method

Ratio Method

Proportion Method

2. $\dfrac{\overset{2}{\cancel{150\ mg}}}{\underset{1}{\cancel{75\ mg}}} \times 7.5\ mL = 15\ mL$

$7.5\ mL : 75\ mg :: x : 150\ mg$

$\dfrac{7.5\ mL}{75\ mg} = \dfrac{x}{150\ mg}$

$7.5 \times 150 = 75x$

$1125 = 75x$

$15\ mL = x$

Dimensional Analysis Method

$\dfrac{\overset{2}{\cancel{150}}\ \cancel{mg}\ \Big|\ 7.5\cancel{(mL)}\ \Big|\ 2 \times 7.5}{\Big|\ \underset{1}{\cancel{75}}\ \cancel{mg}\ \Big|} = 15\ mL$

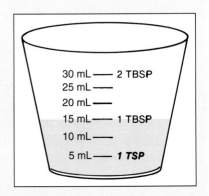

Formula Method

3. $\dfrac{\overset{1}{\cancel{0.125}}\ \text{mg}}{\underset{\underset{1}{2}}{\cancel{0.250}}\ \text{mg}} \times \overset{5}{\cancel{10}} = 5 \text{ mL}$

Ratio Method

$10 \text{ mL} : 0.25 \text{ mg} :: x : 0.125 \text{ mg}$

$10 \times 0.125 = 0.25x$

Proportion Method

$\dfrac{10 \text{ mL}}{0.25 \text{ mg}} = \dfrac{x}{0.125 \text{ mg}}$

$\dfrac{1.25}{0.25} = x$

$5 \text{ mL} = x$

Dimensional Analysis Method

$\dfrac{\overset{1}{\cancel{0.125}}\ \text{mg}}{} \ \left| \ \dfrac{10\ \text{mL}}{\underset{2}{\cancel{0.25}}\ \text{mg}} \ \right| \ \dfrac{10}{2} = 5 \text{ mL}$

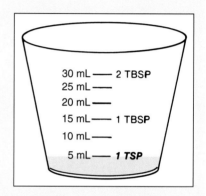

Formula Method

4. $\dfrac{\overset{3}{\cancel{375}}\ \text{mg}}{\underset{1}{\cancel{125}}\ \text{mg}} \times 5 \text{ mL} = 15 \text{ mL}$

Ratio Method

$5 \text{ mL} : 125 \text{ mg} :: x : 375 \text{ mg}$

Proportion Method

$\dfrac{5 \text{ mL}}{125 \text{ mg}} = \dfrac{x}{375 \text{ mg}}$

$\dfrac{1875}{125} = x$

$15 \text{ mL} = x$

Dimensional Analysis Method

$\dfrac{\overset{3}{\cancel{375}}\ \text{mg}}{} \ \left| \ \dfrac{5\ \text{mL}}{\underset{1}{\cancel{125}}\ \text{mg}} \ \right| \ \dfrac{3 \times 5}{} = 15 \text{ mL}$

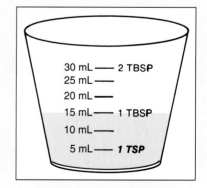

Formula Method

Ratio Method

Proportion Method

5. 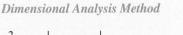 $\dfrac{\overset{2}{\cancel{40}} \text{ mg}}{\underset{1}{\cancel{20}} \text{ mg}} \times 2.5 \text{ mL} = 5 \text{ mL}$

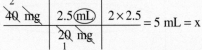
2.5 mL : 20 mg : : x : 40 mg

$\dfrac{2.5 \text{ mL}}{20 \text{ mg}} = \dfrac{x}{40 \text{ mg}}$

$\dfrac{100}{20} = x$

$5 \text{ mL} = x$

Dimensional Analysis Method

$\dfrac{\overset{2}{\cancel{40}} \text{ mg}}{} \left| \dfrac{2.5 \text{ (mL)}}{\underset{1}{\cancel{20}} \text{ mg}} \right| \dfrac{2 \times 2.5}{} = 5 \text{ mL} = x$

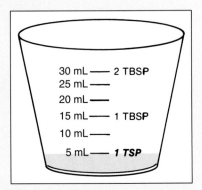

Formula Method

Ratio Method

Proportion Method

6. Rule: $\dfrac{D}{H} \times S = A$

$\dfrac{0.50 \text{ mg}}{0.25 \text{ mg}} \times 1 \text{ tablet} = 0.25 \overline{)0.50}^{\,2.} = 2 \text{ tablets}$

1 tablet : 0.25 mg : : x : 0.5 mg

$\dfrac{1 \text{ tablet}}{0.25 \text{ mg}} = \dfrac{x}{0.50}$

$\dfrac{0.50}{0.25} = x$

2 tablets = x

Dimensional Analysis Method

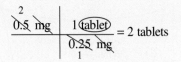 $\dfrac{\overset{2}{\cancel{0.5}} \text{ mg}}{} \left| \dfrac{1 \text{ (tablet)}}{\underset{1}{\cancel{0.25}} \text{ mg}} \right| = 2 \text{ tablets}$

Formula Method   *Ratio Method*   *Proportion Method*

7. Equivalent 0.1 mg = 100 mcg

$\dfrac{\cancel{100}\ \cancel{mcg}}{\cancel{100}\ \cancel{mcg}} \times 1\ \text{capsule} = 1\ \text{capsule}$

1 capsule : 100 mcg : : x : 100 mcg

$\dfrac{1\ \text{capsule}}{100\ \text{mcg}} = \dfrac{x}{100\ \text{mcg}}$

100 mcg = 1 capsule

Dimensional Analysis Method

$\dfrac{\cancel{100}\ \cancel{mcg}}{} \Big| \dfrac{1\ \text{capsule}}{0.1\ \cancel{mg}} \Big| \dfrac{1\ \cancel{mg}}{1000\ \cancel{mcg}} \Big| \dfrac{1}{0.1 \times 10} = \dfrac{1}{1} = 1\ \text{capsule}$

Formula Method   *Ratio Method*   *Proportion Method*

8. $\dfrac{\overset{5}{\cancel{250}\ \text{mg}}}{\underset{2}{\cancel{100}\ \text{mg}}} \times 1\ \text{tablet} = \dfrac{5}{2} = 2\frac{1}{2}\ \text{tablets}$

1 tablet : 100 mg : : x : 250 mg

$\dfrac{1\ \text{tablet}}{100\ \text{mg}} = \dfrac{x}{250\ \text{mg}}$

$\dfrac{250}{100} = x$

2.5 tablet = x

Dimensional Analysis Method

$\dfrac{\overset{2.5}{\cancel{250}\ \cancel{mg}}}{} \Big| \dfrac{1\ \text{tablet}}{\underset{1}{\cancel{100}\ \cancel{mg}}} \Big| \dfrac{2.5 \times 1}{} = 2.5\ \text{tablets}$

Formula Method   *Ratio Method*   *Proportion Method*

9. Equivalent 0.5 g = 500 mg

$\dfrac{\overset{2}{\cancel{500}\ \text{mg}}}{\underset{1}{\cancel{250}\ \text{mg}}} \times 1\ \text{capsule} = 2\ \text{capsule}$

1 capsule : 250 mg : : x : 500 mg

$\dfrac{1\ \text{capsule}}{250\ \text{mg}} = \dfrac{x}{500\ \text{mg}}$

$\dfrac{500}{250} = x$

2 capsules = x

Dimensional Analysis Method

$\dfrac{0.5\ \cancel{g}}{} \Big| \dfrac{1\ \text{capsule}}{\underset{1}{\cancel{250}\ \cancel{mg}}} \Big| \dfrac{\overset{4}{\cancel{1000}\ \cancel{mg}}}{1\ \cancel{g}} \Big| \dfrac{0.5 \times 4}{} = 2\ \text{capsules}$

Formula Method	*Ratio Method*	*Proportion Method*

10. Equivalent 0.3 mg = 300 mcg

$$\frac{\overset{1}{\cancel{300\ mcg}}}{\underset{1}{\cancel{300\ mcg}}} \times 1 \text{ tablet} = 1 \text{ tablet}$$

1 tablet : 300 mcg :: x : 300 mcg

$$\frac{1 \text{ tablet}}{300 \text{ mcg}} = \frac{x}{300 \text{ mcg}}$$

$$\frac{300}{300} = x$$

$$1 \text{ tablet} = x$$

Dimensional Analysis Method

$$\frac{0.3\ \cancel{mg}}{} \left| \frac{1\ \text{(tablet)}}{300\ \cancel{mcg}} \right| \frac{1000\ \cancel{mcg}}{1\ \cancel{mg}} \left| \frac{0.3 \times 10}{3} \right. = 1 \text{ tablet}$$

Test 2: Calculation of Oral Doses (Test 2)

Formula Method	*Ratio Method*	*Proportion Method*

1. Equivalent 0.8 g = 800 mg

$$\frac{\overset{2}{\cancel{800\ mg}}}{\underset{1}{\cancel{400\ mg}}} \times 1 \text{ tablet} = 2 \text{ tablets}$$

1 tablet : 400 mg :: x : 800 mg

$$\frac{1 \text{ tablet}}{400 \text{ mg}} = \frac{x}{800 \text{ mg}}$$

$$\frac{800}{400} = x$$

$$2 \text{ tablets} = x$$

Dimensional Analysis Method

$$\frac{0.8\ \cancel{g}}{} \left| \frac{1\ \text{(tablet)}}{400\ \cancel{mg}} \right| \frac{1000\ \cancel{mg}}{1\ \cancel{g}} \left| \frac{0.8 \times 10}{4} \right. = 2 \text{ tablets}$$

Formula Method	*Ratio Method*	*Proportion Method*

2. Equivalent 0.3 g = 300 mg

$$\frac{\overset{1}{\cancel{300\ mg}}}{\underset{1}{\cancel{300\ mg}}} \times 1 \text{ tablet} = 1 \text{ tablet}$$

1 tablet : 300 mg :: x : 300 mg

$$\frac{1 \text{ tablet}}{300 \text{ mg}} = \frac{x}{300 \text{ mg}}$$

$$\frac{300}{300} = x$$

$$1 \text{ tablet} = x$$

Dimensional Analysis Method

$$\frac{0.3\ \cancel{g}}{} \left| \frac{1\ \text{(tablet)}}{300\ \cancel{mg}} \right| \frac{1000\ \cancel{mg}}{1\ \cancel{g}} \left| \frac{0.3 \times 10}{3} \right. = 1 \text{ tablet}$$

Formula Method   *Ratio Method*   *Proportion Method*

3. $\dfrac{\overset{3}{\cancel{600}}\text{ mg}}{\underset{2}{\cancel{400}}\text{ mg}} \times 1$ tablet $= \frac{3}{2} = 1.5$ or $1\frac{1}{2}$ tablets   1 tablet : 400 mg :: x : 600 mg $\dfrac{1 \text{ tablet}}{400 \text{ mg}} = \dfrac{x}{600 \text{ mg}}$

$$\frac{600}{400} = x$$

$$1.5 \text{ tablets} = x$$

Dimensional Analysis Method

$$\dfrac{\cancel{600}\text{ mg}}{} \left| \dfrac{1\,\widehat{\text{tablet}}}{\cancel{400}\text{ mg}} \right| \dfrac{6}{4} = 1.5 \text{ tablets}$$

Formula Method   *Ratio Method*   *Proportion Method*

4. 0.65 g = 650 mg

$\dfrac{\overset{2}{\cancel{650}}\text{ mg}}{\underset{1}{\cancel{325}}\text{ mg}} \times 1$ tablet $= 2$ tablets   1 tablet : 325 mg :: x : 650 mg $\dfrac{1 \text{ tablet}}{325 \text{ mg}} = \dfrac{x}{650 \text{ mg}}$

$$\frac{650}{325} = x$$

$$2 \text{ tablets} = x$$

Dimensional Analysis Method

$$\dfrac{0.65\,\cancel{g}}{} \left| \dfrac{1\,\widehat{\text{tablet}}}{325\,\cancel{mg}} \right| \dfrac{1000\,\cancel{mg}}{1\,\cancel{g}} \left| \dfrac{0.65 \times 1000}{325} \right. = 2 \text{ tablets}$$

Formula Method   *Ratio Method*   *Proportion Method*

5. $\dfrac{\overset{1}{\cancel{250}}\text{ mg}}{\underset{2}{\cancel{500}}\text{ mg}} \times 1$ tablet $= \frac{1}{2}$ tablet   1 tablet : 500 mg :: x : 250 mg $\dfrac{1 \text{ tablet}}{500 \text{ mg}} = \dfrac{x}{250 \text{ mg}}$

$$\frac{250}{500} = x$$

$$0.5 \text{ tablet} = x$$

Dimensional Analysis Method

$$\dfrac{250\,\cancel{mg}}{} \left| \dfrac{1\,\widehat{\text{tablet}}}{500\,\cancel{mg}} \right| \dfrac{25}{50} = \frac{1}{2} \text{ tablet}$$

Formula Method   *Ratio Method*   *Proportion Method*

6. $\dfrac{750{,}000 \text{ units}}{100{,}000 \text{ units}} \times 1 \text{ mL} = \dfrac{75}{10} = 7.5 \text{ mL}$ $1 \text{ mL} : 100{,}000 \text{ units} :: x : 750{,}000 \text{ units}$ $\dfrac{1 \text{ mL}}{100{,}000 \text{ units}} = \dfrac{x}{750{,}000 \text{ units}}$

$$\dfrac{750{,}000}{100{,}000} = x$$

$$7.5 \text{ mL} = x$$

Dimensional Analysis Method

$$\dfrac{750{,}000 \text{ units}}{} \, \Big| \, \dfrac{1 \text{ mL}}{100{,}000 \text{ units}} \, \Big| \, \dfrac{75}{10} = 7.5 \text{ mL}$$

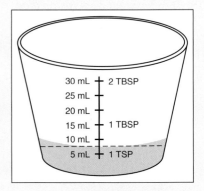

Formula Method   *Ratio Method*   *Proportion Method*

7. Equivalent 0.75 g = 750 mg

$\dfrac{\overset{3}{750} \text{ mg}}{\underset{1}{250} \text{ mg}} \times 5 \text{ mL} = 15 \text{ mL}$ $5 \text{ mL} : 250 \text{ mg} :: x : 750 \text{ mg}$ $\dfrac{5 \text{ mL}}{250 \text{ mg}} = \dfrac{x}{750}$

$$\dfrac{3750}{250} = x$$

$$15 \text{ mL} = x$$

Dimensional Analysis Method

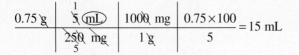

$$0.75 \text{ g} \, \Big| \, \dfrac{\overset{1}{5} \text{ mL}}{\underset{5}{250} \text{ mg}} \, \Big| \, \dfrac{1000 \text{ mg}}{1 \text{ g}} \, \Big| \, \dfrac{0.75 \times 100}{5} = 15 \text{ mL}$$

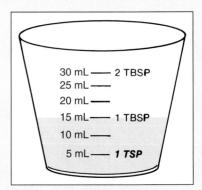

APPENDIX A Proficiency Test Answers **403**

Formula Method

Ratio Method

Proportion Method

8. $\dfrac{\overset{2}{\cancel{500 \text{ mg}}}}{\underset{1}{\cancel{250 \text{ mg}}}} \times 5 \text{ mL} = 10 \text{ mL}$

$5 \text{ mL} : 250 \text{ mg} : : x : 500 \text{ mg}$

$\dfrac{5 \text{ mL}}{250 \text{ mg}} = \dfrac{x}{500 \text{ mg}}$

$\dfrac{2500}{250} = 10 \text{ mL}$

Dimensional Analysis Method

$\dfrac{\overset{2}{\cancel{500 \text{ mg}}}}{} \Bigg| \dfrac{5 \text{ } \cancel{\text{mL}}}{\underset{1}{\cancel{250 \text{ mg}}}} \Bigg| \dfrac{2 \times 5}{} = 10 \text{ mL}$

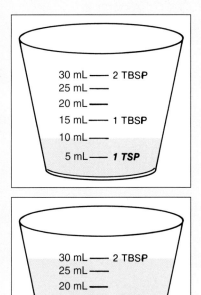

9. No arithmetic necessary. Pour 30 mL.

Formula Method

Ratio Method

Proportion Method

10. $\dfrac{\overset{2}{\cancel{160 \text{ mg}}}}{\underset{1}{\cancel{80 \text{ mg}}}} \times 15 \text{ mL} = 30 \text{ mL}$

$15 \text{ mL} : 80 \text{ mg} : : x : 160 \text{ mg}$

$\dfrac{15 \text{ mL}}{80 \text{ mg}} = \dfrac{x}{160 \text{ mg}}$

$\dfrac{2400}{80} = x$

$30 \text{ mL} = x$

Dimensional Analysis Method

$\dfrac{\overset{2}{\cancel{160 \text{ mg}}}}{} \Bigg| \dfrac{15 \text{ } \cancel{\text{mL}}}{\underset{1}{\cancel{80 \text{ mg}}}} \Bigg| \dfrac{2 \times 15}{} = 30 \text{ mL}$

Test 3: Calculation of Oral Doses (Test 3)

Formula Method   *Ratio Method*   *Proportion Method*

1. $\dfrac{\overset{10}{\cancel{20 \text{ mEq}}}}{\underset{\underset{1}{2}}{\cancel{30 \text{ mEq}}}} \times \overset{1}{\cancel{15}} \text{ mL} = 10 \text{ mL}$

$15 \text{ mL} : 30 \text{ mEq} : : x : 20 \text{ mEq}$

$\dfrac{15 \text{ mL}}{30 \text{ mEq}} = \dfrac{x}{20 \text{ mEq}}$

$\dfrac{300}{30} = x$

$10 \text{ mL} = x$

Dimensional Analysis Method

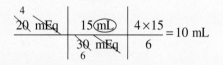

$\dfrac{\overset{4}{\cancel{20}} \text{ mEq}}{} \bigg| \dfrac{15 \,\text{(mL)}}{\underset{6}{\cancel{30}} \text{ mEq}} \bigg| \dfrac{4 \times 15}{6} = 10 \text{ mL}$

Formula Method   *Ratio Method*   *Proportion Method*

2. $\dfrac{\overset{16}{\cancel{80 \text{ mcg}}}}{\underset{25}{\cancel{125 \text{ mcg}}}} \times \overset{1}{\cancel{5}} \text{ mL} = \dfrac{\frac{16}{80}}{\frac{25}{5}} = \dfrac{16}{5} \overset{3.2}{\overline{)16.0}} = 3.2 \text{ mL}$

$5 \text{ mL} : 125 \text{ mg} : : x : 80 \text{ mg}$

$\dfrac{5 \text{mL}}{125 \text{ mg}} = \dfrac{x}{80 \text{ mg}}$

$\dfrac{40}{125} = x$

$3.2 \text{ mL} = x$

Dimensional Analysis Method

$\dfrac{80 \text{ mg}}{} \bigg| \dfrac{\overset{1}{\cancel{5}} \,\text{(mL)}}{\underset{25}{\cancel{125}} \text{ mg}} \bigg| \dfrac{80}{25} = 3.2 \text{ mL}$

If you do not have a dropper bottle, you could use a syringe without the needle to obtain the dose.

Formula Method   *Ratio Method*   *Proportion Method*

3. $0.02 \text{ g} = 20 \text{ mg}$

$\dfrac{\overset{2}{\cancel{20 \text{ mg}}}}{\underset{1}{\cancel{10 \text{ mg}}}} \times 1 \text{ tablet} = 2 \text{ tablets}$

$1 \text{ tablet} : 10 \text{ mg} : : x : 20 \text{ mg}$

$\dfrac{1 \text{ tablet}}{10 \text{ mg}} = \dfrac{x}{20 \text{ mg}}$

$\dfrac{20}{10} = x$

$2 \text{ tablets} = x$

Dimensional Analysis Method

$\dfrac{0.02 \text{ g}}{} \bigg| \dfrac{1 \,\text{(tablet)}}{\underset{1}{\cancel{10}} \text{ mg}} \bigg| \dfrac{\overset{100}{\cancel{1000}} \text{ mg}}{1 \,\cancel{\text{g}}} \bigg| \dfrac{0.02 \times 100}{} = 2 \text{ tablets}$

Formula Method

4. 0.5 g = 500 mg

$$\frac{\overset{2}{\cancel{500}\text{ mg}}}{\underset{1}{\cancel{250}\text{ mg}}} \times 1\text{ capsule} = 2\text{ capsules}$$

Ratio Method

1 capsule : 250 mg : : x : 500 mg

Proportion Method

$$\frac{1\text{ capsule}}{250\text{ mg}} = \frac{x}{500\text{ mg}}$$

$$\frac{500}{250} = x$$

2 capsules = x

Dimensional Analysis Method

$$\frac{0.5\ \cancel{g}}{} \left| \frac{1\ \text{capsule}}{\underset{1}{\cancel{250}\ \text{mg}}} \right| \frac{\overset{4}{\cancel{1000}\ \text{mg}}}{1\ \cancel{g}} \right| 0.5 \times 4 = 2\text{ capsules}$$

Formula Method

5. $$\frac{\overset{2}{\cancel{0.50}\text{ mg}}}{\underset{1}{\cancel{0.25}\text{ mg}}} \times 1\text{ tablet} = 2\text{ tablets}$$

Ratio Method

1 tablet : 0.25 mg : : x : 0.5 mg

Proportion Method

$$\frac{1\text{ tablet}}{0.25\text{ mg}} = \frac{x}{0.5\text{ mg}}$$

$$\frac{0.5}{0.25} = x$$

2 tablets = x

Dimensional Analysis Method

$$\frac{\overset{2}{\cancel{0.5}\ \text{mg}}}{} \left| \frac{1\ \text{tablet}}{\underset{1}{\cancel{0.25}\ \text{mg}}} \right| 2 \times 1 = 2\text{ tablets}$$

Formula Method

6. $$\frac{\overset{}{40\,\text{mg}}}{\underset{1}{\cancel{5}\,\text{mg}}} \times \overset{1}{\cancel{5}}\ \text{mL} = 40\text{ mL}$$

Ratio Method

5 mL : 5 mg : : x : 40 mg

Proportion Method

$$\frac{5\text{ mL}}{5\text{ mg}} = \frac{x}{40\text{ mg}}$$

$$\frac{200}{5} = x$$

40 mL = x

Dimensional Analysis Method

$$\frac{40\ \cancel{\text{mg}}}{} \left| \frac{5\ \text{mL}}{\cancel{5}\ \cancel{\text{mg}}} \right. = 40\text{ mL}$$

Formula Method

7. $\dfrac{\overset{3}{\cancel{75}\text{ mg}}}{\underset{2}{\cancel{50}\text{ mg}}} \times 1 \text{ tablet} = \dfrac{3}{2}\overline{)\dfrac{1.5}{3.0}} = 1\tfrac{1}{2} \text{ tablets}$

Ratio Method

1 tablet : 50 mg : : x : 75 mg

Proportion Method

$\dfrac{1 \text{ tablet}}{50 \text{ mg}} = \dfrac{x}{75 \text{ mg}}$

$\dfrac{75}{50} = x$

1.5 tablets = x

Dimensional Analysis Method

$\dfrac{\overset{15}{\cancel{75}}\text{ mg}}{} \left|\ \dfrac{1\,\boxed{\text{tablet}}}{\underset{10}{\cancel{50}}\text{ mg}}\ \right|\ \dfrac{15}{10} = 1.5 \text{ tablets}$

Formula Method

8. $\dfrac{\overset{1}{\cancel{40}\text{ mg}}}{\underset{2}{\cancel{80}\text{ mg}}} \times 1 \text{ tablet} = \tfrac{1}{2} \text{ tablet}$

Ratio Method

1 tablet : 80 mg : : x : 40 mg

Proportion Method

$\dfrac{1 \text{ tablet}}{80 \text{ mg}} = \dfrac{x}{40 \text{ mg}}$

$\dfrac{40}{80} = x$

0.5 tablet = x

Dimensional Analysis Method

$\dfrac{\overset{1}{\cancel{40}}\text{ mg}}{} \left|\ \dfrac{1\,\boxed{\text{tablet}}}{\underset{2}{\cancel{80}}\text{ mg}}\ \right|\ \dfrac{1}{2} = \tfrac{1}{2} \text{ tablet}$

Formula Method

9. 0.125 mg = 125 mcg

$\dfrac{\overset{1}{\cancel{125}\text{ mcg}}}{\underset{\underset{2}{4}}{\cancel{500}\text{ mcg}}} \times \overset{5}{\cancel{10}} \text{ mL} = \dfrac{5}{2}\overline{)\dfrac{2.5}{5.0}} = 2.5 \text{ mL}$

Ratio Method

10 mL : 500 mcg : : x : 125 mcg

Proportion Method

$\dfrac{10 \text{ mL}}{500 \text{ mcg}} = \dfrac{x}{125}$

$\dfrac{1250}{500} = x$

2.5 mL = x

Dimensional Analysis Method

$\dfrac{0.125\text{ mg}}{} \left|\ \dfrac{10\,\boxed{\text{mL}}}{\underset{1}{\cancel{500}}\text{ mcg}}\ \right|\ \dfrac{\overset{2}{\cancel{1000}}\text{ mcg}}{1\text{ mg}}\ \right|\ 0.125 \times 10 \times 2 = 2.5 \text{ mL}$

Formula Method

10. $\dfrac{\overset{3}{\cancel{75}} \text{ mg}}{\underset{\underset{1}{2}}{\cancel{50}} \text{ mg}} \times \overset{5}{\cancel{10}} \text{ mL} = 15 \text{ mL}$

Ratio Method

$10 \text{ mL} : 50 \text{ mg} : : x : 75 \text{ mg}$

Proportion Method

$\dfrac{10 \text{ mL}}{50 \text{ mg}} = \dfrac{x}{75 \text{ mg}}$

$\dfrac{750}{50} = x$

$15 \text{ mL} = x$

Dimensional Analysis Method

$\dfrac{75 \text{ mg}}{} \left| \dfrac{\overset{1}{\cancel{10}} \text{ \textcircled{mL}}}{\underset{5}{\cancel{50}} \text{ mg}} \right| \dfrac{75}{5} = 15 \text{ mL}$

Formula Method

11. $\dfrac{5 \text{ mg}}{2 \text{ mg}} \times 1 \text{ tablet} = \dfrac{5}{2} \enclose{longdiv}{5.0} \; \begin{smallmatrix}2.5\end{smallmatrix} = 2\tfrac{1}{2} \text{ tablets}$

Ratio Method

$1 \text{ tablet} : 2 \text{ mg} : : x : 5 \text{ mg}$

Proportion Method

$\dfrac{1 \text{ tablet}}{2 \text{ mg}} = \dfrac{x}{5 \text{ mg}}$

$\dfrac{5}{2} = x$

$2.5 \text{ tablets} = x$

Dimensional Analysis Method

$\dfrac{5 \text{ mg}}{} \left| \dfrac{1 \text{ \textcircled{tablet}}}{2 \text{ mg}} \right| \dfrac{5}{2} = 2.5 \text{ tablets}$

Formula Method

12. $0.15 \text{ mg} = 150 \text{ mcg}$

$\dfrac{\overset{1}{\cancel{150}} \text{ mcg}}{\underset{2}{\cancel{300}} \text{ mcg}} \times 1 \text{ tablet} = \tfrac{1}{2} \text{ tablet}$

Ratio Method

$1 \text{ tablet} : 300 \text{ mcg} : : x : 150 \text{ mcg}$

Proportion Method

$\dfrac{1 \text{ tablet}}{300 \text{ mcg}} = \dfrac{x}{150 \text{ mcg}}$

$\dfrac{150}{300} = x$

$0.5 \text{ tablet} = x$

Dimensional Analysis Method

$\dfrac{0.15 \text{ mg}}{} \left| \dfrac{1 \text{ \textcircled{tablet}}}{300 \text{ mcg}} \right| \dfrac{1000 \text{ mcg}}{1 \text{ mg}} \left| \dfrac{0.15 \times 10}{3} \right. = 0.5 \text{ tablet}$

Formula Method

13. $\dfrac{\overset{3}{\cancel{375}} \text{ mg}}{\underset{2}{\cancel{250}} \text{ mg}} \times 1 \text{ tablet} = \dfrac{3}{2} \overset{1.5}{\overline{)3.0}} = 1\tfrac{1}{2}$ tablets

Ratio Method

1 tablet : 250 mg : : x : 375 mg

Proportion Method

$$\dfrac{1 \text{ tablet}}{250 \text{ mg}} = \dfrac{x}{375 \text{ mg}}$$

$$\dfrac{375}{250} = x$$

$$1.5 \text{ tablets} = x$$

Dimensional Analysis Method

$$\dfrac{\overset{15}{\cancel{375}} \text{ mg}}{} \left| \dfrac{1 \text{(tablet)}}{\underset{10}{\cancel{250}} \text{ mg}} \right| \dfrac{15}{10} = 1.5 \text{ tablets}$$

Formula Method

14. 0.6 g = 600 mg

$\dfrac{\overset{2}{\cancel{600}} \text{ mg}}{\underset{1}{\cancel{300}} \text{ mg}} \times 1 \text{ tablet} = 2 \text{ tablets}$

Ratio Method

1 tablet : 300 mg : : x : 600 mg

Proportion Method

$$\dfrac{1 \text{ tablet}}{300 \text{ mg}} = \dfrac{x}{600}$$

$$\dfrac{600}{300} = x$$

$$2 \text{ tablets} = x$$

Dimensional Analysis Method

$$\dfrac{0.6 \text{ g}}{} \left| \dfrac{1 \text{(tablet)}}{\cancel{300} \text{ mg}} \right| \dfrac{\cancel{1000} \text{ mg}}{1 \text{ g}} \left| \dfrac{0.6 \times 10}{3} \right. = 2 \text{ tablets}$$

Formula Method

15. $\dfrac{\overset{3}{\cancel{1.5}} \text{ mg}}{\underset{\underset{1}{2}}{\cancel{1.0}} \text{ mg}} \times \overset{4}{\cancel{8}} \text{ mL} = 12 \text{ mL}$

Ratio Method

8 mL : 1 mg : : x : 1.5 mg

Proportion Method

$$\dfrac{8 \text{ mL}}{1 \text{ mg}} = \dfrac{x}{1.5 \text{ mg}}$$

$$\dfrac{12}{1} = x$$

$$12 \text{ mL} = x$$

Dimensional Analysis Method

$$\dfrac{1.5 \text{ mg}}{} \left| \dfrac{8 \text{(mL)}}{1 \text{ mg}} \right| \dfrac{1.5 \times 8}{} = 12 \text{ mL}$$

Use a syringe without the needle to measure the dose.

Formula Method *Ratio Method* *Proportion Method*

16. $\dfrac{\overset{2}{\cancel{25.0}}\ \cancel{mg}}{\underset{1}{\cancel{12.5}}\ \cancel{mg}} \times 5\ mL = 10\ mL$ 5 mL : 12.5 mg : : x : 25 mg $\dfrac{5\ mL}{12.5\ mg} = \dfrac{x}{25\ mg}$

$\dfrac{125}{12.5} = x$

10 mL = x

Dimensional Analysis Method

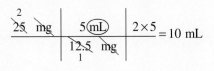

$\dfrac{\overset{2}{\cancel{25}}\ \cancel{mg}}{\begin{array}{c}\underset{1}{\cancel{12.5}}\ \cancel{mg}\end{array}} \ \Big|\ \dfrac{5\ \cancel{mL}}{\ }\ \Big|\ \dfrac{2 \times 5}{} = 10\ mL$

Formula Method *Ratio Method* *Proportion Method*

17. $\dfrac{\overset{3}{\cancel{60}}\ \cancel{mg}}{\underset{2}{\cancel{40}}\ \cancel{mg}} \times 0.6\ mL = \dfrac{1.8}{2} = 0.9\ mL$ 0.6 mL : 40 mg : : x : 60 mg $\dfrac{0.6\ mL}{40\ mg} = \dfrac{x}{60\ mg}$

$\dfrac{36}{40} = x$

0.9 mL = x

Dimensional Analysis Method

$\dfrac{\overset{3}{\cancel{60}}\ \cancel{mg}}{\begin{array}{c}\underset{2}{\cancel{40}}\ \cancel{mg}\end{array}}\ \Big|\ \dfrac{0.6\ \cancel{mL}}{\ }\ \Big|\ \dfrac{3 \times 0.6}{2} = 0.9\ mL$

Formula Method *Ratio Method* *Proportion Method*

18. 0.5 g = 500 mg

$\dfrac{\overset{2}{\cancel{500}}\ \cancel{mg}}{\underset{1}{\cancel{250}}\ \cancel{mg}} \times 5\ mL = 10\ mL$ 5 mL : 250 mg : : x : 500 mg $\dfrac{5\ mL}{250\ mg} = \dfrac{x}{500\ mg}$

$\dfrac{2500}{250} = x$

10 mL = x

Dimensional Analysis Method

$\dfrac{0.5\ \cancel{g}}{\ }\ \Big|\ \dfrac{5\ \cancel{mL}}{\underset{1}{\cancel{250}}\ \cancel{mg}}\ \Big|\ \dfrac{\overset{4}{\cancel{1000}}\ \cancel{mg}}{1\ \cancel{g}}\ \Big|\ \dfrac{0.5 \times 5 \times 4}{} = 10\ mL$

Formula Method *Ratio Method* *Proportion Method*

19. $\dfrac{\overset{3}{\cancel{15}}\ \text{mg}}{\underset{10}{\cancel{50}}\ \text{mg}}\times 5\ \text{mL}=1.5\ \text{mL}$

5 mL : 50 mg : : x : 15 mg

$\dfrac{5\ \text{mL}}{50\ \text{mg}}=\dfrac{\text{x}}{15\ \text{mg}}$

$\dfrac{75}{50}=\text{x}$

1.5 mL = x

Dimensional Analysis Method

$\dfrac{15\ \text{mg}}{}\left|\dfrac{\overset{1}{\cancel{5}}\ \text{\textcircled{mL}}}{\underset{10}{\cancel{50}}\ \text{mg}}\right|\dfrac{15}{10}=1.5\ \text{mL}$

Formula Method *Ratio Method* *Proportion Method*

20. $\dfrac{\overset{2}{\cancel{50}}\ \text{mg}}{\underset{1}{\cancel{25}}\ \text{mg}}\times 5\ \text{mL}=10\ \text{mL}$

5 mL : 25 mg : : x : 50 mg

$\dfrac{5\ \text{mL}}{25\ \text{mg}}=\dfrac{\text{x}}{50\ \text{mg}}$

$\dfrac{250}{25}=\text{x}$

10 mL = x

Dimensional Analysis Method

$\dfrac{\overset{2}{\cancel{50}}\ \text{mg}}{}\left|\dfrac{5\ \text{\textcircled{mL}}}{\underset{1}{\cancel{25}}\ \text{mg}}\right|2\times 5=10\ \text{mL}$

Chapter 7

Test 1: Calculations of Liquid Injections (Test 1)

Formula Method *Ratio Method* *Proportion Method*

1. Equivalent 0.1 g = 100 mg

$\dfrac{\overset{1}{\cancel{100}}\ \text{mg}}{\underset{2}{\cancel{200}}\ \text{mg}}\times 3\ \text{mL}=\dfrac{3}{2}\overset{1.5}{\overline{\smash{\big)}3.0}}$

3 mL : 200 mg : : x : 100 mg

$\dfrac{3\ \text{mL}}{200\ \text{mg}}=\dfrac{\text{x}}{100\ \text{mg}}$

$\dfrac{300}{200}=\text{x}$

Give 1.5 mL IM.

1.5 mL = x

Dimensional Analysis Method

$\dfrac{0.1\ \cancel{\text{g}}}{}\left|\dfrac{3\ \text{\textcircled{mL}}}{\underset{1}{\cancel{200}}\ \text{mg}}\right|\dfrac{\overset{5}{\cancel{1000}}\ \text{mg}}{1\ \cancel{\text{g}}}\left|\ 0.1\times 3\times 5=1.5\ \text{mL}\right.$

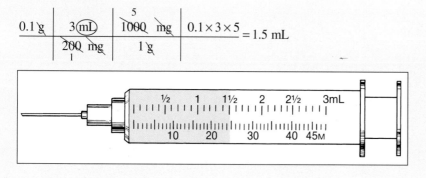

Formula Method   *Ratio Method*   *Proportion Method*

2. $\dfrac{\frac{1}{\cancel{5}}\ \text{mg}}{\frac{\cancel{15}}{3}\ \text{mg}} \times 1\ \text{mL} = \dfrac{1}{3} \overline{)\dfrac{.333}{1.000}}$ $\overset{\curvearrowright}{1\ \text{mL} : 15\ \text{mg} : : x : 5\ \text{mg}}$ $\dfrac{1\ \text{mL}}{15\ \text{mg}} = \dfrac{x}{5\ \text{mg}}$

$\dfrac{5}{15} = x$

Give 0.33 mL IV.   0.333 mL = x

Dimensional Analysis Method

$\dfrac{\frac{1}{\cancel{5}}\ \text{mg} \ \left|\ \dfrac{1\ \text{(mL)}}{\frac{\cancel{15}}{3}\ \text{mg}}\ \right|\ \dfrac{1}{3}\ \right.}{} = 0.33\ \text{mL}$

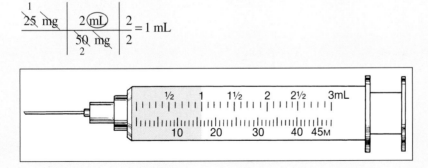

Formula Method   *Ratio Method*   *Proportion Method*

3. $\dfrac{\frac{1}{\cancel{25}}\ \text{mg}}{\frac{\cancel{50}}{2}\ \text{mg}} \times \overset{1}{\cancel{2}}\ \text{mL} = 1\ \text{mL}$ $\overset{\curvearrowright}{2\ \text{mL} : 50\ \text{mg} : : x : 25\ \text{mg}}$ $\dfrac{2\ \text{mL}}{50\ \text{mg}} = \dfrac{x}{25\ \text{mg}}$

$\dfrac{50}{50} = x$

Give 1 mL IM.   1 mL = x

Dimensional Analysis Method

$\dfrac{\frac{1}{\cancel{25}}\ \text{mg} \ \left|\ \dfrac{2\ \text{(mL)}}{\frac{\cancel{50}}{2}\ \text{mg}}\ \right|\ \dfrac{2}{2}\ \right.}{} = 1\ \text{mL}$

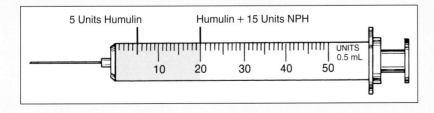

4. 20 units. Remember that Humulin insulin is a type of regular insulin and so must be drawn up first into the syringe.

Formula Method

Ratio Method

Proportion Method

5. 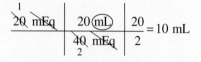 $\dfrac{\cancel{20}^{1} \text{ mEq}}{\cancel{40}_{2}^{1} \text{ mEq}} \times \cancel{20}^{10} \text{ mL} = 10 \text{ mL}$

20 mL : 40 mEq : : x : 20 mEq

$\dfrac{20 \text{ mL}}{40 \text{ mEq}} = \dfrac{x}{20 \text{ mEq}}$

$\dfrac{400}{40} = x$

Add 10 mL to IV.

$10 \text{ mL} = x$

Dimensional Analysis Method

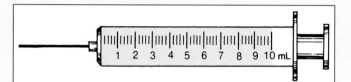 $\dfrac{\cancel{20}^{1} \text{ mEq}}{} \; \bigg| \; \dfrac{20 \,\widehat{\text{mL}}}{\cancel{40}_{2} \text{ mEq}} \; \bigg| \; \dfrac{20}{2} = 10 \text{ mL}$

![syringe marked 1 2 3 4 5 6 7 8 9 10 mL]

Formula Method

Ratio Method

Proportion Method

6. 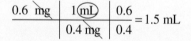 $\dfrac{0.6 \text{ mg}}{\cancel{0.4}_{2} \text{ mg}}^{3} \times 1 \text{ mL} = \dfrac{3}{2}\overline{\smash{)}\begin{array}{r} 1.5 \\ 3.0 \end{array}}$

1 mL : 0.4 mg : : x : 0.6 mg

$\dfrac{1 \text{ mL}}{0.4 \text{ mg}} = \dfrac{x}{0.6 \text{ mg}}$

$\dfrac{0.6}{0.4} = x$

Give 1.5 mL subcutaneous.

$1.5 \text{ mL} = x$

Dimensional Analysis Method

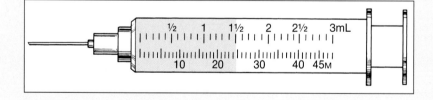 $\dfrac{0.6 \text{ mg}}{} \; \bigg| \; \dfrac{1 \,\widehat{\text{mL}}}{0.4 \text{ mg}} \; \bigg| \; \dfrac{0.6}{0.4} = 1.5 \text{ mL}$

![syringe marked ½ 1 1½ 2 2½ 3mL and 10 20 30 40 45m]

Formula Method   *Ratio Method*   *Proportion Method*

7. $\dfrac{\overset{2}{\cancel{0.8}}\ \cancel{mg}}{\underset{1}{\cancel{0.4}}\ \cancel{mg}} \times 1\ mL = 2\ mL$ $\overset{\longleftrightarrow}{1\ mL : 0.4\ mg :: x : 0.8\ mg}$ $\dfrac{1\ mL}{0.4\ mg} = \dfrac{x}{0.8\ mg}$

$\dfrac{0.8}{0.4} = x$

Give 2 mL IV. $2\ mL = x$

Dimensional Analysis Method

$\dfrac{0.8\ \cancel{mg}}{} \left|\ \dfrac{1\ \cancel{mL}}{0.4\ \cancel{mg}}\ \right|\ \dfrac{0.8}{0.4} = 2\ mL$

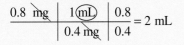

8. Equivalent 0.5 g = 500 mg

Formula Method   *Ratio Method*   *Proportion Method*

$\dfrac{\overset{2}{\cancel{500}}\ \cancel{mg}}{\underset{1}{\cancel{250}}\ \cancel{mg}} \times 1\ mL = 2\ mL$ $\overset{\longleftrightarrow}{1\ mL : 250\ mg :: x : 500\ mg}$ $\dfrac{1\ mL}{250\ mg} = \dfrac{x}{500\ mg}$

$\dfrac{500}{250} = x$

$2\ mL = x$

Dimensional Analysis Method

$\dfrac{0.5\ \cancel{g}}{} \left|\ \dfrac{1\ \cancel{mL}}{250\ \cancel{mg}}\ \right|\ \dfrac{\overset{4}{\cancel{1000}}\ \cancel{mg}}{1\ \cancel{g}}\ \right|\ 0.5 \times 4 = 2\ mL$

Add 2 mL to IV. Were you confused by the 25%? No reason to use it to solve this problem!

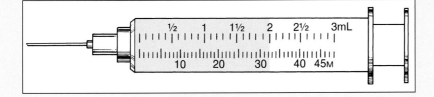

Formula Method   *Ratio Method*   *Proportion Method*

9. $\dfrac{200 \text{ mg}}{300 \text{ mg}} \times 2 \text{ mL} = \dfrac{4}{5} \overline{\smash{\big)}4.0}^{\,.8}$ $2 \text{ mL} : 500 \text{ mg} :: x : 200 \text{ mg}$ $\dfrac{2 \text{ mL}}{500 \text{ mg}} = \dfrac{x}{200 \text{ mg}}$

$$\dfrac{400}{500} = x$$

$$0.8 \text{ mL} = x$$

Dimensional Analysis Method

$$\dfrac{200 \text{ mg}}{} \left| \dfrac{2 \text{ mL}}{500 \text{ mg}} \right| \dfrac{2 \times 2}{5} = 0.8 \text{ mL}$$

Give 0.8 mL IM.

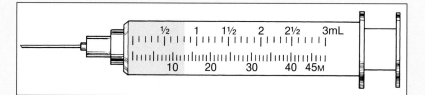

10. Equivalent 1:100 means   1 g in 100 mL

1 g = 1000 mg

Hence, the solution is 1000 mg/100 mL.

Formula Method   *Ratio Method*   *Proportion Method*

$\dfrac{7.5 \text{ mg}}{1000 \text{ mg}} \times 100 \text{ mL} = \dfrac{7.5}{10} \overline{\smash{\big)}7.50}^{\,.75}$ $100 \text{ mL} : 1000 \text{ mg} :: x : 7.5 \text{ mg}$ $\dfrac{100 \text{ mL}}{1000 \text{ mg}} = \dfrac{x}{7.5 \text{ mg}}$

$$\begin{array}{r} 7\ 0 \\ \hline 50 \\ 50 \\ \hline \end{array}$$

$$\dfrac{7500}{1000} = x$$

$$0.75 \text{ or } 0.8 \text{ mL} = x$$

Dimensional Analysis Method

$$\dfrac{7.5 \text{ mg}}{} \left| \dfrac{\overset{1}{100} \text{ mL}}{1 \text{ g}} \right| \dfrac{1 \text{ g}}{\underset{10}{1000} \text{ mg}} \left| \dfrac{7.5}{10} \right. = 0.75 \text{ or } 0.8 \text{ mL}$$

Give 0.8 mL subcutaneous.

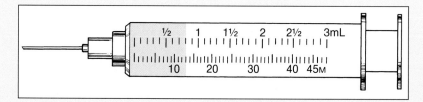

Test 2: Calculations of Liquid Injections (Test 2)

Formula Method   *Ratio Method*   *Proportion Method*

1. $\dfrac{\overset{2}{\cancel{10}} \text{ mg}}{\underset{3}{\cancel{15}} \text{ mg}} \times 1 \text{ mL} = \dfrac{2}{3}\overline{\smash{)}\,0.66}_{\,2.00}$

$1 \text{ mL} : 15 \text{ mg} :: x : 10 \text{ mg}$

$\dfrac{1 \text{ mL}}{15 \text{ mg}} = \dfrac{x}{10 \text{ mg}}$

$\dfrac{10}{15} = x$

$0.66 \text{ or } 0.7 \text{ mL} = x$

Dimensional Analysis Method

$\dfrac{10 \text{ mg}}{\vphantom{x}} \bigg| \dfrac{1 \text{ \textcircled{mL}}}{15 \text{ mg}} \bigg| \dfrac{10}{15} = 0.66 \text{ or } 0.7 \text{ mL}$

Give 0.7 mL IV.

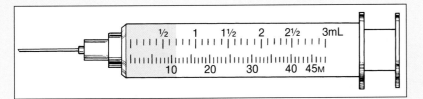

Formula Method   *Ratio Method*   *Proportion Method*

2. $\dfrac{\overset{1}{\cancel{25}} \text{ mg}}{\underset{4}{\cancel{100}} \text{ mg}} \times 1 \text{ mL} = \dfrac{1}{4}\overline{\smash{)}\,0.25}_{\,1.00}$

$1 \text{ mL} : 100 \text{ mg} :: x : 25 \text{ mg}$

$\dfrac{1 \text{ mL}}{100 \text{ mg}} = \dfrac{x}{25 \text{ mg}}$

$\dfrac{25}{100} = x$

$0.25 \text{ mL} = x$

Dimensional Analysis Method

$\dfrac{\overset{1}{\cancel{25}} \text{ mg}}{\vphantom{x}} \bigg| \dfrac{1 \text{ \textcircled{mL}}}{\underset{4}{\cancel{100}} \text{ mg}} \bigg| \dfrac{1}{4} = 0.25 \text{ mL}$

Give 0.25 mL. You are using a 1-mL precision syringe;
therefore, the answer is solved to the nearest hundredth.

3. Equivalent 0.1 g = 100 mg

Formula Method

$$\frac{\overset{1}{\cancel{100}}\ mg}{\underset{2}{\cancel{200}}\ mg} \times 3\ mL = \frac{3}{2} \overset{1.5}{\overline{)3.0}}$$

Ratio Method

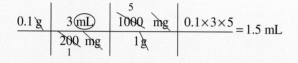

3 mL : 200 mg : : x : 100 mg

Proportion Method

$$\frac{3\ mL}{200\ mg} = \frac{x}{100\ mg}$$

$$\frac{300}{200} = x$$

1.5 mL = x

Dimensional Analysis Method

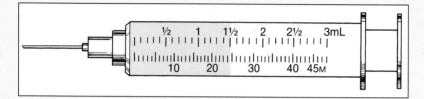

$$\frac{0.1\ \cancel{g}}{} \left| \frac{3\ \text{ⓜⓛ}}{\underset{1}{\cancel{200}}\ \cancel{mg}} \right| \frac{\overset{5}{\cancel{1000}}\ \cancel{mg}}{1\ \cancel{g}} \right| \frac{0.1 \times 3 \times 5}{} = 1.5\ mL$$

Give 1.5 mL IM.

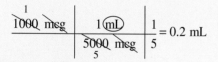

Formula Method

4. $\frac{\overset{1}{\cancel{1000}}\ mcg}{\underset{5}{\cancel{5000}}\ mcg} \times 1\ mL = \frac{1}{5} \overset{0.2}{\overline{)1.0}}$

Ratio Method

1 mL : 5000 mcg : : x : 1000 mcg

Proportion Method

$$\frac{1\ mL}{5000\ mcg} = \frac{x}{1000\ mcg}$$

$$\frac{1000}{5000} = x$$

0.2 mL = x

Dimensional Analysis Method

$$\frac{\overset{1}{\cancel{1000}}\ \cancel{mcg}}{} \left| \frac{1\ \text{ⓜⓛ}}{\underset{5}{\cancel{5000}}\ \cancel{mcg}} \right| \frac{1}{5} = 0.2\ mL$$

Give 0.2 mL IM.

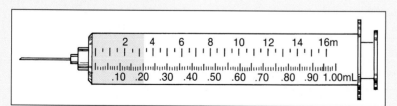

5. Equivalent 1% means   1 g in 100 mL

$$1 \text{ g} = 1000 \text{ mg}$$

Hence, the solution is 1000 mg in 100 mL.

Formula Method

$$\frac{\overset{5}{\cancel{25}} \text{ mg}}{\underset{\underset{2}{10}}{\cancel{1000}} \text{ mg}} \times \overset{1}{\cancel{100}} \text{ mL} = \frac{5}{2} \overset{2.5}{\overline{)5.0}}$$

Ratio Method

100 mL : 1000 mg : : x : 25 mg

Proportion Method

$$\frac{100 \text{ mL}}{1000 \text{ mg}} = \frac{\text{x}}{25 \text{ mg}}$$

$$\frac{2500}{1000} = \text{x}$$

$$2.5 \text{ mL} = \text{x}$$

Dimensional Analysis Method

$$\frac{25 \,\cancel{\text{mg}}}{} \left| \frac{\overset{1}{\cancel{100}} \text{ (mL)}}{\cancel{1} \text{ g}} \right| \frac{\cancel{1} \text{ g}}{\underset{10}{\cancel{1000}} \text{ mg}} \left| \frac{25}{10} \right. = 2.5 \text{ mL}$$

Prepare 2.5 mL.

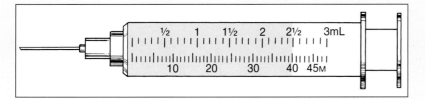

Formula Method

6. $\frac{0.5 \,\text{mg}}{0.4 \,\text{mg}} \times 1 \text{ mL} = \frac{5}{4} \overset{1.25}{\overline{)5.00}}$

Ratio Method

1 mL : 0.4 mg : : x : 0.5 mg

Proportion Method

$$\frac{1 \text{ mL}}{0.4 \text{ mg}} = \frac{\text{x}}{0.5 \text{ mg}}$$

$$\frac{0.5 \text{ mg}}{0.4 \text{ mg}} = \text{x}$$

1.25 or 1.3 mL = x

Dimensional Analysis Method

$$\frac{0.5 \,\cancel{\text{mg}}}{} \left| \frac{1 \text{ (mL)}}{0.4 \,\cancel{\text{mg}}} \right| \frac{0.5}{0.4} = 1.25 \text{ or } 1.3 \text{ mL}$$

Give 1.3 mL subcutaneous.

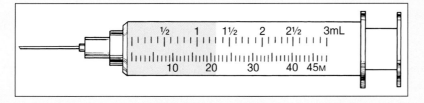

7. 13 units. Remember that Humulin insulin is a type of regular insulin and so must be drawn up first into the syringe!

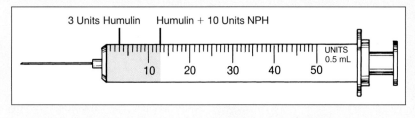

Formula Method

8. $\dfrac{1.2\ \cancel{mEq}}{0.5\ \cancel{mEq}} \times 1\ mL = 0.5\overline{)\begin{array}{c}2.4\\1.20\end{array}}$ ← 1.2

Ratio Method

1 mL : 0.5 mEq : : x : 1.2 mEq

Proportion Method

$\dfrac{1\ mL}{0.5\ mEq} \times \dfrac{x}{1.2\ mEq}$

$\dfrac{1.2}{0.5} = x$

$2.4\ mL = x$

Dimensional Analysis Method

$\dfrac{1.2\ \cancel{mEq}}{} \left|\ \dfrac{1\ \cancel{mL}}{0.5\ \cancel{mEq}}\ \right|\ \dfrac{1.2}{0.5} = 2.4\ mL$

Add 2.4 mL to the IV stat.

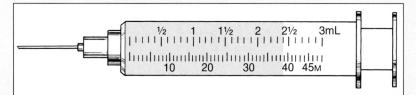

Formula Method

9. $\dfrac{\overset{3}{\cancel{75\ mg}}}{\underset{2}{\cancel{50\ mg}}} \times 1\ mL = 2\overline{)\begin{array}{c}1.5\\3.0\end{array}}$

Ratio Method

1 mL : 50 mg : : x : 75 mg

Proportion Method

$\dfrac{1\ mL}{50\ mg} \times \dfrac{x}{75\ mg}$

$\dfrac{75}{50} = x$

1.5 mL = x

Dimensional Analysis Method

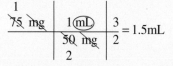 = 1.5mL

Give 1.5 mL IM.

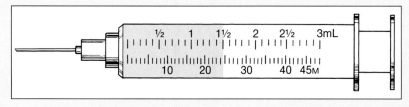

10. Equivalent 1:1000 means   1 g in 1000 mL

                                      1 g = 1000 mg

Hence, the solution is 1000 mg in 1000 mL.

500 mcg = 0.5 mg

Formula Method	*Ratio Method*	*Proportion Method*

Formula Method

$$\frac{0.5\,\text{mg}}{\cancel{1000}\,\text{mg}} \times \overset{1}{\cancel{1000}}\ \text{mL} = 0.5\ \text{mL}$$

Ratio Method

1000 mL : 1000 mg : : x : 0.5 mg

Proportion Method

$$\frac{1000\ \text{mL}}{1000\ \text{mg}} = \frac{x}{0.5\ \text{mg}}$$

$$1000 \times 0.5\ \text{mg} = 1000\text{x}$$

$$\frac{500}{1000} = \text{x}$$

$$0.5\ \text{mL} = \text{x}$$

Dimensional Analysis Method

$$\frac{1}{\cancel{500}\ \cancel{\text{mcg}}} \left| \frac{\cancel{1000}\ \cancel{\text{mL}}}{1\ \cancel{\text{g}}} \right| \frac{1\ \cancel{\text{g}}}{\cancel{1000}\ \cancel{\text{mg}}} \left| \frac{1\ \cancel{\text{mg}}}{\cancel{1000}\ \cancel{\text{mcg}}} \right| \frac{1}{2} = 0.5\ \text{mL}$$

Give 0.5 mL subcutaneous stat.

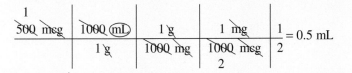

Test 3: Calculations of Liquid Injections (Test 3)

Formula Method

1. $\dfrac{\overset{1}{\cancel{0.25}}\ \text{mg}}{\underset{\underset{1}{2}}{\cancel{0.50}}\ \text{mg}} \times \overset{1}{\cancel{2}}\ \text{mL} = 1\ \text{mL}$

Ratio Method

2 mL : 0.5 mg : : x : 0.25 mg

Proportion Method

$$\frac{2\ \text{mL}}{0.5\ \text{mg}} \times \frac{x}{0.25\ \text{mg}}$$

$$\frac{0.50}{0.50} = \text{x}$$

$$1\ \text{mL} = \text{x}$$

Dimensional Analysis Method

$$\frac{1}{\cancel{0.25}\ \text{mg}} \left| \frac{2\ \cancel{\text{mL}}}{\underset{2}{\cancel{0.5}}\ \text{mg}} \right| \frac{2}{2} = 1\ \text{mL}$$

Formula Method   *Ratio Method*   *Proportion Method*

2. $\dfrac{40 \text{ mg}}{50 \text{ mg}} \times 2 \text{ mL} = \dfrac{8}{5}\overline{)8.0}^{1.6} = 1.6 \text{ mL}$

2 mL : 50 mg : : x : 40 mg

$\dfrac{2 \text{ mL}}{50 \text{ mg}} = \dfrac{x}{40 \text{ mg}}$

$\dfrac{80}{50} = x$

$1.6 \text{ mL} = x$

Dimensional Analysis Method

$\dfrac{40 \text{ mg}}{} \left|\dfrac{2 \text{ mL}}{50 \text{ mg}}\right|\dfrac{4 \times 2}{5} = \dfrac{8}{5} = 1.6 \text{ mL}$

Formula Method   *Ratio Method*   *Proportion Method*

3. $\dfrac{8 \text{ mg}}{15 \text{ mg}} \times 1 \text{ mL} = \dfrac{8}{15}\overline{)8.00}^{0.53} = 0.5 \text{ mL}$

$\dfrac{7\ 5}{50}$
$\dfrac{}{45}$

1 mL : 15 mg : : x : 8 mg

$\dfrac{1 \text{ mL}}{15 \text{ mg}} \times \dfrac{x}{8 \text{ mg}}$

$\dfrac{8}{15} = x$

0.53 or 0.5 mL = x

Dimensional Analysis Method

$\dfrac{8 \text{ mg}}{} \left|\dfrac{1 \text{ mL}}{15 \text{ mg}}\right|\dfrac{8}{15} = 0.53 \text{ or } 0.5 \text{ mL}$

Formula Method   *Ratio Method*   *Proportion Method*

4. $\dfrac{\frac{1}{25} \text{ mg}}{\frac{100}{4} \text{ mg}} \times 1 \text{ mL} = \dfrac{1}{4}\overline{)1.00}^{0.25} = 0.25 \text{ mL}$

1 mL : 100 mg : : x : 25 mg

$\dfrac{1 \text{ mL}}{100 \text{ mg}} \times \dfrac{x}{25 \text{ mg}}$

$\dfrac{25}{100} = x$

0.25 mL = x

Dimensional Analysis Method

$\dfrac{\frac{1}{25} \text{ mg}}{} \left|\dfrac{1 \text{ mL}}{\frac{100}{4} \text{ mg}}\right|\dfrac{1}{4} = 0.25 \text{ mL}$

Use the 1-mL precision syringe.

Formula Method   *Ratio Method*   *Proportion Method*

5. $\dfrac{200 \text{ mg}}{500 \text{ mg}} \times 2 \text{ mL}$ $\overset{4}{} \dfrac{0.8}{5 \overline{)4.0}} = 0.8 \text{ mL}$ $2 \text{ mL} : 500 \text{ mg} :: x : 200 \text{ mg}$ $\dfrac{2 \text{ mL}}{500 \text{ mg}} = \dfrac{x}{200 \text{ mg}}$

$$\dfrac{400}{500} = x$$

$$0.8 \text{ mL} = x$$

Dimensional Analysis Method

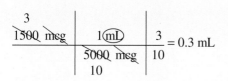

$$\dfrac{200 \text{ mg}}{} \Bigg| \dfrac{2 \text{ mL}}{500 \text{ mg}} \Bigg| \dfrac{2 \times 2}{5} = \dfrac{4}{5} = 0.8 \text{ mL}$$

Formula Method   *Ratio Method*   *Proportion Method*

6. $\dfrac{\overset{3}{1500 \text{ mcg}}}{\underset{10}{5000 \text{ mcg}}} \times 1 \text{ mL} = \overset{3}{} \dfrac{0.3}{10 \overline{)3.0}} = 0.3 \text{ mL}$ $1 \text{ mL} : 5000 \text{ mcg} :: x : 1500 \text{ mcg}$ $\dfrac{1 \text{ mL}}{5000 \text{ mcg}} = \dfrac{x}{1500 \text{ mcg}}$

$$\dfrac{1500}{5000} = x$$

$$0.3 \text{ mL} = x$$

Dimensional Analysis Method

$$\dfrac{\overset{3}{1500 \text{ mcg}}}{} \Bigg| \dfrac{1 \text{ mL}}{\underset{10}{5000 \text{ mcg}}} \Bigg| \dfrac{3}{10} = 0.3 \text{ mL}$$

Formula Method   *Ratio Method*   *Proportion Method*

7. $\dfrac{\overset{3}{0.6 \text{ mg}}}{\underset{2}{0.4 \text{ mg}}} \times 1 \text{ mL} = \overset{3}{} \dfrac{1.5}{2 \overline{)3.0}} = 1.5 \text{ mL}$ $1 \text{ mL} : 0.4 \text{ mg} :: x : 0.6 \text{ mg}$ $\dfrac{1 \text{ mL}}{0.4 \text{ mg}} = \dfrac{x}{0.6 \text{ mg}}$

$$\dfrac{0.6}{0.4} = x$$

$$1.5 \text{ mL} = x$$

Dimensional Analysis Method

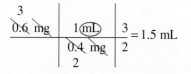

$$\dfrac{\overset{3}{0.6 \text{ mg}}}{} \Bigg| \dfrac{1 \text{ mL}}{\underset{2}{0.4 \text{ mg}}} \Bigg| \dfrac{3}{2} = 1.5 \text{ mL}$$

Formula Method *Ratio Method* *Proportion Method*

8. $0.1\ g = 100\ mg$

$$\frac{\overset{1}{\cancel{100\ mg}}}{\underset{2}{\cancel{200\ mg}}} \times 3\ mL = \overset{3}{2}\overline{)3.0}^{\,1.5} = 1.5\ mL$$

$3\ mL : 200\ mg :: x : 100\ mg$

$$\frac{3\ mL}{200\ mg} = \frac{x}{100\ mg}$$

$$\frac{300}{200} = x$$

$$1.5\ mL = x$$

Dimensional Analysis Method

$$\frac{0.1\ \cancel{g}}{} \left|\ \frac{3\ \cancel{mL}}{200\ \cancel{mg}}\ \right|\ \frac{\overset{5}{\cancel{1000}}\ \cancel{mg}}{1\ \cancel{g}}\ \right|\ \frac{0.1 \times 3 \times 5}{} = 1.5\ mL$$

Formula Method *Ratio Method* *Proportion Method*

9. $$\frac{\overset{3}{\cancel{1.5\ mg}}}{\underset{4}{\cancel{2.0\ mg}}} \times 1\ mL = \overset{3}{4}\overline{)3.00}^{\,0.75} = 0.75\ mL$$

$1\ mL : 2\ mg :: x : 1.5\ mg$

$$\frac{1\ mL}{2\ mg} = \frac{x}{1.5\ mg}$$

$$\frac{1.5}{2} = x$$

$$0.75 = x$$

Dimensional Analysis Method

$$\frac{1.5\ \cancel{mg}}{}\ \left|\ \frac{1\ \cancel{mL}}{2\ \cancel{mg}}\ \right|\ \frac{1.5}{2} = 0.75\ mL$$

Use a 1-mL precision syringe.

Formula Method *Ratio Method* *Proportion Method*

10. $\dfrac{600,000\ \cancel{units}}{500,000\ \cancel{units}} \times 1\ mL$

$1\ mL : 500,000\ units :: x : 600,000\ units$

$$\frac{1\ mL}{500,000\ units} = \frac{x}{600,000\ units}$$

$= \overset{6}{5}\overline{)6.0}^{\,1.2} = 1.2\ mL$

$$\frac{6\cancel{00,000}}{5\cancel{00,000}} = x$$

$$1.2\ mL = x$$

Dimensional Analysis Method

$$\frac{6\cancel{00,000}\ \cancel{units}}{}\ \left|\ \frac{1\ \cancel{mL}}{5\cancel{00,000}\ \cancel{units}}\ \right|\ \frac{6}{5} = 1.2\ mL$$

Formula Method   *Ratio Method*   *Proportion Method*

11. 200 mcg = 0.2 mg

$$\frac{\overset{1}{0.\cancel{2}\text{ mg}}}{\underset{4}{0.\cancel{8}\text{ mg}}}\times 1\text{ mL} = \overset{1}{4}\overline{)\overset{0.25}{1.00}} = 0.25\text{ mL}$$

$\overset{\longleftrightarrow}{1\text{ mL} : 0.8\text{ mg} :: x : 0.2\text{ mg}}$

$$\frac{1\text{ mL}}{0.8\text{ mg}} = \frac{x}{0.2\text{ mg}}$$

$$\frac{0.2}{0.8} = x$$

$$0.25\text{ mL} = x$$

Dimensional Analysis Method

$$\frac{1}{\underset{}{\cancel{200}\text{ mcg}}}\Bigg|\frac{1\,\text{mL}}{0.8\text{ mg}}\Bigg|\frac{1\text{ mg}}{\underset{5}{\cancel{1000}\text{ mcg}}}\Bigg|\frac{1}{0.8\times 5}\Bigg|\frac{1}{4} = 0.25\text{ mL}$$

12. 1:4000 means   1 g in 4000 mL

                   1 g = 1000 mg

                   500 mcg = 0.5 mg

Formula Method   *Ratio Method*   *Proportion Method*

$$\frac{0.5\text{ mg}}{\underset{1}{1000\text{ mg}}}\times\overset{4}{\cancel{4000}}\text{ mL} = \frac{\begin{array}{c}0.5\\ \times 4\end{array}}{2.0\text{ mL}}$$

$\overset{\longleftrightarrow}{4000\text{ mL} : 1000\text{ mg} :: x : 0.5\text{ mg}}$

$$\frac{4000\text{ mL}}{1000\text{ mg}}\times\frac{x}{0.5\text{ mg}}$$

$$\frac{2000}{1000} = 2\text{ mL}$$

Dimensional Analysis Method

$$\frac{1}{\cancel{500}\text{ mcg}}\Bigg|\frac{\overset{4}{\cancel{4000}}\,\text{mL}}{1\text{ g}}\Bigg|\frac{1\text{ g}}{\underset{2}{\cancel{1000}\text{ mg}}}\Bigg|\frac{1\text{ mg}}{\underset{1}{\cancel{1000}\text{ mcg}}}\Bigg|\frac{4}{2} = 2\text{ mL}$$

Formula Method   *Ratio Method*   *Proportion Method*

13. $\dfrac{3\text{ mg}}{2\text{ mg}}\times 1\text{ mL} = \overset{3}{2}\overline{)\overset{1.5}{3.0}} = 1.5\text{ mL}$

$\overset{\longleftrightarrow}{1\text{ mL} : 2\text{ mg} :: x : 3\text{ mg}}$

$$\frac{1\text{ mL}}{2\text{ mg}} = \frac{x}{3\text{ mg}}$$

$$\frac{3}{2} = x$$

$$1.5\text{ mL} = x$$

Dimensional Analysis Method

$$\frac{3\text{ mg}}{}\Bigg|\frac{1\,\text{mL}}{2\text{ mg}}\Bigg|\frac{3}{2} = 1.5\text{ mL}$$

14. 1:1000 means   1 g = 1000 mL

1 g = 1000 mg

Formula Method

$$\frac{0.4\,\text{mg}}{1000\,\text{mg}} \times \overset{1}{1000}\,\text{mL} = 0.4\,\text{mL}$$

Ratio Method

1000 mL : 1000 mg : : x : 0.4 mg

Proportion Method

$$\frac{1000\,\text{mL}}{1000\,\text{mg}} = \frac{x}{0.4\,\text{mg}}$$

$$\frac{400}{1000} = x$$

$$0.4\,\text{mL} = x$$

Dimensional Analysis Method

$$\frac{0.4\,\text{mg}}{} \left| \frac{\overset{1}{1000\,\text{mL}}}{1\,\text{g}} \right| \frac{1\,\text{g}}{1000\,\text{mg}} \left| \frac{0.4}{1} \right. = 0.4\,\text{mL}$$

Use a 1-mL precision syringe.

15. 50% means   50 g in 100 mL

500 mg = 0.5 g

Formula Method

$$\frac{0.5\,\text{g}}{\underset{1}{50\,\text{g}}} \times \overset{2}{100}\,\text{mL} = 1\,\text{mL}$$

Ratio Method

100 mL : 50 g : : x : 0.5 g

Proportion Method

$$\frac{100\,\text{mL}}{50\,\text{g}} = \frac{x}{0.5\,\text{g}}$$

$$\frac{50\,\text{g}}{50\,\text{g}} = x$$

$$1\,\text{mL} = x$$

Dimensional Analysis Method

$$\frac{1}{500\,\text{mg}} \left| \frac{\overset{2}{100\,\text{mL}}}{\underset{1}{50\,\text{g}}} \right| \frac{1\,\text{g}}{\underset{2}{1000\,\text{mg}}} \left| \frac{2}{2} \right. = 1\,\text{mL}$$

Formula Method

16. $\dfrac{\overset{1}{\cancel{0.75 \text{ mg}}}}{\underset{2}{\cancel{1.50 \text{ mg}}}} \times 1 \text{ mL} = \frac{1}{2} \text{ mL or } 0.5 \text{ mL}$

Ratio Method

1 mL : 1.5 mg : : x : 0.75 mg

Proportion Method

$\dfrac{1 \text{ mL}}{1.5 \text{ mg}} = \dfrac{\text{x}}{0.75 \text{ mg}}$

$\dfrac{0.75}{1.5} = \text{x}$

0.5 mL = x

Dimensional Analysis Method

$\dfrac{\overset{1}{\cancel{0.75}} \text{ mg}}{} \left| \dfrac{1 \text{ mL}}{\underset{2}{\cancel{1.5}} \text{ mg}} \right| \dfrac{1}{2} = 0.5 \text{ mL}$

Use a 1-mL precision syringe.

17. 20% means   20 g in 100 mL

100 mg = 0.1 g

Formula Method

$\dfrac{0.1 \text{ g}}{\underset{1}{\cancel{20}} \text{ g}} \times \overset{5}{\cancel{100}} \text{ mL} = 0.5 \text{ mL}$

Ratio Method

100 mL : 20 g : : x : 0.1 g

Proportion Method

$\dfrac{100 \text{ mL}}{20 \text{ g}} = \dfrac{\text{x}}{0.1 \text{ g}}$

$\dfrac{10}{20} = \text{x}$

0.5 mL = x

Dimensional Analysis Method

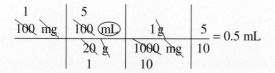

$\dfrac{1}{\cancel{100} \text{ mg}} \left| \dfrac{\overset{5}{\cancel{100}} \text{ mL}}{\underset{1}{\cancel{20}} \text{ g}} \right| \dfrac{1 \text{ g}}{\underset{10}{\cancel{1000}} \text{ mg}} \left| \dfrac{5}{10} \right. = 0.5 \text{ mL}$

Use a 1-mL precision syringe.

Formula Method

18. $\dfrac{\overset{1}{\cancel{0.125 \text{ mg}}}}{\underset{\underset{1}{2}}{\cancel{0.250 \text{ mg}}}} \times \overset{1}{\cancel{2}} \text{ mL} = 1 \text{ mL}$

Ratio Method

2 mL : 0.25 mg : : x : 0.125 mg

Proportion Method

$\dfrac{2 \text{ mL}}{0.25 \text{ mg}} = \dfrac{x}{0.125 \text{ mg}}$

$\dfrac{0.25}{0.25} = x$

$1 \text{ mL} = x$

Dimensional Analysis Method

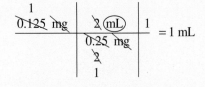

$= 1 \text{ mL}$

Formula Method

19. $\dfrac{\overset{6}{\cancel{12 \text{ mg}}}}{\underset{5}{\cancel{10 \text{ mg}}}} \times 1 \text{ mL} = \dfrac{\cancel{6}}{5} \overset{1.2}{\cancel{)6.0}} = 1.2 \text{ mL}$

Ratio Method

1 mL : 10 mg : : x : 12 mg

Proportion Method

$\dfrac{1 \text{ mL}}{10 \text{ mg}} = \dfrac{x}{12 \text{ mg}}$

$\dfrac{12}{10} = x$

$1.2 \text{ mL} = x$

Dimensional Analysis Method

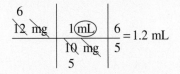

$= 1.2 \text{ mL}$

Formula Method

20. $\dfrac{\overset{5}{\cancel{10 \text{ mEq}}}}{\underset{\underset{1}{2}}{\cancel{40 \text{ mEq}}}} \times \overset{1}{\cancel{20}} \text{ mL} = 5 \text{ mL}$

Ratio Method

20 mL : 40 mEq : : x : 10 mEq

Proportion Method

$\dfrac{20 \text{ mL}}{40 \text{ mEq}} = \dfrac{x}{10 \text{ mEq}}$

$\dfrac{200}{40} = x$

$5 \text{ mL} = x$

Dimensional Analysis Method

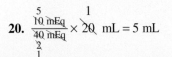

$= 5 \text{ mL}$

This is correct because the route is IV.

Test 4: Mental Drill in Liquids-for-Injection Problems

1. 2 mL IM

2. 5 mL IV

3. 2 mL IM

4. 1 mL IM

5. 0.5 mL IM

6. 1 mL IM

7. 0.75 mL or 0.8 mL subcutaneous

8. 1 mL subcutaneous

9. 20 mL IV

10. 2.5 mL IM

11. 0.8 mL IM

12. 2 mL IM

13. 2 mL IV

14. 1.5 mL IM

15. 1.5 mL IM

16. 0.35 mL or 0.4 mL IM

17. 1.5 mL subcutaneous

18. 1.5 mL IM

Test 5: Injections from Powders

1. a. 1.5 mL, sterile water

b. 280 mg/mL

c. *Formula Method*

$$\frac{250 \text{ mg}}{280 \text{ mg}} \times 1 \text{ mL} = A$$

$$0.89 \times 1 \text{ mL} = A$$

$$0.89 \text{ or } 0.9 \text{ mL} = A$$

Ratio Method

$$1 \text{ mL} : 280 \text{ mg} :: x : 250 \text{ mg}$$

Proportion Method

$$\frac{1 \text{ mL}}{280 \text{ mg}} = \frac{x}{250 \text{ mg}}$$

$$\frac{250}{280} = x$$

$$0.89 \text{ mL} = x$$

or

$$0.9 \text{ mL} = x$$

Dimensional Analysis Method

$$\frac{\overset{50}{\cancel{250}} \text{ mg}}{} \left| \frac{1 \text{(mL)}}{\underset{56}{\cancel{280}} \text{ mg}} \right| \frac{50}{56} = 0.89 \text{ or } 0.9 \text{ mL}$$

d. 0.9 mL

e. 280 mg/mL, date, time, initials

f. Refrigerate; stable for 7 days

2. a. 2 mL sterile water for injection

b. 1 g/2.6 mL

c. *Formula Method*

$$\frac{\cancel{1} \text{g}}{\cancel{1} \text{g}} \times 2.6 \text{ mL} = 2.6 \text{ mL}$$

Ratio Method

$$2.6 \text{ mL} : 1 \text{ g} :: x : 1 \text{ g}$$

Proportion Method

$$\frac{2.6 \text{ mL}}{1 \text{ g}} = \frac{x}{1 \text{ g}}$$

$$x = 2.6 \text{ mL}$$

Dimensional Analysis Method

$$\frac{1 \cancel{g}}{} \left| \frac{2.6 \text{(mL)}}{1 \cancel{g}} \right| \frac{2.6}{} = 2.6 \text{ mL}$$

   d. 2.6 mL

   e. Nothing is left in the vial.

   f. Discard the vial in a proper receptacle.

3. a. 1.8 mL sterile water for injection

   b. 250 mg/mL

   c. *Formula Method*

$$\frac{D}{H} \times S = A$$

$$\frac{\overset{6}{\cancel{300 \text{ mg}}}}{\underset{5}{\cancel{250 \text{ mg}}}} \times 1 \text{ mL} = \frac{6}{5}\overline{\smash{\big)}6.0}^{\,1.2}$$

Ratio Method

$$1 \text{ mL} : 250 \text{ mg} : : x : 300 \text{ mg}$$

Proportion Method

$$\frac{1 \text{ mL}}{250 \text{ mg}} = \frac{x}{300 \text{ mg}}$$

$$\frac{300}{250} = x$$

$$1.2 \text{ mL} = x$$

Dimensional Analysis Method

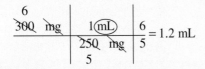

$$\frac{\overset{6}{\cancel{300}} \text{ mg}}{} \left| \frac{1 \text{ mL}}{\underset{5}{\cancel{250}} \text{ mg}} \right| \frac{6}{5} = 1.2 \text{ mL}$$

   d. 1.2 mL

   e. Nothing! Discard the vial. Directions say solution must be used within 1 hour.

   f. No. Discard the vial in an appropriate receptacle.

4. a. 2 mL sterile water for injection

   b. 400 mg/mL

   c. *Formula Method*

$$\frac{D}{H} \times S = A$$

$$\frac{300 \text{ mg}}{400 \text{ mg}} \times 1 \text{ mL} = \frac{3}{4}\overline{\smash{\big)}3.00}^{\,0.75} \text{ or } 0.8 \text{ mL}$$

Ratio Method

$$1 \text{ mL} : 400 \text{ mg} : : x : 300 \text{ mg}$$

Proportion Method

$$\frac{1 \text{ mL}}{400 \text{ mg}} = \frac{x}{300 \text{ mg}}$$

$$\frac{\cancel{300}}{\cancel{400}} = x$$

$$0.75 = x$$

or

$$0.8 \text{ mL}$$

Dimensional Analysis Method

$$\frac{\cancel{300} \text{ mg}}{} \left| \frac{1 \text{ mL}}{\cancel{400} \text{ mg}} \right| \frac{3}{4} = 0.75 \text{ or } 0.8 \text{ mL}$$

   d. 0.8 mL

   e. 400 mg/mL, date, time, initials

   f. Refrigerate; stable for 1 week

5. a. 2.5 mL sterile water for injection

   b. 330 mg/mL

   c. *Formula Method*

$$\frac{D}{H} \times S = A$$

0.33 g is 330 mg.

Ratio Method

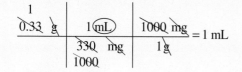

1 mL : 330 mg : : x : 330 mg

Proportion Method

$$\frac{1 \text{ mL}}{330 \text{ mg}} = \frac{x}{330 \text{ mg}}$$

$$\frac{330}{330} = x$$

$$1 \text{ mL} = x$$

Dimensional Analysis Method

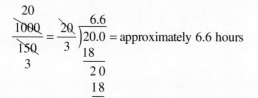

$$\frac{1}{0.33 \text{ g}} \left| \frac{1 \text{ mL}}{330 \text{ mg}} \right| \frac{1000 \text{ mg}}{1 \text{ g}} = 1 \text{ mL}$$

   d. 1 mL IM

   e. 330 mg/mL, date, time, initials

   f. Refrigerate; stable for 96 hours

Chapter 8

Test 1: Basic IV Problems

1. a. You have 1000 mL running at 150 mL/hr, therefore

$$\frac{1000}{150} = \frac{20}{3} \overset{\displaystyle 6.6}{\big)20.0} = \text{approximately 6.6 hours}$$

Dimensional Analysis Method

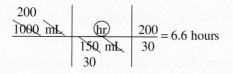

$$\frac{1000 \text{ mL}}{} \left| \frac{\text{hr}}{150 \text{ mL}} \right| \frac{200}{30} = 6.6 \text{ hours}$$

   b. $\frac{\# \text{mL} \times \text{TF}}{\# \text{min}} = \text{gtt/min}$

$$\frac{150 \times 10}{60} = 25 \text{gtt/min macro}$$

$$\frac{150 \times 60}{60} = 150 \text{gtt/min micro}$$

Choose macrotubing.

Dimensional Analysis Method

$$\frac{150 \text{ mL}}{\text{hr}} \left| \frac{\overset{1}{10} \text{ gtt}}{\text{mL}} \right| \frac{1 \text{ hr}}{\underset{6}{60} \text{ min}} \right| \frac{150}{6} = 25 \text{ gtt/min macro}$$

$$\frac{150 \text{ mL}}{\text{hr}} \left| \frac{60 \text{ gtt}}{\text{mL}} \right| \frac{1 \text{ hr}}{60 \text{ min}} = 150 \text{ gtt/min micro}$$

c. 25 gtt/min macro

Note: You could choose microtubing; however, the drip rate is hard to count.

2. a. Because the amount is small and will run over 6 hours, choose *microdrip tubing*.

b. Step 1.

$$\frac{\#\text{mL}}{\text{hr}} = \text{mL/hr} = 6\overset{16.6}{\overline{)100.0}} = 17 \text{ mL/hr}$$

$$\begin{array}{r} \underline{6} \\ 40 \\ \underline{36} \\ 4\,0 \\ \underline{3\,6} \end{array}$$

Step 2. $\dfrac{\#\text{mL/hr} \times \text{TF}}{\#\text{min}} = \dfrac{17 \times 60}{60} = 17 \text{ gtt/min}$

Dimensional Analysis Method

$$\frac{100 \text{ mL}}{6 \text{ hr}} \left| \frac{\overset{1}{60} \text{ gtt}}{\text{mL}} \right| \frac{1 \text{ hr}}{\underset{1}{60} \text{ min}} \right| \frac{100}{6} = 16.6 \text{ or } 17 \text{ gtt/min}$$

3. a. Because the stock bag is 250 mL NS, you would aseptically allow 100 mL to run off. This will leave 150 mL NS.

b. *Microdrip* because

Step 1. $\dfrac{\#\text{mL}}{\#\text{hr}} = \text{mL/hr}$ $\qquad \dfrac{150 \text{ mL}}{\underset{1}{3} \text{ hr}} = 50 \text{ mL/hr}$

Step 2. $\dfrac{\#\text{mL/hr} \times \text{TF}}{\#\text{min}} = \text{gtt/min}$

With microdrip, the # mL/hr = gtt/min; hence, microdrip would be 50 gtt/min.

Proof: $\dfrac{50 \times 60}{60} = 50 \text{ gtt/min}$

Macrodrip would be $\dfrac{50 \times \overset{1}{15}}{\underset{4}{60}}$

$$= 4\overset{12.5}{\overline{)50.0}} = 13 \text{ gtt/min}$$

$$\begin{array}{r} \underline{4} \\ 10 \\ \underline{8} \\ 20 \\ 20 \end{array}$$

c. 50 gtt/min (microdrip)

Note: It would not be incorrect to choose the macrodrip. However, 50 gtt/min provides a better flow.

Dimensional Analysis Method

$$\frac{50}{\cancel{150} \text{ mL}} \Bigg| \frac{\cancel{15} \text{gtt}}{\text{mL}} \Bigg| \frac{1 \text{ hr}}{\cancel{60} \text{ min}} \Bigg| \frac{50}{4} = 12.5 \text{ or } 13 \text{ gtt/min}$$

$$\frac{50}{\cancel{150} \text{ mL}} \Bigg| \frac{\cancel{60} \text{ gtt}}{\text{mL}} \Bigg| \frac{1 \text{ hr}}{\cancel{60} \text{ min}} \Bigg| \frac{50}{1} = 50 \text{ gtt/min}$$

4. 21 mL/hr

Logic Step 1. $\frac{\#\text{mL}}{\#\text{hr}} = \text{mL/hr}$

$$\frac{500 \text{ mL}}{24 \text{ hr}} \quad \begin{array}{r} 20.8 \\ 24\overline{)500.0} \\ \underline{48} \\ 20\ 0 \\ \underline{19\ 2} \end{array} = 21 \text{ mL/hr}$$

Step 2 is not necessary because you have an infusion pump that delivers milliliters per hour.

Dimensional Analysis Method

$$\frac{500 \text{ mL}}{24 \text{ hr}} \Bigg| \frac{500}{24} = 20.8 \text{ or } 21 \text{ mL/hr}$$

5. Use a reconstitution device to add 100 mg powder to 250 mL D5W and give IVPB over 1 hour (60 min); TF = 10 gtts/mL.

$\frac{\# \text{ mL} \times \text{TF}}{\#\text{min}} = \text{gtt/min}$

$$\frac{250 \times \cancel{10}}{\cancel{60}} = \frac{250}{6} \quad \begin{array}{r} 41.6 \\ 6\overline{)250.0} \end{array} = 42 \text{ gtt/min}$$

Label the IVPB.
Set the rate at 42 gtt/min.

Dimensional Analysis Method

$$\frac{250 \text{ mL}}{1 \text{ hr}} \Bigg| \frac{\cancel{10} \text{gtt}}{\text{mL}} \Bigg| \frac{1 \text{ hr}}{\cancel{60} \text{ min}} \Bigg| \frac{250}{6} = 41.6 \text{ or } 42 \text{ gtt/min}$$

6 a. Order is 500 mg. Stock is 1 g in 10 mL.

1 g = 1000 mg

Formula Method

$\frac{D}{H} \times S = A$ $\frac{500 \text{ mg}}{1000 \text{ mg}} \times 10 \text{ mL} = 5 \text{ mL}$

Ratio Method

10 mL : 1000 mg : : x : 500 mg

Proportion Method

$\frac{10 \text{ mL}}{1000 \text{ mg}} = \frac{x}{500}$

$\frac{5000}{1000} = x$

5 mL = x

Dimensional Analysis Method

$\frac{1}{50\!\!\!/0 \text{ mg}} \left| \frac{\overset{1}{10} \text{ } \cancel{(mL)}}{1 \cancel{g}} \right| \frac{1 \cancel{g}}{10\!\!\!/0\!\!\!/0 \text{ mg}} \left| \frac{\overset{10}{10}}{2} \right. = 5 \text{ mL}$

Add 5 mL aminophylline to make 500 mg in 250 mL D5W.

b. $\frac{\text{\# mL}}{\text{\# hr}} = \text{mL/hr}$

$\frac{250 \text{ mL}}{8 \text{ hr}} = 31.2 = 31 \text{ mL/hr}$

mL/hr = microgtt/min

No math necessary.

31 mL/hr = 31 gtt/min

Label IV.

Set the rate at 31 gtt/min.

Dimensional Analysis Method

$\frac{\overset{125}{25\!\!\!/0} \text{ } \cancel{(mL)}}{\underset{4}{8} \text{ } \cancel{(hr)}} \left| \frac{125}{4} \right. = 31 \text{ mL/hr}$

7.   2800 mL

Logic: The patient gets 125 mL/hr and there are 24 hours in a day; four times a day the patient receives Cefoxitin. That leaves 20 hours (24 − 4) times 125 mL/hr:

$\begin{array}{r} 125 \\ \times\ 20 \\ \hline 2500 \text{ mL} \end{array}$

The patient gets 75 mL q6h and, therefore, is receiving 75 mL four times in 24 hours.

So $\begin{array}{r} 75 \\ \times\ 4 \\ \hline 300 \end{array}$

$\begin{array}{r} 2500 \text{ mL} \\ +\ 300 \text{ mL} \\ \hline 2800 \text{ mL} \end{array}$

8. a. 90 mL/hr—no math necessary—pump

b.

$\frac{\text{total \# mL}}{\text{mL/hr}} = \text{hr}$

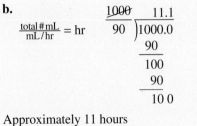

Dimensional Analysis Method

$\frac{1}{\cancel{(hr)}} \left| \frac{100\!\!\!/0 \text{ } \cancel{mL}}{9\!\!\!/0 \text{ } \cancel{mL}} \right| \frac{100}{9} = 11.1 \text{ hr}$

Approximately 11 hours

9. 50 mg

Logic: Have 0.5 g in 500 mL. Substitute milligrams for grams: 0.5 g = 500 mg. The solution is 500 mg in 500 mL. Reducing this means 1 mg in 1 mL. Because the patient is receiving 50 mL/hour, the patient is receiving 50 mg aminophylline per hour.

10. **a.** Need 75 mL D5W. Take a 100-mL bag of D5W and aseptically remove 25 mL. Add 5 mL Bactrim to the 75 mL. Time is 60 minutes. The order is 75 mL/hour. No math is necessary. You have a pump in milliliters per hour.

    Label the IVPB.

  b. Set the pump:

    Secondary volume (mL): 75

    Secondary rate (mL/hr): 75

    For 90 minutes: $\dfrac{75 \times 60}{90} = 50$ mL/hr

    Secondary volume (mL): 75

    Secondary rate (mL/hr): 50

Chapter 9

Test 1: Special IV Calculations

1. *Formula Method*

$$\frac{D}{H} \times S = A$$

$$\frac{15 \ \overline{units}/hr}{\underset{1}{\cancel{125} \ \overline{units}}} \times \overset{2}{\cancel{250}} \ mL = A$$

$15 \times 2 = 30$ mL/hr on a pump

Set the pump.

Total # mL: 250

mL/hr: 30

Ratio Method

250 mL : 125 units : : x : 15 units

Proportion Method

$$\frac{x \ mL}{15 \ units} = \frac{250 \ mL}{125 \ units}$$

$$\frac{3750}{125} = x$$

30 mL/hr

Dimensional Analysis Method

$$\frac{15 \ \overline{units}}{\cancel{hr}} \bigg| \frac{\overset{2}{\cancel{250}} \ \cancel{mL}}{\underset{1}{\cancel{125} \ \overline{units}}} \bigg| \ 15 \times 2 = 30 \ mL/hr$$

2. *Formula Method*

$$\frac{D}{H} \times S = A$$

$$\frac{\overset{3}{\cancel{1500}} \ \overline{units}/hr}{\underset{\underset{1}{50}}{\cancel{25000} \ \overline{units}}} \times \overset{10}{\cancel{500}} = 30 \ mL/hr$$

Ratio Method

500 mL : 25000 units : : x : 1500 units

Proportion Method

$$\frac{x \ mL}{1500 \ units} = \frac{500 \ mL}{\underset{50}{\cancel{25000}}}$$

$$\frac{750,000}{25,000} = x$$

30 mL/hr = x

Dimensional Analysis Method

$$\frac{30 \quad \cancel{1500} \text{ units}}{\cancel{\text{hr}}} \Bigg| \frac{1}{\cancel{500} \text{ (mL)}} \Bigg| \frac{30}{1} = 30 \text{ mL/h}$$
$$\frac{\cancel{25000} \text{ units}}{\cancel{50}}$$

Set the pump.

Total # mL = 500 mL

mL/hr = 30

3. Logic: Infusion pumps are set in milliliters per hour so multiply

2 mg/min × 60 minutes = 120 mg/hr

2 g = 2000 mg

Formula Method

$$\frac{D}{H} \times S = A$$

$$\frac{\overset{1}{\cancel{120} \text{ mg/hr}}}{\underset{4}{\cancel{2000} \text{ mg}}} \times \cancel{500} \text{ mL} = 30 \text{ mL/hr on a pump}$$

Ratio Method

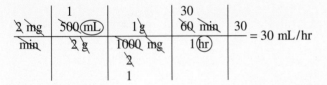

500 mL : 2000 mg : : x : 120 mg

Proportion Method

$$\frac{500 \text{ mL}}{2000 \text{ mg}} = \frac{x}{120 \text{ mg}}$$

$$\frac{60000}{2000} = x$$

$$\frac{120}{4} = x$$

30 mL = x

Dimensional Analysis Method

$$\frac{\cancel{2} \text{ mg}}{\cancel{\text{min}}} \Bigg| \frac{1}{\cancel{500} \text{ (mL)}} \Bigg| \frac{1 \text{ g}}{\cancel{1000} \text{ mg}} \Bigg| \frac{30}{60 \text{ min}} \Bigg| \frac{30}{1 \text{ (hr)}} = 30 \text{ mL/hr}$$

Set the pump.

Total # mL: 500

mL/hr: 30

4. Add diltiazem to the IV.

Formula Method

$$\frac{D}{H} \times S = A$$

$$\frac{\overset{25}{\cancel{125} \text{ mg}}}{\underset{1}{\cancel{5} \text{ mg}}} \times 1 \text{ mL} = 25 \text{ mL drug}$$

Ratio Method

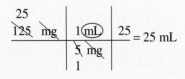

1 mL : 5 mg : : x : 125 mg

Proportion Method

$$\frac{1 \text{ mL}}{5 \text{ mg}} = \frac{x}{125 \text{ mg}}$$

$$\frac{125}{5} = x$$

25 mL

Dimensional Analysis Method

$$\frac{25}{\cancel{125} \text{ mg}} \Bigg| \frac{1 \text{ (mL)}}{\cancel{5} \text{ mg}} \Bigg| \frac{25}{1} = 25 \text{ mL}$$

Remove 25 mL IV fluid from the IV bag and add 25 mL diltiazem = 100 mL altogether.

Formula Method

$$\frac{D}{H} \times S = A$$

$$\frac{\overset{1}{\cancel{5}} \text{ mg}}{\underset{25}{\cancel{125}} \text{ mg}} \times \overset{4}{\cancel{100}} \text{ mL} = 4 \text{ mL/hr}$$

Ratio Method

$$100 \text{ mL} : 125 \text{ mg} :: x : 5 \text{ mg}$$

Proportion Method

$$\frac{100 \text{ mL}}{125 \text{ mg}} = \frac{x}{5 \text{ mg}}$$

$$\frac{500}{125} = x$$

$$4 \text{ mL/hr}$$

Dimensional Analysis Method

$$\frac{\overset{1}{\cancel{5}} \text{ mg}}{\textcircled{hr}} \left| \frac{100 \text{ (mL)}}{\underset{25}{\cancel{125}} \text{ mg}} \right| \frac{100}{25} = 4 \text{ mL/hr}$$

Second way: If you add 25 mL of drug to the 100 mL D5W, you make 125 mL (a 1:1 solution). Because the order is 5 mg/hour, set the pump at 5 mL/hr.

Formula Method

Proof: $\frac{D}{H} \times S = A$

$$\frac{\overset{1}{\cancel{5}} \text{ mg}}{\underset{25}{\cancel{125}} \text{ mg}} \times \overset{5}{\cancel{125}} \text{ mL} = 5 \text{ mL/hr}$$

Ratio Method

$$125 \text{ mL} : 125 \text{ mg} :: x : 5 \text{ mg}$$

Proportion Method

$$\frac{125 \text{ mL}}{125 \text{ mg}} = \frac{x}{5 \text{ mg}}$$

$$\frac{625}{125} = x$$

$$5 \text{ mL/hr} = x$$

Dimensional Analysis Method

$$\frac{5 \text{ mg}}{\textcircled{hr}} \left| \frac{\cancel{125} \text{ (mL)}}{\cancel{125} \text{ mg}} \right| \frac{5}{} = 5 \text{ mL/hr}$$

It is considered better to remove fluid from the IV bag so the volume remains the same.

5. 2 g = 2000 mg

Order calls for 4 mg/min. Pumps are set in mL/hr. Multiply 4 mg/min × 60 min = 240 mg/hr.

Formula Method

$$\frac{D}{H} \times S = A$$

$$\frac{\overset{60}{\cancel{240}} \text{ mg/hr}}{\underset{4}{\underset{1}{\cancel{2000}}} \text{ mg}} \times \overset{1}{\cancel{500}} \text{ mL} = 60 \text{ mL/hr}$$

Ratio Method

$$500 \text{ mL} : 2000 \text{ mg} :: x : 240 \text{ mg}$$

Proportion Method

$$\frac{500 \text{ mL}}{2000 \text{ mg}} = \frac{x}{240 \text{ mg}}$$

$$\frac{120,000}{2000} = x$$

$$\frac{240}{4} = x$$

$$60 \text{ mL} = x$$

Dimensional Analysis Method

$$\frac{\overset{2}{\cancel{4}}\ \text{mg}}{\text{min}}\ \left|\ \frac{\overset{1}{500}\ \text{(mL)}}{\underset{1}{\cancel{2}}\ \text{g}}\ \right|\ \frac{1\ \text{g}}{1000\ \text{mg}}\ \left|\ \frac{\overset{30}{\cancel{60}}\ \text{min}}{1\ \text{hr}}\ \right|\ \frac{2\ \times\ 30}{}\ =\ 60\ \text{mL/hr}$$

Set the pump.

Total # mL: 500

mL/hr: 60

6. a. Add KCl to the IV.

Formula Method

$$\frac{D}{H} \times S = A$$

$$\frac{\overset{2}{\cancel{40}}\ \cancel{\text{mEq}}}{\underset{1}{\cancel{20}}\ \cancel{\text{mEq}}} \times 10\ \text{mL} = 20\ \text{mL}$$

Ratio Method

10 mL : 20 mEq : : x : 40 mEq

Proportion Method

$$\frac{10\ \text{mL}}{20\ \text{mEq}} = \frac{x}{40\ \text{mEq}}$$

$$\frac{400}{20} = x$$

$$20\ \text{mL} = x$$

Dimensional Analysis Method

$$\frac{\overset{2}{\cancel{40}}\ \cancel{\text{mEq}}}{}\ \left|\ \frac{10\ \text{(mL)}}{\underset{1}{\cancel{20}}\ \cancel{\text{mEq}}}\ \right|\ \frac{2\ \times\ 10}{}\ =\ 20\ \text{mL}$$

b. Remove 20 mL IV fluid and add the 20 mL of KCl to make 1000 mL.

Formula Method

$$\frac{D}{H} \times S = A$$

1 L = 1000 mL

$$\frac{\overset{1}{\cancel{10}}\ \cancel{\text{mEq/hr}}}{\underset{\underset{1}{\cancel{4}}}{\cancel{40}}\ \cancel{\text{mEq}}} \times \overset{250}{\cancel{1000}}\ \text{mL} = 250\ \text{mL/hr}$$

Ratio Method

1000 mL : 40 mEq : : x : 10 mEq

Proportion Method

$$\frac{1000\ \text{mL}}{40\ \text{mEq}} = \frac{x}{10\ \text{mEq}}$$

$$\frac{10000}{40} = x$$

$$250\ \text{mL} = x$$

Dimensional Analysis Method

$$\frac{10\ \text{mEq}}{\text{(hr)}}\ \left|\ \frac{\cancel{1}\ \cancel{L}}{\underset{1}{\cancel{40}}\ \text{mEq}}\ \right|\ \frac{\overset{25}{\cancel{1000}}\ \text{(mL)}}{\cancel{1}\ \cancel{L}}\ \right|\ \frac{10\ \times\ 25}{}\ =\ 250\ \text{mL/hr}$$

Set pump at 250 mL/hr. This is a large volume and KCl is a potent electrolyte; therefore, the patient must be on a cardiac monitor for safety. Check the order with the doctor.

Total # mL: 1000

mL/hr: 250

7. 2 g = 2000 mL

Order calls for 1 mg/min. Pumps are set in mL/hr. Multiply 1 mg/min × 60 mg = 60 mg/hr.

Formula Method

$$\frac{D}{H} \times S = A$$

$$\frac{\overset{15}{\cancel{60}\ \text{mg/hr}}}{\underset{\underset{1}{4}}{\cancel{2000}\ \text{mg}}} \times \overset{1}{\cancel{500}}\ \text{mL} = 15\ \text{mL/hr}$$

Ratio Method

500 mL : 2000 mg : : x : 60 mg

Proportion Method

$$\frac{500\ \text{mL}}{2000\ \text{mg}} = \frac{x}{60\ \text{mg/hr}}$$

$$\frac{30000}{2000} = x$$

15 mL/hr

Dimensional Analysis Method

$$\frac{1\ \text{mg}}{\text{min}} \left| \frac{\overset{1}{\cancel{500}}\ \cancel{\text{mL}}}{2\ \cancel{\text{g}}} \right| \frac{1\ \cancel{\text{g}}}{\underset{\underset{1}{\cancel{2}}}{\cancel{1000}\ \cancel{\text{mg}}}} \left| \frac{\overset{30}{\cancel{60}\ \cancel{\text{min}}}}{1\ \cancel{\text{hr}}} \right| \frac{30}{2} = 15\ \text{mL/hr}$$

Set the pump.

Total # mL: 500

mL/hr: 15

8. Use a reconstitution device (see Chapter 8) to add 50 mg of drug to 500 mL D5W.

$$\frac{\#\,\text{mL}}{\#\,\text{hr}} = \text{mL/hr}$$

$$\frac{500\ \text{mL}}{6\ \text{hr}} \quad 6\,\overline{)500.0} = 83\ \text{mL/hr}$$

with long division:
83.0
500.0
48
20
18
2 0
1 8

Dimensional Analysis Method

$$\frac{500\ \cancel{\text{mL}}}{6\ \cancel{\text{hr}}} \left| \frac{500}{6} \right. = 83.33\ \text{or } 83\ \text{mL/hr}$$

Set the pump.

Total # mL: 500

mL/hr: 83

9. Add vasopressin to the IV.

Formula Method

$$\frac{D}{H} \times S = A$$

$$\frac{\overset{10}{\cancel{200}\ \text{units}}}{\underset{1}{\cancel{20}\ \text{units}}} \times 1\ \text{mL} = 10\ \text{mL}$$

Ratio Method

1 mL : 20 units : : x : 200 units

Proportion Method

$$\frac{1\ \text{mL}}{20\ \text{units}} = \frac{x}{200\ \text{units}}$$

$$\frac{200}{20} = x$$

$$10\ \text{mL} = x$$

Dimensional Analysis Method

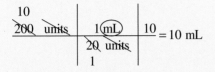

$$\frac{\overset{10}{\cancel{200}\ \text{units}}}{} \mid \frac{1\ \text{mL}}{\underset{1}{\cancel{20}\ \text{units}}} \mid \frac{10}{} = 10\ \text{mL}$$

Remove 10 mL fluid from the IV and add 10 mL drug = 500 mL.

Formula Method

$$\frac{D}{H} \times S = A$$

$$\frac{\overset{9}{\cancel{18}\ \text{units/hr}}}{\underset{1}{\cancel{200}\ \text{units}}} \times \cancel{500}\ \text{mL} = 45\ \text{mL/hr}$$

Ratio Method

500 mL : 200 units : : x : 18 units

Proportion Method

$$\frac{500\ \text{mL}}{200\ \text{units}} = \frac{x}{18\ \text{units}}$$

$$\frac{900}{20} = x$$

$$45\ \text{mL} = x$$

Dimensional Analysis Method

$$\frac{18\ \text{units}}{\cancel{\text{hr}}} \mid \frac{500\ \cancel{\text{mL}}}{\cancel{200}\ \text{units}} \mid \frac{18 \times 5}{2} = 45\ \text{mL/hr}$$

Set the pump.

Total # mL: 500

mL/hr: 45

10. Order: 250 mcg/min

Solution: 500 mg in 500 mL D5W

Step 1. $\dfrac{500\ \text{mg}}{500\ \text{mL}} = 1\ \text{mg/mL}$

Step 2. 1 mg = 1000 mcg/mL

Step 3. Not needed

Step 4. 1000 mcg/60 gtt

Step 5. $\dfrac{\overset{1}{\cancel{250}\ \text{mcg/min}}}{\underset{\underset{1}{4}}{\cancel{1000}\ \text{mcg}}} \times \overset{15}{\cancel{60}}\ \text{gtt}$

15 gtt/min = 15 mL/hr

Set the pump.

Total # mL: 500

mL/hr: 15

Dimensional Analysis Method

$$\frac{\cancel{1}}{\cancel{250}\ \cancel{mcg}} \left| \frac{\cancel{500}\ \cancel{(mL)}}{\cancel{500}\ \cancel{mg}} \right| \frac{1\ \cancel{mg}}{\cancel{1000}\ \cancel{mcg}} \left| \frac{\cancel{60}\ \cancel{min}}{1\cancel{(hr)}} \right| \frac{60}{4} = 15\ mL/hr$$

11. Order: 2.5 mcg/kg/min

    Solution: 400 mg in 250 mL

    Weight: 60 kg

    Multiply 60 kg × 2.5 mg = 150 mcg.

    Step 1. $\dfrac{\overset{8}{\cancel{400}}\ mg}{\underset{5}{\cancel{250}}\ mL} = 8\ mg/5\ mL$

    Step 2. 8 mg = 8000 mcg. Solution is 8000 mcg/5 mL.

    Step 3. $\dfrac{8000\ mcg}{5\ mL} = 1600\ mcg/mL$

    Step 4. 1600 mcg/60 gtt

    Step 5. $\dfrac{150\ mcg/min}{1600\ mL} \times \cancel{60}\ gtt = \dfrac{\overset{90}{\cancel{60}}}{16}$

$$16\ \overline{)90.0\ } = 6 \qquad \begin{array}{r} 5.6 \\ \hline \underline{80} \\ 10\ 0 \\ \underline{9\ 6} \end{array}$$

    6 gtt/min = 6 mL/hr

    Set the pump.

    Total # mL: 250

    # mL/hr: 6

Dimensional Analysis Method

$$\frac{2.5\ \cancel{mcg}}{\cancel{kg}\ /\ \cancel{min}} \left| \frac{\overset{1}{\cancel{250}}\ \cancel{(mL)}}{\cancel{600}\ \cancel{mg}} \right| \frac{1\ \cancel{mg}}{\cancel{1000}\ \cancel{mcg}} \left| \frac{\cancel{60}\ \cancel{min}}{1\cancel{(hr)}} \right| \cancel{60}\ \cancel{kg} \left| \frac{2.5 \times 6 \times 6}{4 \times 4} = 5.625\ or\ 6\ mL/hr\right.$$

12. Order: 2 milliunits/min

    Solution: 9 units in 150 mL NS

    Step 1. $\dfrac{9\ units}{150\ mL} = 0.06\ units/mL$

    Step 2. 1 unit = 1000 milliunits

    Step 3. 0.06 units = 60 milliunits/mL

    Step 4. 60 milliunits/60 gtt

Step 5. $\dfrac{2 \text{ milliunits /min}}{60 \text{ milliunits}} \times 60 \text{ gtt} = 2 \text{ gtt/min}$

2 gtt/min = 2 mL/hr

Set the pump.

Total # mL: 150 mL

mL/hr: 2

Dimensional Analysis Method

$$\dfrac{2 \text{ milliunits}}{\text{minute}} \left| \dfrac{150 \text{ mL}}{9 \text{ units}} \right| \dfrac{1 \text{ unit}}{10\,00 \text{ milliunits}} \left| \dfrac{60 \text{ minute}}{1 \text{ hr}} \right| \dfrac{2 \times 15 \times 6}{9 \times 10} = 2 \text{ mL/hr}$$

13. a. Correct; $100 \text{ mg/m}^2 \times 1.7 = 170 \text{ mg}$

b. 1 L = 1000 mL

$\dfrac{\# \text{ mL}}{\# \text{ hr}} = \text{mL/hr}$

$$\dfrac{100}{24} \overset{41.6}{\overline{)1000.0}} = 42 \text{ mL/hr}$$
$$\underline{96}$$
$$40$$
$$\underline{24}$$
$$160$$
$$\underline{144}$$

Set the pump.

Total # mL: 1000

mL/hr: 42

Dimensional Analysis Method

$$\dfrac{1 \text{ L}}{24 \text{ hr}} \left| \dfrac{1000 \text{ mL}}{1 \text{ L}} \right| \dfrac{1000}{24} = 41.66 \text{ or } 42 \text{ mL/hr}$$

14. Order: 5 mcg/kg/min

Solution: 50 mg in 250 mL

Weight: 90 kg

Multiply: $5 \times 90 = 450 \text{ mcg/min}$

Step 1. $\dfrac{\overset{1}{50} \text{ mg}}{\underset{5}{250} \text{ mL}} = 0.2 \text{ mg/mL}$

Step 2. 0.2 mg = 200 mcg

Step 3. Solution is 200 mcg/mL.

Step 4. 200 mcg/60 gtt

Step 5. $\dfrac{450 \text{ mcg/min}}{200 \text{ mcg}} \times 60 \text{ gtt} = \dfrac{45 \times 6}{2} = 135 \text{ gtt/min} = 135 \text{ mL/hr}$

Set the pump.

Total # mL: 250 mL

mL/hr: 135 mL/hr

Dimensional Analysis Method

$$\dfrac{1}{\cancel{5} \text{ mcg}}{\dfrac{1}{\cancel{250}\,\text{(mL)}}}\Bigg|\dfrac{1 \text{ mg}}{\cancel{50}\text{ mg}}\Bigg|\dfrac{60 \text{ min}}{\cancel{1000}\text{ mcg}}\Bigg|\dfrac{90 \text{ kg}}{1\,\text{(hr)}}\Bigg|\dfrac{60 \times 90}{10 \times 4} = 135 \text{ mL/hr}$$

15. Order: 2 mcg/min

Solution: 4 mg in 250 mL

Step 1. $\dfrac{4 \text{ mg}}{250 \text{ mL}} = 0.016 \text{ mg/mL}$

Step 2. 0.016 mg = 16 mcg

Step 3. 16 mcg/mL

Step 4. 16 mcg/60 gtt

$\dfrac{\overset{1}{\cancel{2}} \text{ mcg/min}}{\underset{8}{\cancel{16}} \text{ mcg}} \times 60 \text{ gtt} = \dfrac{60}{8} = 7.5 \text{ or } 8 \text{ gtt/min} = 8 \text{ mL/hr}$

Set the pump.

Total # mL: 250 mL

mL/hr: 8 mL/hr

Dimensional Analysis Method

$$\dfrac{1}{\cancel{2}\text{ mcg}}\Bigg|\dfrac{1}{\cancel{250}\,\text{(mL)}}\Bigg|\dfrac{1 \text{ mg}}{\cancel{1000}\text{ mcg}}\Bigg|\dfrac{\overset{15}{\cancel{60}}\text{ minute}}{1\,\text{(hr)}}\Bigg|\dfrac{15}{2} = 7.5 \text{ or } 8 \text{ mL/hr}$$

Chapter 10

Test 1: Infants and Children Dosage Problems

1. Safe dose 0.5 mg to 1 mg/dose IM. The order is safe.

Formula Method

$\frac{D}{H} \times S = A$

$\frac{1 \text{ mg}}{10 \text{ mg}} \times 1 \text{ mL}$

$= 0.1 \text{ mL IM}$

Ratio Method

1 mL : 10 mg : : x : 1 mg

Proportion Method

$\frac{1 \text{ mL}}{10 \text{ mg}} = \frac{x}{1 \text{ mg}}$

$\frac{1}{10} = x$

$0.1 \text{ mL} = x$

Dimensional Analysis Method

$\frac{1 \text{ mg}}{} \bigg| \frac{1 \text{ mL}}{10 \text{ mg}} \bigg| \frac{1}{10} = 0.1 \text{ mL}$

Use a precision syringe.

2. Safe dose: 20 to 40 mg/kg/24 hours given q8h.

Low Range

$\begin{array}{r} 20 \text{ mg} \\ \times\ 10 \text{ kg} \\ \hline 200 \text{ mg/24 h} \end{array}$

High Range

$\begin{array}{r} 40 \text{ mg} \\ \times\ 10 \text{ kg} \\ \hline 400 \text{ mg/24 h} \end{array}$

Order is 125 mg q8h (3 doses).

125 mg × 3 doses = 375. Dose is safe.

No math necessary. Stock is 125 mg/5 mL.

Give 5 mL.

3. Safe dose: 50,000 units/kg × 1 dose

$\begin{array}{r} 50,000 \text{ units} \\ \times\quad 10 \text{ kg} \\ \hline 500,000 \text{ units} \end{array}$

The order is safe.

Formula Method

$\frac{D}{H} \times S = A$

$\frac{500,000 \text{ units}}{600,000 \text{ units}} \times 1 \text{ mL} = \frac{5}{6} = 0.83 \text{ mL}$

Ratio Method

1 mL : 600,000 units : : x : 500,000 units

Proportion Method

$\frac{1 \text{ mL}}{600,000 \text{ units}} = \frac{x}{500,000 \text{ units}}$

$\frac{500,000}{600,000} = x$

0.83 mL

Dimensional Analysis Method

$\frac{500,000 \text{ units}}{} \bigg| \frac{1 \text{ mL}}{600,000 \text{ units}} \bigg| \frac{5}{6} = 0.83 \text{ mL}$

Use a precision syringe. Give 0.83 mL IM.

4. Step 1. Safe dose: 2.5 mg/kg/dose q8h

$$\begin{array}{r} 2.5 \text{ mg} \\ \times\ 3.6 \text{ kg} \\ \hline 9 \text{ mg} \end{array}$$

Order is safe.

Step 2. Minimum safe dilution: 2 mg/mL

$$2 \text{ mg}\overline{)\ 9 \text{ mg}}^{\ 4.5 \text{ mL}}\ \text{is the minimum safe dilution. 10 mL is safe.}$$

Formula Method

Step 3: $\frac{D}{H} \times S = A$

$$\frac{9\,\text{mg}}{40\,\text{mg}} \times 1 \text{ mL} = 40\overline{)9.000}^{\ .225} = 0.23 \text{ mL}$$

Ratio Method

1 mL : 40 mg : : x : 9 mg

Proportion Method

$$\frac{1 \text{ mL}}{40 \text{ mg}} = \frac{x}{9 \text{ mg}}$$

$$\frac{9}{40} = x$$

0.23 mL

Dimensional Analysis Method

$$\frac{9\,\text{mg}}{} \ \left|\ \frac{1\,\text{mL}}{40\,\text{mg}}\ \right|\ \frac{9}{40} = 0.23 \text{ mL}$$

Use a precision syringe to draw up 0.23 mL.

Step 4. Add about 5 mL D5¼NS to the Buretrol. Add the 0.23 mL drug. Add more D5¼NS to make 10 mL.

Step 5. Set the pump at 20 because 20 mL in 1 hour will deliver the 10 mL in 30 min.

Step 6. When the IV is completed, add a flush of 20 mL D5¼NS to the Buretrol to clear the tubing of medication.

5. Safe dose: infants and children younger than 3 years: 10 to 40 mg. The dose is safe.

Formula Method

$$\frac{D}{H} \times S = A \qquad \frac{10\,\text{mg}}{20\,\text{mg}} \times 5 \text{ mL} = \frac{5}{2} = 2.5 \text{ mL po}$$

Ratio Method

5 mL : 20 mg : : x : 10 mg

Proportion Method

$$\frac{5 \text{ mL}}{20 \text{ mg}} = \frac{x}{10 \text{ mg}}$$

$$50 = 20x$$

$$\frac{50}{20} = x$$

$$\frac{10}{4} = x$$

2.5 mL = x

Dimensional Analysis Method

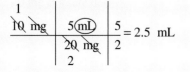

Formula Method

$$\frac{D}{H} \times S = A \qquad \frac{20 \text{ mg}}{50 \text{ mg}} \times 1 \text{ mL} = \frac{2}{5} = 0.4 \text{ mL IV}$$

Ratio Method

1 mL : 50 mg : : x : 20 mg

Proportion Method

$$\frac{1 \text{ mL}}{50 \text{ mg}} = \frac{x}{20 \text{ mg}}$$

$$\frac{20}{50} = x$$

0.4 mL

Dimensional Analysis Method

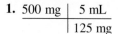

$$\frac{20 \text{ mg}}{} \quad \frac{1 \text{ (mL)}}{50 \text{ mg}} \quad \frac{2}{5} = 0.4 \text{ tablets}$$

Use a precision syringe.

Chapter 11

Test 1: Dimensional Analysis

1. $\dfrac{500 \text{ mg}}{} \quad \dfrac{5 \text{ mL}}{125 \text{ mg}}$

$$\frac{\overset{4}{500 \text{ mg}}}{} \quad \frac{5 \text{ (mL)}}{\underset{1}{125 \text{ mg}}} \quad \frac{4 \times 5}{} = 20 \text{ mL}$$

2. $\dfrac{5000 \text{ units}}{} \quad \dfrac{1 \text{ mL}}{10000 \text{ units}}$

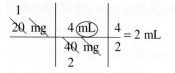

$$\frac{\overset{1}{5000 \text{ units}}}{} \quad \frac{1 \text{ (mL)}}{\underset{2}{10000 \text{ units}}} \quad \frac{1}{2} = \frac{1}{2} \text{ or } 0.5 \text{ mL}$$

3. $\dfrac{20 \text{ mg}}{} \quad \dfrac{4 \text{ mL}}{40 \text{ mg}}$

$$\frac{\overset{1}{20 \text{ mg}}}{} \quad \frac{4 \text{ (mL)}}{\underset{2}{40 \text{ mg}}} \quad \frac{4}{2} = 2 \text{ mL}$$

4. $\dfrac{0.25 \text{ mg}}{} \quad \dfrac{1 \text{ tablet}}{0.125 \text{ mg}}$

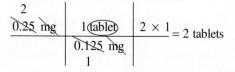

$$\frac{\overset{2}{0.25 \text{ mg}}}{} \quad \frac{1 \text{ (tablet)}}{\underset{1}{0.125 \text{ mg}}} \quad \frac{2 \times 1}{} = 2 \text{ tablets}$$

5. $\dfrac{650 \text{ mg}}{} \bigg| \dfrac{5 \text{ mL}}{325 \text{ mg}}$

$\dfrac{\overset{2}{\cancel{650}} \text{ mg}}{} \bigg| \dfrac{5 \,\textcircled{mL}}{\underset{1}{\cancel{325}} \text{ mg}} \bigg| \dfrac{2 \times 5}{} = 10 \text{ mL}$

6. 10% = 10 g in 100 mL

$\dfrac{0.5 \text{ g}}{} \bigg| \dfrac{100 \text{ mL}}{10 \text{ g}}$

$\dfrac{\overset{1}{\cancel{0.5}} \text{ g}}{} \bigg| \dfrac{100 \,\textcircled{mL}}{\underset{20}{\cancel{10} \text{ g}}} \bigg| \dfrac{100}{20} = 5 \text{ mL}$

7. $\dfrac{125 \text{ mcg}}{} \bigg| \dfrac{1 \text{ mL}}{0.25 \text{ mg}} \bigg| \dfrac{1 \text{ mg}}{1000 \text{ mcg}}$

$\dfrac{\overset{1}{\cancel{125}} \text{ mcg}}{} \bigg| \dfrac{1 \,\textcircled{mL}}{0.25 \text{ mg}} \bigg| \dfrac{1 \text{ mg}}{\underset{8}{\cancel{1000}} \text{ mcg}} \bigg| \dfrac{1 \times 1 \times 1}{0.25 \times 8} = \dfrac{1}{2} \text{ or } 0.5 \text{ mL}$

8. $\dfrac{375 \text{ mg}}{} \bigg| \dfrac{5 \text{ mL}}{125 \text{ mg}} \bigg| \dfrac{1 \text{ tsp}}{5 \text{ mL}}$

$\dfrac{\overset{15}{\cancel{375}} \text{ mg}}{} \bigg| \dfrac{5 \text{ mL}}{\underset{5}{\cancel{125}} \text{ mg}} \bigg| \dfrac{1 \,\textcircled{tsp}}{5 \text{ mL}} \bigg| \dfrac{15 \times 5 \times 1}{5 \times 5} = \dfrac{75}{25} \text{ or } 3 \text{ tsp}$

9. $\dfrac{\tfrac{1}{150} \text{ g}}{} \bigg| \dfrac{1 \text{ tablet}}{0.4 \text{ mg}} \bigg| \dfrac{60 \text{ mg}}{1 \text{ grain}}$

$\dfrac{\tfrac{1}{150} \text{ g}}{} \bigg| \dfrac{1 \,\textcircled{tablet}}{0.4 \text{ mg}} \bigg| \dfrac{60 \text{ mg}}{1 \text{ grain}} \bigg| \dfrac{\tfrac{1}{150} \times 60}{0.4} = \dfrac{\tfrac{60}{150}}{0.4} = \dfrac{0.4}{0.4} = 1 \text{ tablet}$

10. Use 1 gr = 65 mg for Tylenol

$\dfrac{5 \text{ g}}{} \bigg| \dfrac{5 \text{ mL}}{325 \text{ mg}} \bigg| \dfrac{65 \text{ mg}}{1 \text{ grain}}$

$\dfrac{\overset{1}{\cancel{5}} \text{ g}}{} \bigg| \dfrac{5 \,\textcircled{mL}}{\underset{65}{\underset{1}{\cancel{325}}} \text{ mg}} \bigg| \dfrac{\overset{1}{\cancel{65}} \text{ mg}}{1 \text{ grain}} \bigg| \dfrac{1 \times 5 \times 1}{1 \times 1} = 5 \text{ mL}$

11.
$$\frac{40 \text{ mg}}{\text{m}^2} \left| \frac{0.44 \text{ m}^2}{} \right.$$

$$\frac{40 \text{ mg}}{\cancel{\text{m}^2}} \left| \frac{0.44 \ \cancel{\text{m}^2}}{} \right| \frac{40 \times 0.44}{} = 17.6 \text{ mg}$$

12.
$$\frac{0.1 \text{ mg}}{\text{kg}} \left| \frac{1 \text{ mL}}{10 \text{ mg}} \right| \frac{32 \text{ lb}}{} \left| \frac{1 \text{ kg}}{2.2 \text{ lb}} \right.$$

$$\frac{0.2 \text{ mg}}{\text{kg}} \left| \frac{1 \text{ mL}}{10 \text{ mg}} \right| \frac{32 \text{ lb}}{} \left| \frac{1 \text{ kg}}{2.2 \text{ lb}} \right.$$

$$\frac{0.1 \text{ mg}}{\cancel{\text{kg}}} \left| \frac{1 \ \cancel{\text{mL}}}{10 \ \cancel{\text{mg}}} \right| \frac{32 \ \cancel{\text{lb}}}{} \left| \frac{1 \ \cancel{\text{kg}}}{2.2 \ \cancel{\text{lb}}} \right| \frac{0.1 \times 1 \times 32 \times 1}{10 \times 2.2} \left| \frac{3.2}{22} = \frac{3.2}{22} = 0.15 \text{ mL} \right.$$

$$\frac{\overset{1}{0.2} \ \cancel{\text{mcg}}}{\cancel{\text{kg}}} \left| \frac{1 \ \cancel{\text{mL}}}{10 \ \cancel{\text{mg}}} \right| \frac{32 \ \cancel{\text{lb}}}{} \left| \frac{1 \ \cancel{\text{kg}}}{\underset{11}{2.2} \ \cancel{\text{lb}}} \right| \frac{1 \times 1 \times 32}{10 \times 11} = \frac{32}{110} = 0.29 \text{ mL or } 0.3 \text{ mL}$$

13.
$$\frac{0.44 \text{ g}}{} \left| \frac{1 \text{ mL}}{330 \text{ mg}} \right| \frac{1000 \text{ mg}}{1 \text{ g}} \right.$$

$$\frac{0.44 \ \cancel{\text{g}}}{} \left| \frac{1 \ \cancel{\text{mL}}}{330 \ \cancel{\text{mg}}} \right| \frac{1000 \ \cancel{\text{mg}}}{1 \ \cancel{\text{g}}} \right| \frac{0.44 \times 100}{33} = \frac{44}{33} = 1.33 \text{ mL}$$

14.
$$\frac{1{,}000{,}000 \text{ units}}{} \left| \frac{1 \text{ mL}}{500{,}000 \text{ units}} \right.$$

$$\frac{\overset{2}{\cancel{1{,}000{,}000}} \ \cancel{\text{units}}}{} \left| \frac{1 \ \cancel{\text{mL}}}{\underset{1}{\cancel{500{,}000}} \ \cancel{\text{units}}} \right| \frac{2 \times 1}{1} = 2 \text{ mL}$$

15.
$$\frac{500 \text{ mL}}{6 \text{ hr}}$$

$$\frac{500 \ \cancel{\text{mL}}}{6 \ \cancel{\text{hr}}} \left| \frac{500}{6} = 83.3 \text{ or } 83 \text{ mL/hr} \right.$$

16.
$$\frac{1000 \text{ mL}}{16 \text{ hr}}$$

$$\frac{1000 \ \cancel{\text{mL}}}{16 \ \cancel{\text{hr}}} \left| \frac{1000}{16} = 62.5 \text{ or } 63 \text{ mL/hr} \right.$$

17. $\dfrac{1000\ \text{mL}}{10\ \text{hr}}\ \bigg|\ \dfrac{60\ \text{gtt}}{1\ \text{mL}}\ \bigg|\ \dfrac{1\ \text{hr}}{60\ \text{min}}$

$$\frac{\overset{100}{\cancel{1000}\ \cancel{\text{mL}}}}{\underset{}{\cancel{10}\ \cancel{\text{hr}}}}\ \bigg|\ \frac{\overset{1}{60}\ \cancel{\text{gtt}}}{1\ \cancel{\text{mL}}}\ \bigg|\ \frac{1\ \cancel{\text{hr}}}{\underset{1}{\cancel{60}\ \cancel{\text{min}}}}\ \bigg|\ \frac{100 \times 1 \times 1}{1 \times 1 \times 1} = 100\ \text{gtt/min}$$

18. $\dfrac{250\ \text{mL}}{2\ \text{hr}}\ \bigg|\ \dfrac{15\ \text{gtt}}{1\ \text{mL}}\ \bigg|\ \dfrac{1\ \text{hr}}{60\ \text{min}}$

$$\frac{250\ \cancel{\text{mL}}}{2\ \cancel{\text{hr}}}\ \bigg|\ \frac{\overset{1}{\cancel{15}}\ \cancel{\text{gtt}}}{1\ \cancel{\text{mL}}}\ \bigg|\ \frac{1\ \cancel{\text{hr}}}{\underset{4}{\cancel{60}\ \cancel{\text{min}}}}\ \bigg|\ \frac{250 \times 1 \times 1}{2 \times 1 \times 4} = \frac{250}{8} = 31.25\ \text{or}\ 31\ \text{gtt/min}$$

19.

$$\frac{5\ \cancel{\text{units}}}{\cancel{\text{hr}}}\ \bigg|\ \frac{\overset{1}{125}\ \cancel{\text{mL}}}{\underset{1}{\cancel{125}\ \cancel{\text{units}}}}\ \bigg|\ \frac{5}{} = 5\ \text{mL/hr}$$

20. $\dfrac{1500\ \text{units}}{\text{hr}}\ \bigg|\ \dfrac{500\ \text{mL}}{25{,}000\ \text{units}}$

$$\frac{1500\ \cancel{\text{units}}}{\cancel{\text{hr}}}\ \bigg|\ \frac{\overset{1}{\cancel{500}}\ \cancel{\text{mL}}}{\underset{50}{\cancel{25{,}000}\ \cancel{\text{units}}}}\ \bigg|\ \frac{1500}{50} = 30\ \text{mL/hr}$$

21. $\dfrac{30\ \text{mL}}{\text{hr}}\ \bigg|\ \dfrac{25{,}000\ \text{units}}{250\ \text{mL}}$

$$\frac{30\ \cancel{\text{mL}}}{\cancel{\text{hr}}}\ \bigg|\ \frac{\overset{100}{\cancel{25{,}000}}\ \cancel{\text{units}}}{\underset{1}{\cancel{250}\ \cancel{\text{mL}}}}\ \bigg|\ \frac{30 \times 100}{} = 3000\ \text{units/hr}$$

22. $\dfrac{15\ \text{mcg}}{\text{min}}\ \bigg|\ \dfrac{250\ \text{mL}}{50\ \text{mg}}\ \bigg|\ \dfrac{1\ \text{mg}}{1000\ \text{mcg}}\ \bigg|\ \dfrac{60\ \text{min}}{1\ \text{hr}}$

$$\frac{15\ \cancel{\text{mcg}}}{\cancel{\text{min}}}\ \bigg|\ \frac{\overset{5}{250}\ \cancel{\text{mL}}}{\underset{1}{\cancel{50}\ \cancel{\text{mg}}}}\ \bigg|\ \frac{1\ \cancel{\text{mg}}}{1000\ \cancel{\text{mcg}}}\ \bigg|\ \frac{60\ \cancel{\text{min}}}{1\ \cancel{\text{hr}}}\ \bigg|\ \frac{15 \times 5 \times 60}{1000} = \frac{4500}{1000} = 4.5\ \text{or}\ 5\ \text{mL}$$

23.

$$\frac{2\ mg}{min} \left| \frac{500\ mL}{2\ g} \right| \frac{1\ g}{1000\ mg} \left| \frac{60\ min}{1\ hr} \right.$$

$$\frac{\overset{1}{\cancel{2}}\ mg}{\cancel{min}} \left| \frac{\overset{1}{500}\ \cancel{(mL)}}{\underset{1}{\cancel{2}\ \cancel{g}}} \right| \frac{1\ \cancel{g}}{\underset{2}{\cancel{1000}\ \cancel{mg}}} \left| \frac{60\ \cancel{min}}{1\ \cancel{(hr)}} \right| \frac{60}{2} = 30\ mL/hr$$

24.

$$\frac{10\ mcg}{kg/min} \left| \frac{500\ mL}{500\ mg} \right| \frac{1\ mg}{1000\ mcg} \left| \frac{100\ kg}{} \right| \frac{60\ min}{1\ hr}$$

$$\frac{10\ \cancel{mcg}}{kg\ /\ \cancel{min}} \left| \frac{\overset{1}{500}\ \cancel{(mL)}}{\underset{1}{500}\ \cancel{mg}} \right| \frac{1\ \cancel{mg}}{\underset{10}{\cancel{1000}}\ \cancel{mcg}} \left| \frac{\overset{1}{100}\ \cancel{kg}}{} \right| \frac{60\ \cancel{min}}{1\ \cancel{(hr)}} \left| \frac{10\times1\times1\times1\times60}{1\times10\times1} = \frac{600}{10} = 60\ mL/hr \right.$$

25.

$$\frac{5\ mcg}{kg/min} \left| \frac{250\ mL}{50\ mg} \right| \frac{1\ mg}{1000\ mcg} \left| \frac{60\ min}{1\ hr} \right| \frac{220\ lb}{} \left| \frac{1\ kg}{2.2\ lb} \right.$$

$$\frac{\overset{1}{\cancel{5}}\ \cancel{mcg}}{kg\ /\ \cancel{min}} \left| \frac{\overset{1}{250}\ \cancel{(mL)}}{\underset{10}{50}\ \cancel{mg}} \right| \frac{1\ \cancel{mg}}{\underset{4}{\cancel{1000}}\ \cancel{mcg}} \left| \frac{60\ \cancel{min}}{1\ \cancel{(hr)}} \right| \frac{220\ \cancel{lb}}{} \left| \frac{1\ kg}{2.2\ \cancel{lb}} \right. = \frac{1\times1\times1\times60\times220\times1}{10\times4\times1\times2.2}$$

$$= \frac{13,200}{88}$$

$$= 150\ mL/hr$$

Chapter 12
Test 1: Basic Drug Information

1. a	**5.** b	**9.** a	**13.** a	**17.** b
2. c	**6.** a	**10.** b	**14.** a	**18.** d
3. d	**7.** a	**11.** d	**15.** b	**19.** d
4. b	**8.** d	**12.** c	**16.** a	**20.** a

Chapter 13
Test 1: Administration Procedures

Part A

1. d	**5.** c	**9.** d	**13.** b	**17.** b
2. d	**6.** b	**10.** a	**14.** a	**18.** d
3. b	**7.** a	**11.** c	**15.** d	**19.** c
4. d	**8.** d	**12.** a	**16.** b	**20.** c

Part B

1. Correct. As the needle or catheter is removed, there is a possibility of bleeding at the site. In addition, the nurse should use a clamp to carry the needle or catheter to a puncture-proof container.

2. Incorrect. The nurse must wash his or her hands before leaving the room.

3. Incorrect. It is not necessary to wear gloves to prepare an IV because there is no contact at this time with the patient's blood or body fluids.

4. Correct. Universal safeguards state that a mask must be worn when the patient is on strict or respiratory isolation precautions.

5. Correct. There is a potential risk of exposure to hepatitis B virus and HIV. Laboratory testing may not show the presence of the virus or antibodies to the virus.

6. Incorrect. Transdermal pads are applied to intact skin. There is no danger of contact with the patient's blood or body fluids.

7. Correct. In carrying out the vaginal douche there is a possibility of exposure to vaginal secretions.

8. Incorrect. The nurse should squeeze the finger and, after washing hands with soap and water, scrub the area with povidone–iodine (Betadine) or another accepted antiseptic. In addition, the needlestick should be reported to the proper authority and the protocol for exposure to blood should be carried out. Universal safeguards apply to all patients regardless of the diagnosis.

9. Incorrect. There is always a possibility or risk when doing an invasive procedure such as an injection.

10. Incorrect. Because the patient is alert and can take the medicine cup from the nurse, handwashing is adequate.

11. Incorrect. The CDC guidelines advise the nurse not to recap a needle, but to place it immediately in a puncture-proof container.

12. Correct. Nitroglycerin ointment is a potent vasodilator. Wearing gloves protects the nurse against the drug's effect.

13. Incorrect. The nurse's fingers may come in contact with mucous membrane in administering eye drops.

Glossary

Absorption   the passing of a drug in the body across tissue into the general circulation and becomes active in the body

ac   before meals

ad lib   as desired

Adverse effects   nontherapeutic effects that may be harmful

Ampule (ampoule)   a sealed glass container for powdered or liquid drugs

Amt   amount

Antagonism   the interaction between two drugs in which the combined effect is less than the sum of the effects of the drugs acting separately

Apothecary system   a measurement system using grains and minims, introduced into the United States from England in colonial times

AS, AD, AU   left ear, right ear, both ears; JCAHO states do not use, but write out "left ear," "right ear," or "both ears" as appropriate

Avoirdupois system   a measurement system using ounces and pounds; used for patient weight and some drugs

Bactericidal   a drug action that kills an organism

Bacteriostatic   a drug action that inhibits an organism's ability to grow and reproduce

bid   twice a day

Bioavailability   the availability of a drug once it is absorbed and transported in the body to the site of its action

Biotransformation   the conversion of an active drug to an inactive compound

Body surface area, or BSA   calculation of meters squared based on height and weight, as shown in a nomogram

BP   blood pressure

Buccal   the route of administration in which a drug is placed in the pouch between the teeth and cheek

C   Centigrade, Celsius

Cap or Capsule   a gelatin container that holds a drug in a solid or liquid form

CC or cc   cubic centimeter; equal to 1 mL; JCAHO states do not use this abbreviation; use "mL"

CDC   Centers for Disease Control and Prevention

Chemical name   the drug name derived from its chemical structure

Civil law   statutes concerned with the rights and duties of individuals

Clark's Rule   a way to determine dosage of medications for children older than 2 years of age; based on weight

Cm   centimeter

Common factor   a number that is a factor of two different numbers (ie, 3 is a factor of 6 and 9)

Common fraction   a fraction with a whole number in the numerator and denominator (ie, 7/9)

Concentration   the amount of drug in a solution; in fraction, decimal, or percentage form

Contraindication   a situation in which a drug should be avoided

Controlled drug   a drug controlled by federal, state, and local law; a drug that may be lead to drug abuse or dependence

Cream   a semisolid drug preparation applied externally to the skin or mucous membrane

CR   controlled release

Criminal law   statutes that protect the public again actions harmful to society

CSF   cerebrospinal fluid

Cumulation or Accumulation   the inability of the body to metabolize one dose of a drug before another dose is administered; cumulation leads to increased concentration of the drug in the body and possible toxicity

d   day

DEA   US Drug Enforcement Administration

Denominator   the bottom number in a fraction

Dermal route   the topical application of a drug to the skin

Diluent   a liquid used to dissolve a solid, usually a powder, into a solution

Disch   discharge

D/C   discharge or discontinue; JCAHO states do not use; write out "discharge" or "discontinue" as appropriate

Displacement   the increase in the volume of fluid added to a powder, when the powder dissolves and goes into solution

Distribution   the movement of a drug through body fluids, chiefly blood, to cells

Dividend   the number to be divided (eg, 40 divided by 5, 40 is the dividend)

Divisor   the number by which the dividend is divided; in the previous example, 5 is the divisor

dL   deciliter, 100 mL

Dose   the amount of drug to be administered at one time or the total amount to be given

DR   delayed release

dr   dram

Drip or Drop factor   the number of drops of an IV fluid in 1 mL; listed on the IV tubing set or package

Drip rate   the number of drops of an IV solution to be infused per minute

Drop   a minute sphere of liquid

Drug   a chemical agent used in the treatment, diagnosis, or prevention of disease

Elixir   a clear, aromatic, sweetened alcoholic preparation

Emulsion   suspension of a fat or oil in water with the aid of an agent to reduce surface tension

Enteral   refers to the small intestine

Enteric coating   a layer placed over a tablet or capsule to prevent dissolution in the stomach; used to protect the drug from gastric acid or to protect the stomach from drug irritation

Epidural route   medication is administered into the space around the dura mater of the spinal column

ER   extended release

Ethics   a system of values and morals

Excretion   the physiologic elimination of substances from the body

Expiration date   a drug cannot be administered after the last day of the month stamped on the label

F   Fahrenheit

FDA   Food and Drug Administration

Film-coated tablets   compressed, powdered drugs that are smooth and easy to swallow because of their outer shell covering

First-pass effect   drugs that are administered orally that pass from the intestine to the liver and are partially metabolized before entering the circulation

Flow rate   number of milliliters per hour of IV fluid to be infused

fl. oz.   fluid ounce; equal to 30 mL

Fluid extract or fluidextract   potent alcoholic liquid concentration of a drug

Fraction   division of one number by another

Fried's rule   a rule to calculate drug dosages for infants younger than 1 year; based on age

g or Gm   gram

Gauge   the diameter or width of a needle; the higher the gauge number, the finer the needle

Gel   an aqueous suspension of small particles of an insoluble drug in a hydrated form

Generic name   the official name of a drug as listed in the United States or other pharmacopoeia

Gram   weight of 1 mL of water at 4°C; basic unit of weight in metric system

gr   grain; approximately equal to 60 or 65 mg

gtt   drop or drops

h or hr   hour

Half-life   the time that a drug is metabolized by 50% in the body

Hepatotoxic   a drug or side effects of a drug that may affect the liver

Household system   a measurement system based on household items of measurement; uses teaspoon, tablespoon, cups

hs   hour of sleep, at bedtime; JCAHO states not to use this abbreviation; write out "at bedtime"

hypo   hypodermic syringe or injection

I & O   intake and output

IM   intramuscular

Improper fraction a fraction with the numerator larger or equal to the denominator

Incompatibility a mixture of two or more drugs that results in a harmful chemical or physical interaction

Inhalant vapors that are inhaled via the nose, lungs, or trachea

Inhaler a device used to spray liquid or powder in a fine mist into the lungs during inspiration

inj injection

Interaction either desirable or undesirable effects produced by giving two or more drugs together

IU international unit; JCAHO states do not use, write out "international units"

Intraarticular medication injected into the joints

Intradermal or ID an injection given into the upper layers of the skin

Intramuscular or IM an injection given into the muscle

Intrathecal administration into the cerebrospinal fluid via the subarachnoid space

Intravenous or IV medication given by injection or infusion into a vein

Isotonic solutions that have the same osmotic pressure as physiologic body fluids

IV intravenous

IVPB intravenous piggyback; a medication placed in an infusion set and attached to the main line IV for delivery to the patient

JCAHO Joint Commission on Accreditation of Healthcare Organizations; an organization responsible for safety in hospitals and other health care settings; in 2004, the JCAHO issued a list of abbreviations "not to be used" to decrease errors

k or kg kilogram

lb pounds

Liter or L unit of fluid volume in the metric system; equal to one tenth of a cubic meter

Lotion liquid suspension intended for external use

Lowest common denominator the smallest number that is a multiple of all denominators

Lowest terms the smallest numbers possible in the numerator and denominator of a fraction; reducing a fraction to lowest terms means the numerator and denominator cannot be reduced further

Lozenge a flat, round, or rectangular preparation held in the mouth until it dissolves

Magma a bulky suspension of an insoluble preparation in water that must be shaken before pouring

mcg microgram; previously abbreviated as μg; however, this is not an approved abbreviation by the JCAHO

MDI metered dose inhaler; an aerosol device that consists of two parts: a canister under pressure and a mouthpiece; finger pressure on the mouthpiece opens a valve that discharges one dose

Meniscus the curved surface of a liquid in a container

Metabolism the chemical biotransformation of a drug to a form that can be excreted

Meter or m a unit of length in the metric system; equals 39.27 in

Metric System a measurement system that uses meters, liters, grams; common system used worldwide except in the United States; widely used system in dosages of drugs; based on units of 10

mg milligram

MgSO$_4$ magnesium sulfate; JCAHO states do not use; write out "magnesium sulfate" because this abbreviation can be confused with MSO$_4$

Military time time based on a 24-hour clock rather than the traditional 12-hour clock

Milliequivalent or mEq the number of grams of solute in a 1-mL solution; used to measure electrolytes and some medications

min minute

Mixed number a whole number and a fraction (eg, 1 ½)

ML or mL milliliter

mm millimeter

mo month

MS, MSO$_4$ morphine sulfate; JCAHO states do not use; write out morphine sulfate; this abbreviation can be confused with MgSO$_4$

Multidose large stock containers of medication

NDC national drug code; a number used by pharmacists to identify a drug and the packaging method

Nephrotoxic a drug or side effects of a drug that may affect the renal system

Nomogram a tabular illustration of body surface area based on height and weight

Nonparenteral drugs drugs administered by topical, rectal, or oral route

Nonprescription drug   a drug obtained without a prescription; also called *over the counter* or OTC

NPO   nothing by mouth

Numerator   the top number in a fraction

OD   right eye (suggested "do not use"—write out "right eye")

Official name   a drug's official name as listed in the *United States Pharmacopoeia* and the National Formulary

Ointment   a semisolid preparation in a petroleum or lanolin base for external use

Ophthalmic   pertaining to the eye

Oral route   abbreviated po; drugs given through the mouth

OS   left eye (suggested "do not use"—write out "left eye")

OTC   over the counter

Otic   pertaining to the ear

Ototoxic   a drug or side effects of the drug that may affect the ear

OU   both eyes (suggested "do not use"—write out "both eyes")

oz   ounce

Parenteral   a general term that means administration by injection (IV, IM, or subcutaneous)

Paste   a thick ointment used to protect the skin

Pastille   a disklike solid that slowly dissolves in the mouth

Patch   a small adhesive that releases medication over an extended period of time; applied topically

pc   after meals

Percentage   parts per hundred, designated by a percent sign (%)

Percentage solution   the solid that is dissolved in a liquid represents a percentage of the total weight of the solution; measured in grams per 100 mL solution

Pharmacodynamics   the study of the chemical and physical effects of drugs in the body

Pharmacokinetics   the science of the factors that determine how much drug reaches the site of action in the body and is excreted

Pharmacology   the study of the origin, nature, chemistry effects, and uses of drugs

Pharmacotherapeutics   the study of the use of drugs to treat, prevent, and diagnose diseases

Piggyback   medication placed in an IV infusion set attached to the mainline IV for delivery to the patient

Placebo   an inert substance used in place of a drug to determine its psychological effect and the physiologic changes caused by the psychological response

PO   by mouth, oral

Powder   a finely ground solid drug or mixture of drugs for internal or external use

Prefilled cartridge   a small vial with a needle attached that fits into a metal or plastic holder for injection

Prefilled syringe   a liquid, sterile medication that is ready to administer without further preparation

Prescription   an order for medication written by an authorized prescriber

Prescription drug   a drug that requires a prescription; regulated usually by state laws

Prime number   a whole number only divisible by one and itself; a whole number that cannot be reduced any further (ie, 3, 5, 7)

PR   per rectum

PRN   when required

Product   the answer in multiplication

Prolonged-release or slow-release tablet   a powdered, compressed drug that disintegrates more slowly and has a longer duration of action

Proper fraction   a fraction with a numerator smaller than the denominator

Proportion   a set of ratios or fractions

pt   patient or pint

q   each, every

qd   every day; JCAHO states not to use this abbreviation; write out "every day"

q4h   every 4 hours

q6h   every 6 hours

q8h   every 8 hours

q12h   every 12 hours

qid   four times a day

qod   every other day; JCAHO states not to use this abbreviation; write out "every other day"

qt   quart

Quotient   the answer in division

Ratio   a way to compare numbers; numbers are separated by a colon, such as 1:5, which reads one is to five

Reconstitution dissolving a powder to a liquid form

Rectal route or PR medication administered through the rectum

Reduce to simplify

Rounding reducing decimal places in a number; a number may be rounded off to the nearest tenth, hundredth, thousandth, etc.; a number may also be reduced to the nearest whole number

Rx a prescription

SC or SQ subcutaneous; JCAHO states not to use this abbreviation; write out "subcutaneous" or "subq"

Scored tablet a compressed, powdered drug with a line down the center so that the tablet can be broken in half

SI units System International d'Unites; a measurement adapted from the metric system, used in most developed countries to provide a standard language

Solution or sol a clear liquid that contains a drug dissolved in water

Spansule a long-acting capsule that contains drug particles coated to dissolve at different times

Spirits concentrated alcoholic solutions of volatile substances

SR sustained release

Stat immediately

Subcutaneous the tissue between the skin and muscle

Sublingual tablet a powdered drug that is compressed or molded into a solid shape that dissolves quickly under the tongue

Suppository a mixture of a drug with a firm base molded into a shape to be inserted into a body cavity

Suspension solid particles of a drug dispersed in a liquid that must be shaken to obtain an accurate dose

Syrup or syr a solution of sugar in water to disguise the unpleasant taste of a medication

Tablet or tab a powdered drug that is compressed or molded into a solid shape; may contain additives that bind the powder or aid in its absorption

Tbsp tablespoon

tid three times a day

Timed release small beads of drug in a capsule coated to delay absorption

Tincture alcoholic or hydroalcoholic solution of a drug

Tolerance a decreased responsiveness to a drug after repeated exposure

Topical route of administration in which a drug is applied to the skin or mucous membrane

Toxicity a nontherapeutic effect that may result in damage to tissues or organs

TPN total parenteral nutrition

Trade name a brand or proprietary name identified by the symbol that follows the name

Transcribe rewriting; in nursing and hospitals, a drug order is transcribed usually to another form that is used to record and document administration of medications

Transdermal medicated drug molecules contained in a unique polymer patch applied to the skin for slow absorption

Troche a flat, round, or rectangular preparation held in the mouth (or placed in the vagina) until it dissolves

Tsp or tsp teaspoon

U units; JCAHO states not to use this abbreviation; write out "unit"

Unit dose an individually wrapped and labeled dose of a drug

Unit system a measurement system using units to measure amounts of drugs; drugs that use this system include heparin, penicillin, and insulin

Universal precautions procedures to protect against infection that are used where caring for all patients and when handling contaminated equipment

Ung ointment

Vaginal route medication inserted or injected into the vagina

Vial a glass container with a rubber stopper containing one or more doses of a drug

wt weight

Young's rule a rule used to calculate drug dosages for children ages 1 to 12 years; based on the age of the child

Index

Note: Page numbers followed by *f* indicate figures; those followed by *t* indicate tables.